Contemporary Cardiology

Series Editor

Peter P. Toth
Ciccarone Center for the Prevention of Cardiovascular Disease
Johns Hopkins University School of Medicine
Baltimore, MD
USA

For more than a decade, cardiologists have relied on the Contemporary Cardiology series to provide them with forefront medical references on all aspects of cardiology. Each title is carefully crafted by world-renown cardiologists who comprehensively cover the most important topics in this rapidly advancing field. With more than 75 titles in print covering everything from diabetes and cardiovascular disease to the management of acute coronary syndromes, the Contemporary Cardiology series has become the leading reference source for the practice of cardiac care.

More information about this series at http://www.springer.com/series/7677

Gianluca Iacobellis
Editor

Epicardial Adipose Tissue

From Cell to Clinic

Humana Press

Editor
Gianluca Iacobellis
Division of Endocrinology, Diabetes and Metabolism
Department of Medicine
University of Miami
Miller School of Medicine
Miami, FL
USA

ISSN 2196-8969 ISSN 2196-8977 (electronic)
Contemporary Cardiology
ISBN 978-3-030-40572-4 ISBN 978-3-030-40570-0 (eBook)
https://doi.org/10.1007/978-3-030-40570-0

This Humana imprint is published by the registered company Springer Nature Switzerland AG
The registered company address is: Gewerbestrasse 11, 6330 Cham, Switzerland

The more you reveal the secrets
about it
the more I stay loyal
to the legends of the heart

Gianfranco Iacobellis

Preface

The idea of looking at the epicardial adipose tissue hit me about 20 years ago. At the beginning, it was purely an observation. I was completing my fellowship in endocrinology but had an obvious passion for the heart and its potential as an endocrine organ. When my father, a professor of cardiology, was performing echocardiograms, I started noticing a consistent link between the patient's belly and that echo-free space in the echocardiographic imaging. The more abdominally obese the patient, the bigger the echo-free space. That would have been the epicardial fat.

So, first, I developed and validated the ultrasound technique to measure epicardial fat. However, my curiosity was not yet satisfied. I searched the literature on the epicardial adipose tissue but found scarce and dusty information, mostly from old textbooks of human and comparative anatomy. It was clearly a neglected adipose tissue, just silently standing by the heart. At least, it was so believed. Few anatomists from the nineteenth century were questioning the meaning and causes of the fatty heart. The comparative anatomy was actually more intriguing, as I learned that some animals, particularly those who hibernate, had a large fat cushion that could protect the heart during the hibernation. I thought that was fascinating but basically unexplored in humans.

So my pioneering work in this field began. This book's intent is to summarize the enormous and continuously growing scientific-based evidence on the multifaceted aspects of epicardial fat and its clinical applications. Novel discoveries regarding epicardial fat occur on an almost daily basis. I have done my best to present the most updated literature and to report the newest findings in this book. The purpose of this volume is not only to provide an overview of the anatomical, biomolecular, genetic, imaging, and clinical features of epicardial fat but also to stimulate further research and any clinical implications generated by current research. The book will literally take you from cell to clinic, from the lab to your patient.

I have had the privilege to be accompanied by renowned colleagues and friends who greatly contributed to this book with their expertise and dedication. You will read that epicardial fat is actually a very active endocrine (or, better, paracrine) organ that cross-talks with the myocardium and the coronary arteries, as no muscle fascia separates the fat from these contiguous structures. You will be amused by the unique transcriptome of the epicardial fat, so enriched with genes encoding for pro-inflammatory, pro-fibrotic, and atherogenic factors. This volume wants to reach out to a broad spectrum of readers and specialists. Having a biomarker that is peculiar, unique, measurable, and ultimately modifiable is appealing to any basic scientist and clinician. Epicardial fat can play a key role in the development and progression of eliminating diseases such as the coronary artery disease and atrial fibrillation, as nicely described here by worldwide experts in these fields.

We can now, quantitatively and qualitatively, measure this fat depot with routine, noninvasive imaging procedures and predict the cardiovascular risk, as comprehensively discussed in three focused chapters. Experts in the field will guide you through the neuromodulation of the epicardial fat. A beautiful chapter is dedicated to the perivascular fat, so different but also so similar to the epicardial fat. You will also read and learn about the dual role of the epicardial fat, both detrimental and protective. As a *Janus Bifrons*, epicardial fat will show you its dichotomous face.

The topic is certainly innovative, the results are promising, but further investigations are necessary to address key questions. In my view, future research on epicardial fat will take two main streams—causality and utility. First, it will be focused on understanding the independent causative role of epicardial fat in coronary artery disease and atrial fibrillation. Currently, we have evidence that epicardial fat is a sensitive target of drugs modulating the fat. Future studies will explore how the pharmacological manipulation of epicardial fat could eventually restore its physiological and protective properties. Breaking from traditional schemes, the research on the epicardial adipose tissue can open new and important avenues. This book will guide you through this exciting journey.

Miami, FL, USA Gianluca Iacobellis

Contents

Contributors

Charalambos Antoniades, MD, PhD Division of Cardiovascular Medicine, Radcliffe Department of Medicine, University of Oxford, Oxford, UK

Oxford Academic Cardiovascular CT Core Laboratory, John Radcliffe Hospital, Headley Way, Oxford, UK

Bastian Balcer, MD Department of Cardiology and Vascular Medicine, West German Heart and Vascular Center Essen, University Hospital Essen, Essen, Germany

Vladimir Camarena, PhD John P. Hussman Institute for Human Genomics, Department of Human Genetics, University of Miami Miller School of Medicine, Miami, FL, USA

Antonio Concistrè, MD Secondary Arterial Hypertension Unit, Department of Translational and Precision Medicine, "Sapienza" University of Rome, Rome, Italy

Jeffrey J. Goldberger, MD, MBA University of Miami Miller School of Medicine, Department of Medicine, Cardiovascular Division, Miami, FL, USA

Tyler C. Huff, BA John P. Hussman Institute for Human Genomics, Department of Human Genetics, University of Miami Miller School of Medicine, Miami, FL, USA

Gianluca Iacobellis, MD, PhD Division of Endocrinology, Diabetes and Metabolism, Department of Medicine, University of Miami, Miller School of Medicine, Miami, FL, USA

Gino Iannucci, MD Secondary Arterial Hypertension Unit, Department of Translational and Precision Medicine, "Sapienza" University of Rome, Rome, Italy

Christos P. Kotanidis, MD, MSc Division of Cardiovascular Medicine, Radcliffe Department of Medicine, University of Oxford, Oxford, UK

Claudio Letizia, MD Secondary Arterial Hypertension Unit, Department of Translational and Precision Medicine, "Sapienza" University of Rome, Rome, Italy

Anastasios Lymperopoulos, BPharm, MSc, PhD Laboratory for the Study of Neurohormonal Control of the Circulation, Department of Pharmaceutical Sciences, College of Pharmacy, Nova Southeastern University, Fort Lauderdale, FL, USA

Amir Abbas Mahabadi, MD Department of Cardiology and Vascular Medicine, West German Heart and Vascular Center Essen, University Hospital Essen, Essen, Germany

Jennifer Maning, DO Laboratory for the Study of Neurohormonal Control of the Circulation, Department of Pharmaceutical Sciences, College of Pharmacy, Nova Southeastern University, Fort Lauderdale, FL, USA

Luigi Petramala, MD, PhD Secondary Arterial Hypertension Unit, Department of Translational and Precision Medicine, "Sapienza" University of Rome, Rome, Italy

Celina M. Pollard, BS (PharmD candidate) Laboratory for the Study of Neurohormonal Control of the Circulation, Department of Pharmaceutical Sciences, College of Pharmacy, Nova Southeastern University, Fort Lauderdale, FL, USA

Tienush Rassaf, MD Department of Cardiology and Vascular Medicine, West German Heart and Vascular Center Essen, University Hospital Essen, Essen, Germany

David W. Sant, PhD Biomedical Informatics, Department of Biological Engineering, Utah State University, Salt Lake City, UT, USA

Alexandra C. Villasante Fricke, MD Department of Diabetes, Endocrinology, and Metabolism, University of Miami, Miami, FL, USA

Gaofeng Wang, PhD John P. Hussman Institute for Human Genomics, Dr. John T. Macdonald Foundation Department of Human Genetics, Sylvester Comprehensive Cancer Center, Miller School of Medicine, University of Miami, Miami, FL, USA

Ghaith Zaatari, MD University of Miami Miller School of Medicine, Department of Medicine, Cardiovascular Division, Miami, FL, USA

About the Editor

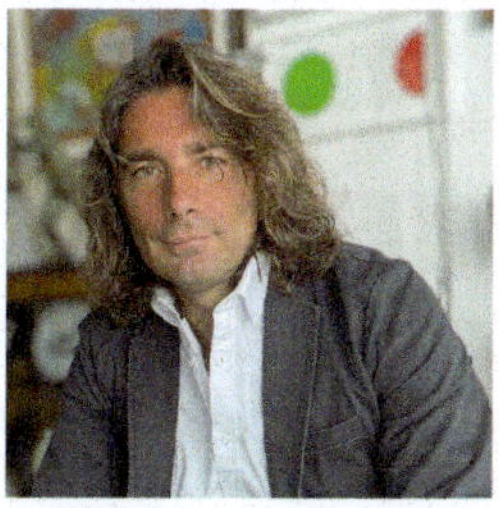

Gianluca Iacobellis is a physician-scientist, M.D., Ph.D., with international academic reputation and research and clinical expertise in obesity, diabetes, and cardiovascular risk.

He is currently full professor of Clinical Medicine and director of the University of Miami Hospital Diabetes Service at the University of Miami, FL, USA.

He has authored 128 scientific articles and 10 textbooks, with a current *h* index of 40 and 6888 citations.

He is considered the worldwide leading expert in the epicardial fat, a new cardiovascular risk [factor. He pioneered the research in the epicardial fat and developed the echocardiographic epicardial fat quantification as a new marker of visceral fat and therapeutic target. His studies suggest the active role of epicardial fat in coronary artery disease and atrial fibrillation. Dr Iacobellis is leading several clinical trials on emerging diabetes/obesity pharmacotherapy targeting the epicardial fat. Results of these studies have been published in high-ranked journals, such as *Nature Reviews Endocrinology* and *Nature Reviews Cardiology*, and presented at important meetings such as the American Diabetes Association, American Heart Association, and Endocrine Society.

Dr. Iacobellis is a co-investigator of a recently awarded NIH R01 grant entitled "Liraglutide Effect in Atrial Fibriallation (LEAF) RHL145165A".

A native of Rome, Italy, Dr. Iacobellis received his M.D. degree cum laude in 1994 from the University of Roma, La Sapienza; he was a research fellow at the Centrum for Metabolism and Endocrinology, Karolinska University, Stockholm, Sweden, in 1999; he became specialist in endocrinology in 2000 and obtained his Ph.D. in Endocrinology, Metabolic, and Cardiovascular Disorders in 2004.

In 2004, he was then an invited postdoctoral clinical research fellow at the Center for Human Nutrition, Southwestern Medical Center, University of Texas, Dallas, USA. In 2005, he moved to Canada as clinical research fellow in the Cardiovascular Obesity Research and Management Department, McMaster University, Hamilton, Ontario.

Since 2006 to 2010, he was appointed associate professor of endocrinology, Department of Medicine, McMaster University, and director of bariatric endocrinology at St. Joseph's Hospital, Hamilton, Ontario, Canada.

In 2010, he moved to the University of Miami, FL, USA, as associate professor of clinical medicine, Division of Endocrinology, and director of the ACC Diabetes Clinic at Jackson Memorial Hospital, Miami.

In 2013, he was promoted professor of clinical medicine and director of the University of Miami Hospital Diabetes Service.

Dr. Iacobellis' clinical activity as endocrinologist is at the Diabetes Research Institute (DRI), University of Miami.

1 Anatomy of the Epicardial Adipose Tissue

Gianluca Iacobellis

Key Points

- Epicardial adipose tissue (EAT) is the visceral fat depot located between the myocardium and the visceral layer of the pericardium. No fascia separates the EAT from the underlying myocardium; the two tissues share the same microcirculation.
- EAT derives from the splanchnopleuric mesoderm, along with mesenteric and omental fat.
- EAT can be located directly within the myocardium or around the coronary artery adventitia. EAT is commonly found in the atrioventricular and interventricular grooves.

Introduction

The role and presence of adipose tissue in humans are intriguing, but far to be completely understood. Until the early 2000s, the adipose tissue of the human heart was considered an innocent and somehow irrelevant bystander. This previously neglected fat depot emerged to the attention of pathologists, clinicians, and scientists only very recently [1]. Understanding the anatomy and pathology of the cardiac fat depots played a key role in highlighting the peculiar features of the epicardial fat (EAT) and their clinical implications. The perception of the potential role of the adipose tissue in humans is therefore profoundly changed.

G. Iacobellis (✉)
Division of Endocrinology, Diabetes and Metabolism, Department of Medicine, University of Miami, Miller School of Medicine, Miami, FL, USA
e-mail: giacobellis@med.miami.edu

Comparative Anatomy

Anatomy, genes, and metabolic pathways of adipose tissues have been studied from their invertebrate origins through lower vertebrates to mammals and birds. Comparative studies have suggested similarities in anatomical sites of cardiac fat depot between animals and humans. For example, bovine heart presents a large cardiac fat resembling the pathological EAT accumulation in humans (Fig. 1.1).

Embryologically, EAT has been detected in the fetus of sheep [2] and also in mice [3]. Primary epicardial cells can be grown from embryonic heart tissue explants. The presence of epicardial fat in the mouse atrioventricular (AV) groove starts around 2 weeks after birth and represents a unique postnatal aspect of epicardial differentiation [3]. Interestingly when human and mouse epicardial fat cells are treated with palmitate, the human line showed prominent adipocyte

G. Iacobellis (ed.), *Epicardial Adipose Tissue*, Contemporary Cardiology,
https://doi.org/10.1007/978-3-030-40570-0_1

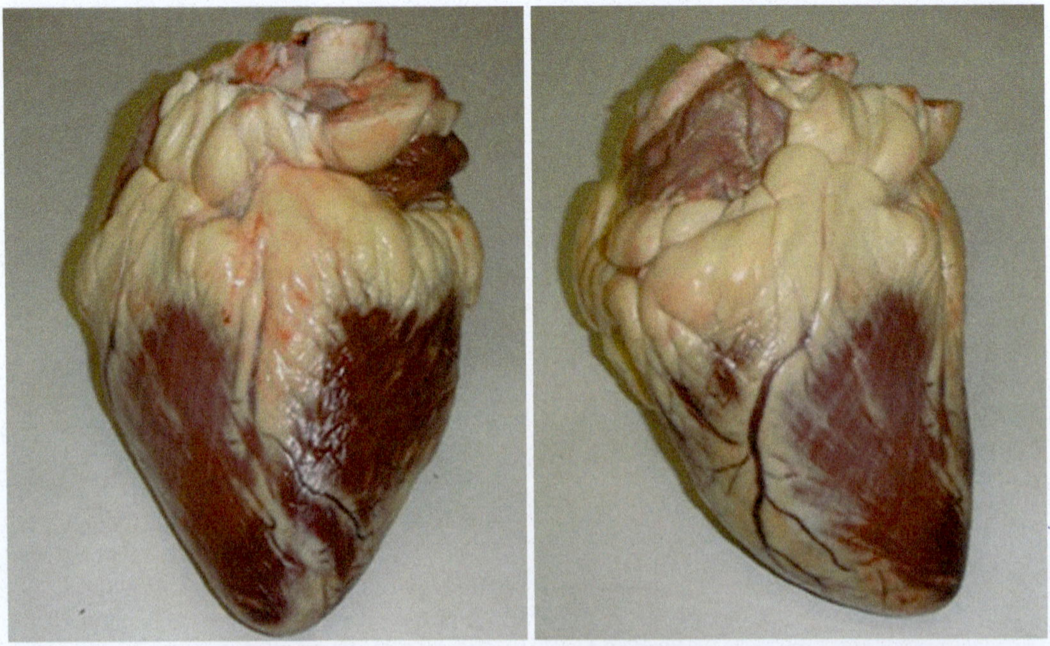

Fig. 1.1 Bovine heart with large fat accumulation resembling human fatty heart. (From author's own collection)

differentiation, whereas mouse cells had not. Peroxisome proliferator-activated receptor gamma (PPARγ) activity is necessary for the development of mouse AV EAT [3]. Comparing human epicardial adipocytes and myocardium with the developmental origins and maturation of homologous tissues in mice explains its appearance early in life and much of the contrasts between species [3]. Epicardial and pericardial fat depots can be also found in mammals, especially large species, and in large birds, such as swans [4] (Fig. 1.2).

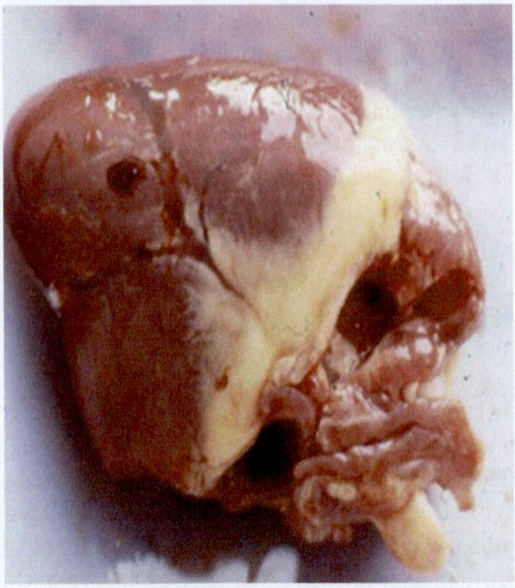

Fig. 1.2 Cardiac fat in swan. (From author's own collection)

Guinea pigs have a small but variable amount, and the tissue is well known in domestic livestock (sheep, pigs, etc.), but there is little epicardial fat in laboratory rats and mice, so the tissue has not been thoroughly studied experimentally. The epicardial fat mass is highly variable among individuals, especially in nidifugous species such as ungulates, and in very lean and emaciated animals.

Epicardial fat depot amounts to only 0.02% of the total adipose mass and is unrelated to total fatness or body mass. The lack of relationship between the epicardial adipose tissue and general adiposity has been confirmed in human studies, in which it was found that body mass index (BMI) was not the main determinant of EAT thickness [1].

Both epicardial and pericardial adipose tissue are found in most lean, healthy wild mammals,

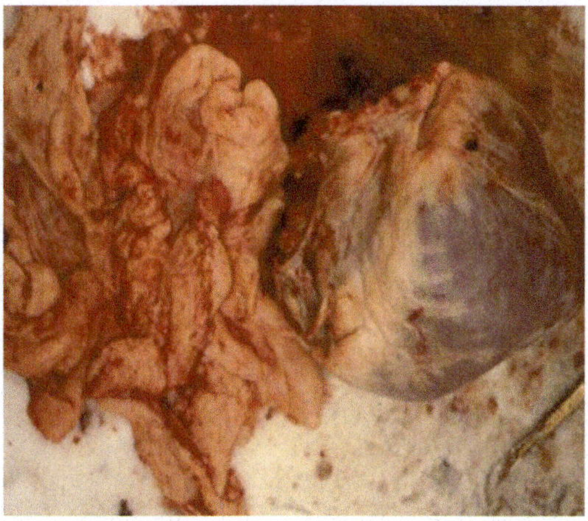

Fig. 1.3 Large cardiac fat accumulation in polar artic bear. (From author's own collection)

especially large species, such as polar artic bears (Fig. 1.3), and large birds such as swans (*Cygnus olor*) [5] but are absent in the huge marine turtles [6] and probably other lower vertebrates. They are selectively spared in starvation, so both emaciated and very lean, healthy specimens may have lipid-filled adipocytes only in the cardiac and perinodal depots. Interestingly, artic polar bears can use the large epicardial depot as fuel of energy to the myocardium during their long periods of hibernation. This is likely an example as EAT in some animals can serve as brown fat to release heat to the heart in conditions of high demand, such as starvation and cold temperatures. As in humans, epicardial adipocytes are not bounded by fascia and always adhere tightly to the myocardium. In species that naturally become obese, no correlation between the masses of these depots and those elsewhere in the body is found [4].

EAT is minimally represented in murid rodents so can be mostly studied experimentally in guinea pigs or larger animals [4, 5]. The difficulties of developing commonly used experimental animal models have been a limitation in understanding the physiology and pathophysiology of EAT. Rodents are generally considered to not have much epicardial fat, although they have paracardial fat, an anatomically and functionally different noncardiac fat depot. However, more recent studies have shown that EAT is actually present in mice and can therefore be used as experimental model [3]. Using genetic fate mapping approaches, Yagamuchi et al. showed that EAT in mice is derived by mesenchymal transformation of the epicardium.

While human hearts show a significant amount of adipose tissue covering the entire surface or a large portion of the ventricles, adult hearts from mice and rats show no ventricular EAT and have direct contact of the epicardium to the myocardium. EAT in mouse, histologically defined as subepicardial, is limited to specific location between the atrial and ventricular chambers on the dorsal to dorsolateral sides of the heart, also known as the AV groove. Remarkably, mouse EAT is perfused by coronary vasculature rather than from systemic vessels [3]. By performing a retroaortic ink perfusion of isolated adult mouse hearts, Yamaguchi found an ink perfusion into the small vessels of the EAT located in the AV groove and into the major and minor coronary vessels of the ventricle [3]. This finding is of great importance as it confirms the crosstalk between the fat and the heart throughout a shared microcirculation.

Rodent EAT is not well predictable in amount. Given the intrinsic metabolism of EAT is very fast in mice, its accumulation is commonly very small. The development of experimental mouse model of EAT in response to diet is therefore challenging. However, Ace22/y mutant mice (ACE2KO) were recently used to evaluate EAT in response to different diet [7]. Male wild-type and ACE2KO mice were fed either a high-fat diet or a control diet from weaning to 6 months of age. EAT was collected under a stereo microscope after removal of the pericardium and pericardial fat [7].

There is a compelling need for animal models to study dynamics of the EAT that could not be analyzed in humans, such as pre- and postsurgical changes. The Ossabaw miniature swine, which naturally represents human components of metabolic syndrome and coronary artery disease, have been used to study EAT [8]. This animal's coronary arterial supply more closely resembles that of humans compared to rodent research models. Ossabaw pig's epicardial fat can be visualized macroscopically and potentially surgically removed [8].

Sheep, specifically Bluefaced Leicester cross Swaledale ewes were used to evaluate postnatal changes within the function and development of EAT [9]. At 7 days of life, EAT exhibited modules enriched with genes associated with cardiomyocyte cell differentiation.

Human Anatomy

Embryology

EAT is the fat depot located between the myocardium and the epicardium including the surroundings of the epicardial coronary vessels (subepicardial fat), while the pericardial fat is located over the extrinsic leaf of the pericardium, corresponding to the tissue located within the pericardial sac [10]. EAT and pericardial fat are two different cardiac fat depots. Their embryology and vascular irrigation are completely different [11]. EAT derives from the splanchnopleuric mesoderm, along with mesenteric and omental fat. This common embryogenesis has been confirmed by genomic studies in animals such as chick [12] and mouse [13]. Starting at the 4th week of gestation, the heart is suspended in a mesh of tubes from its cranial and caudal side [5]. The myocardial cells start to secret hyaluronic acid (cardiac gel) which separates them from the endothelium. The mesothelial cells that are located in the septum transversum will become part of the epicardium once they have migrated near the venous sinus. The pericardial fat comes from the thoracic mesenchyme which also originates the parietal pericardium [5]. The epicardium is the outer noncontractile mesothelium of the heart. Once formed, the epicardium serves as a source of secreted factors that influence mitogenic expansion of the ventricular myocardium and assembly of coronary blood vessels [14, 15]. Interestingly, the epicardium is a multipotent progenitor cell population. The epicardium undergoes transformation to generate mesenchymal cells that first reside in the subepicardial space between the epicardium and myocardium [16, 17].

A recent study looked at the gene pathway development in human EAT during early life [18]. EAT was collected from children, aged from 6 days to 7 years, with congenital cardiomyopathies who required cardiac surgery [18]. This elegant study highlighted the complexity of the processes implicated in the control of thermogenesis in EAT of neonates and the way in which these gene-to-gene interactions shift towards lipogenesis through infancy. Of note, the authors noted that EAT in the neonate has limited flexibility and responsiveness. With aging, epicardial adipocytes become more susceptible to environmental factors. These activate transcriptional regulatory pathways that gradually change epicardial fat function from thermogenic to energy storage.

Microscopic Anatomy

EAT lies between the myocardium and the visceral layer of the pericardium. Remarkably, no fascia (as found on skeletal muscle) separates the fat from the underlying myocardium (Fig. 1.4). The absence of anatomical separation between the fat and the myocardium is unique to EAT. EAT can be located directly within the myocardium or around the coronary artery adventitia. Hence, its contiguity to the adventitia and the absence of muscle fascia suggest the possibility of a paracrine or vasocrine crosstalk between EAT and the myocardium. Although EAT and myocardium share a common blood supply, as coronary artery supplies both, a direct microcirculatory interconnection between the two tissues has not been fully proven, yet. However, there are stronger evidences of a microcirculatory connection between the EAT in the AV groove and the coronary wall via *vasa vasora* [3, 5, 10].

Microscopically, EAT is composed of mainly adipocytes, but also inflammatory, stromovascular and immune cells, ganglia, and interconnecting nerves [10]. Intrinsic cardiac neurons and ganglionated plexuses, containing adrenergic and cholinergic neurons, are embedded in EAT [19, 20].

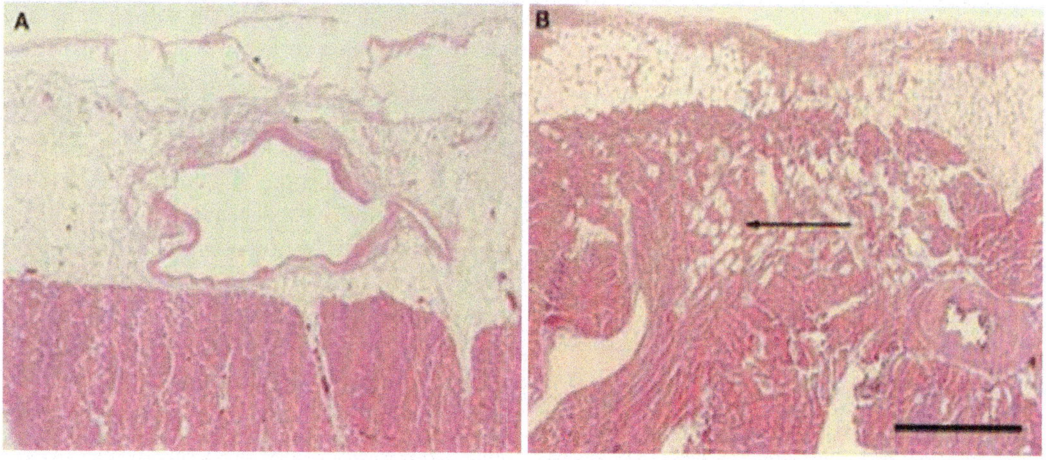

Fig. 1.4 (a) Microscopic appearance of the epicardial layer in the left ventricle. (b) Microscopic appearance of the epicardial layer in the right ventricle. The arrow shows the isles of mature adipocytes. No fascial structure divides the epicardial adipose tissue from the underlying myocardium. Mature adipocytes are more frequent in the right-hand side than the left and might be seen within the subepicardic myocardium. Scale bar = 1 mm. (From Iacobellis et al. [10], with permission)

When compared to other visceral fat depots, including the pericardial, epicardial adipocytes are generally smaller, possibly due to the peculiar anatomical location, the larger number of pre-adipocytes than mature adipocytes, but also due to a high-consuming metabolism that may prevent large lipid storage [21]. This latter finding may also explain why it is poorly represented in fast-metabolic animals such as mice. EAT is generally thought to be a white adipose tissue. However, recent findings suggest epicardial adipocyte may have brown fatlike or beige fat features. In fact, small unilocular adipocytes without uncoupling protein- 1 (UCP-1) immuno-staining have been described in EAT suggesting some histological similarities with those described in vitro in beige lineage adipocytes [22].

Beige cells were originally described as a distinct group of brown adipocytes derived from a subpopulation of progenitors in murine predominantly white subcutaneous fat [23]. Beige adipocytes express low amounts of UCP-1 under basal conditions but could be induced to differentiate and proliferate in vivo or in vitro into mature multilocular thermogenically active brown adipocytes with high amounts of UCP-1 after stimulation by cold exposure, drugs such as β3 adrenergic agents, and PPARγ agonists. These cells had a different cellular lineage from classical, constitutive brown adipocytes in the interscapular fat pad of mice. Human beige fat cells have been identified in mesenteric and retroperitoneal fat as well as posterior mediastinal fat from newborn infants, children, and teenagers, and more recently in human EAT. Adult EAT exhibits beige cell characteristics while simultaneously expressing low levels of some genes typifying white adipocytes [24].

Macroscopic Anatomy

EAT constitutes a significant cardiac component. The heart and great vessels are enclosed by epicardial tissue comprised of a mesothelium covering fibroelastic tissue corresponding to the tunica adventitia. It is important to distinguish the epicardial from the pericardial adipose tissue [11]. In fact, the two fat depots are embryologically, anatomically, and functionally different. The anatomical difference between epicardial and pericardial adipose tissue depots is clearly depicted in Fig. 1.5 [25]. The presence of fatty heart has been reported from the eighteenth century [26]. In the early nineteenth century, Dr. Latham described the case of a patient who died by rup-

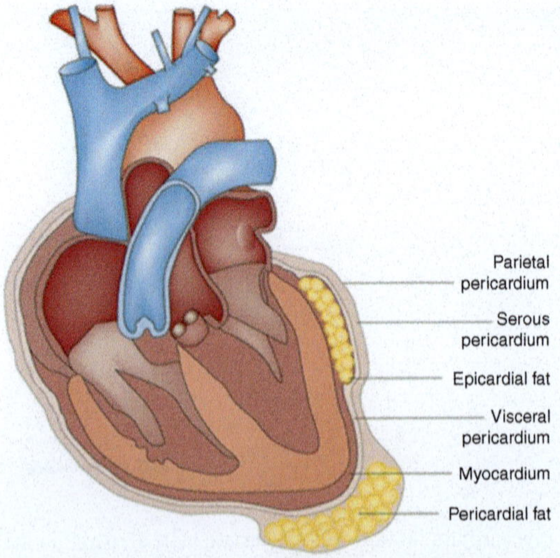

Fig. 1.5 Schematic of the heart and its fat depots. Epicardial fat is located between the myocardium and the visceral layer of the epicardium, whereas the pericardial fat is between the visceral and parietal pericardium, so it is external to the myocardium. (From Iacobellis [25], with permission)

ture of the heart. In his autoptical examination [27], Dr. Latham reported that "the fat in some parts occupied the place of the muscular fibers, the external layers especially"; he also noted that the heart rupture could have occurred "for no other reason rather than because the heart is fat." The presence of EAT has been described at the end of the nineteenth century. However that first observation could not be totally correct. In 1884 The German anatomist Rindfleisch described an abundance of adipose tissue in the ascending aorta fold [28]. Rindfleisch reported the presence of a previously unrecognized fibrofatty epicardial fold on the side of the human ascending aorta, and then called the fold of Rindfleisch. Rindfleisch hypothesized that the large lobular pads of fat enhanced the elasticity of the visceral pericardium and suggested that they played a significant role in the pathogenesis of aortic arch aneurysms. He also named this apparatus *vincula aortae*. Nevertheless, later in 1927 Davis reported this fat depot as periaortic fat, rather than epicardial fat that extended from the tunica adventitia [29]. The histological and ultrastructural demonstration of type I and type II cells similar to those of the carotid body suggests that the fold is probably a homologue of the mammalian aortic bodies and carotid body also enriched in ganglia and paraganglia [30–33]. Hence, Rindfleisch's fold is indeed surrounded by adipose tissue, but this could be a peri-aortic fat rather than myocardial epicardial fat. Also, the fold or plica reflects the structure on the aorta depending upon the diameter of the aorta. As soon as the aorta enlarges (e.g., in aortic diseases), the fold flattens or disappears and cannot be seen.

EAT is located between the myocardium and the visceral layer of the epicardium, whereas the pericardial fat is between the visceral and parietal pericardium [25]. The pericardial fat is therefore situated outside the visceral pericardium, on the external surface of the parietal pericardium, originates from the primitive thoracic mesenchyme, and is supplied by non-coronary arteries. EAT is physiologically represented within the human heart and is commonly found in the atrioventricular and interventricular grooves, but it could expand from the epicardial surface into the myocardium as represented in Fig. 1.6 [10]. EAT fills the adjacent atrioventricular groove, surrounding the circumflex coronary artery and the coronary sinus.

Recent radiological studies using steady-state free precession (SSFP) cardiac magnetic resonance (CMR) imaging showed the presence of EAT in anatomical areas of the heart that were not previously well described [34]. Excessive EAT can deeply infiltrate into the interatrial groove. Externally, this fold (also called Waterston's groove) is filled with EAT and contains the artery supplying the sinus node. EAT surrounds the *fossa ovalis* extending superiorly, posteriorly, and inferiorly. The presence of EAT in the interatrial groove may have important clinical implications in the genesis of arrhythmias. Abundant EAT can accumulate between the atrioventricular junction and the inferior pyramidal space, also called *crux cordis*. EAT can accumulate below the atrioventricular junction or merge the fat depot within the inferior pyramidal space. The inferior pyramidal space includes arteries, veins, and nerves [35].

EAT can also be located between the two atrial walls in a region called left lateral ridge, a fold between the orifice of the left atrial appendage and the left pulmonary veins. Remarkably, as

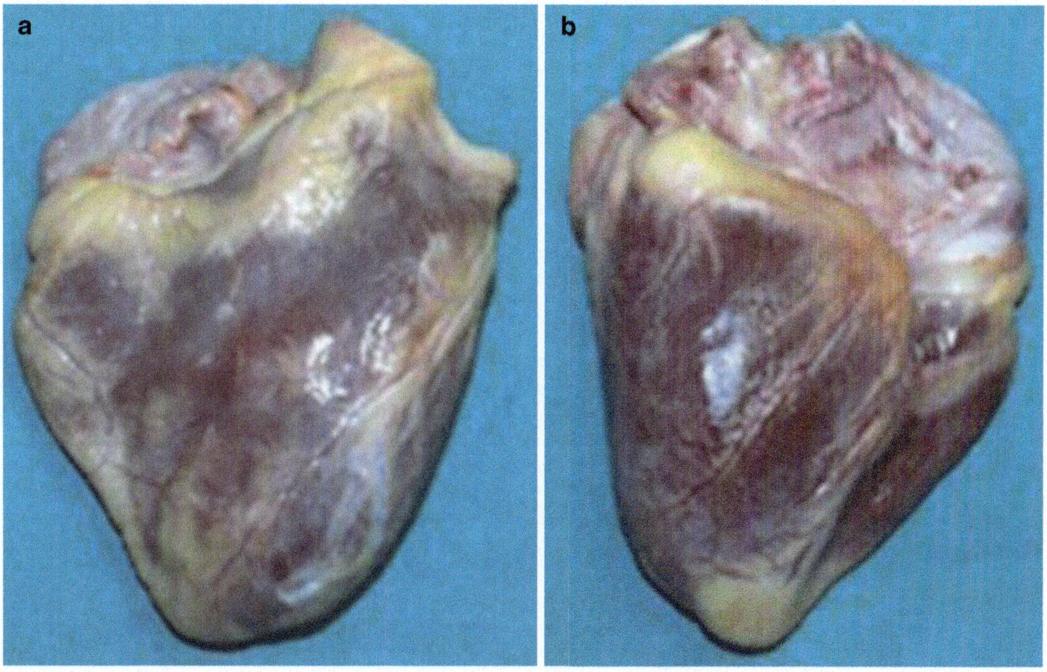

Fig. 1.6 Macroscopic appearance of epicardial fat in physiology. (**a**) Anterior view of a normal (210 g) heart. (**b**) Posterior view of a normal (210 g) heart. In the normal heart, the fat distribution is limited to the atrioventricular and interventricular grooves, and along the major coronary branches. Scale bar = 4 cm. (From Iacobellis et al. [10], with permission)

EAT reaches the hinge of the mitral valve posterior leaflets, it can serve as electrical insulator between left atrium and ventricle [34]. EAT can also cover the entire AV groove around the tricuspid valve orifice [36]. An excessive amount of EAT can also invade the transverse pericardial sinus, separating the aortic sinuses from the atrial walls. The presence of EAT in the transverse pericardial sinus helps to better understand the aortic-mitral fibrous continuity, as elegantly discovered by Leo et al. [34].

EAT can be further differentiated in pericoronary and myocardial epicardial fat [37]. Coronary epicardial adipose tissue is the adipose tissue depot located on the surface of the heart, encasing the epicardial coronary arteries. Peri-coronary epicardial adipose tissue (cEAT) is directly around or on the coronary artery adventitia, whereas myocardial epicardial fat (mEAT) is the fat depot over the myocardium since the two components may be functionally distinct, despite their anatomic contiguity. Epicardial blood supply comes from the coronary arteries (the same microcirculation as the myocardium), while pericardial fat derives from branches of the internal mammary gland. Hence we can summarize that, macroscopically, human EAT is located and visible on the free wall of the right ventricle, in the left ventricular apex, in the atrioventricular and interatrial grooves, around the two appendages, between the atrioventricular junction and the inferior pyramidal space, around and between the atria walls, directly over the myocardium and also following the adventitia of the coronary arteries [33, 34, 38].

References

1. Iacobellis G, Assael F, Ribaudo MC, Zappaterreno A, Alessi G, Di Mario U, et al. Epicardial fat from echocardiography: a new method for visceral adipose tissue prediction. Obes Res. 2003;11:304–10.
2. Henry BA, Pope M, Birtwistle M, Loughnan R, Alagal R, Fuller-Jackson JP, et al. Ontogeny and thermogenic role for sternal fat in female sheep. Endocrinology. 2017;158:2212–25.
3. Yamaguchi Y, Cavallero S, Patterson M, Shen H, Xu J, Kumar SR, et al. Adipogenesis and epicardial adipose tissue: a novel fate of the epicardium induced by mesenchymal transformation and PPARγ activation. Proc Natl Acad Sci U S A. 2015;112:2070–5.

4. Pond CM. The contribution of wild animal biology to human physiology and medicine: adipose tissue associated with lymphoid and cardiac tissues. Ecoscience. 2003;10:1–9.
5. Marchington JM, Mattacks CA, Pond CM. Adipose tissue in the mammalian heart and pericardium: structure, fetal development and biochemical properties. Comp Biochem Physiol B. 1989;94:225–32.
6. Braz JKFS, Freitas ML, Magalhães MS. Histology and immunohistochemistry of the cardiac ventricular structure in the green turtle (*Chelonia mydas*). Anat Histol Embryol. 2016;45:277–84.
7. Patel VB, Mori J, McLean BA, Basu R, Das SK, Ramprasath T, et al. ACE2 deficiency worsens epicardial adipose tissue inflammation and cardiac dysfunction in response to diet-induced obesity. Diabetes. 2016;65:85–95.
8. McKenney-Drake ML, Rodenbeck SD, Bruning RS, Kole A, Yancey KW, Alloosh M, et al. Epicardial adipose tissue removal potentiates outward remodeling and arrests coronary atherogenesis. Ann Thorac Surg. 2017;103:1622–30.
9. Fainberg HP, Birtwistle M, Alagal R, Alhaddad A, Pope M, Davies G, et al. Transcriptional analysis of adipose tissue during development reveals depot-specific responsiveness to maternal dietary supplementation. Sci Rep. 2018;8:9628.
10. Iacobellis G, Corradi D, Sharma AM. Epicardial adipose tissue: anatomic, biomolecular and clinical relationships with the heart. Nat Clin Pract Cardiovasc Med. 2005;2:536–43.
11. Iacobellis G. Epicardial and pericardial fat: close, but very different. Obesity (Silver Spring). 2009;17:625; author reply 626–7.
12. Ho E, Shimada Y. Formation of the epicardium studied with the scanning electron microscope. Dev Biol. 1978;66:579–85.
13. Walden TB, Hansen IR, Timmons JA, Cannon B, Nedergaard J. Recruited vs. nonrecruited molecular signatures of brown, "brite," and white adipose tissues. Am J Physiol Endocrinol Metab. 2012;302:E19–31.
14. Virágh S, Challice CE. The origin of the epicardium and the embryonic myocardial circulation in the mouse. Anat Rec. 1981;201:157–68.
15. Sucov HM, Gu Y, Thomas S, Li P, Pashmforoush M. Epicardial control of myocardial proliferation and morphogenesis. Pediatr Cardiol. 2009;30:617–25.
16. Riley PR. An epicardial floor plan for building and rebuilding the mammalian heart. Curr Top Dev Biol. 2012;100:233–51.
17. Acharya A. The bHLH transcription factor Tcf21 is required for lineage-specific EMT of cardiac fibroblast progenitors. Development. 2012;139:2139–49.
18. Ojha S, et al. Gene pathway development in human epicardial adipose tissue during early life. JCI Insight. 2016;1:e87460.
19. Arora RC, Waldmann M, Hopkins DA, Armour JA. Porcine intrinsic cardiac ganglia. Anat Rec A Discov Mol Cell Evol Biol. 2003;271:249–58.
20. White IA. Cardiac sympathetic denervation in the failing heart: a role for epicardial adipose tissue. Circ Res. 2016;118:1189–91.
21. Bambace C. Adiponectin gene expression and adipocyte diameter: a comparison between epicardial and subcutaneous adipose tissue in men. Cardiovasc Pathol. 2011;20:e153–6.
22. Sacks HS, Fain JN, Bahouth SW, Ojha S, Frontini A, Budge H, et al. Human epicardial fat exhibits beige features. J Clin Endocrinol Metab. 2013;98:E1448–55.
23. Wu J, Boström P, Sparks LM, Ye L, Choi JH, Giang AH, et al. Beige adipocytes are a distinct type of thermogenic fat cell in mouse and human. Cell. 2012;150:366–76.
24. Company JM, Booth FW, Laughlin MH, Arce-Esquivel AA, Sacks HS, Bahouth SW, et al. Epicardial fat gene expression after aerobic exercise training in pigs with coronary atherosclerosis: relationship to visceral and subcutaneous fat. J Appl Physiol. 2010;109:1904–1.
25. Iacobellis G. Local and systemic effects of the multifaceted epicardial adipose tissue depot. Nat Rev Endocrinol. 2015;11:363–71.
26. Bedford E. The story of fatty heart. A disease of Victorian times. Br Heart J. 1972;34:23–8.
27. The collected works of Dr. P. M. Latham, with memoir by Sir Thomas Watson. Edited for the society by R. Martin. Vol. 69; London: The New Sydenham Society; 1876–78.
28. Rindfleisch E. Ueber klammenartige Verbindungen zwischen Aorta und Pulmonalis. Virchows Arch Pathol Anat Physiol Klin Med. 1884;96:302–6.
29. Davis DJ. The periaortic fat bodies. Arch Pathol Lab Med. 1927;4:937–42.
30. Robertson HF. The vascularization of the epicardial and periaortic fat pads. Am J Pathol. 1930;6:209–15.
31. De Kock LL. Histology of the carotid body. Nature. 1951;67:661.
32. De Kock LL, Dunn AE. An electron microscope study of the carotid body. Acta Anat (Basel). 1966;64:163–78.
33. Ross LL. Electron microscopic observations of the carotid body of the cat. J Biophys Biochem Cytol. 1959;6:253–61.
34. Leo LA, Paiocchi VL, Schlossbauer SA, Ho SY, Faletra FF. The intrusive nature of epicardial adipose tissue as revealed by cardiac magnetic resonance. J Cardiovasc Echography. 2019;29:45–51.
35. Faletra FF, Leo LA, Paiocchi VL, Schlossbauer SA, Borruso MG, Pedrazzini G, et al. Imaging-based tricuspid valve anatomy by computed tomography, magnetic resonance imaging, two and three-dimensional echocardiography: correlation with anatomic specimen. Eur Heart J Cardiovasc Imaging. 2019;20:1–3.
36. Dean JW, Ho SY, Rowland E, Mann J, Anderson RH. Clinical anatomy of the atrioventricular junctions. J Am Coll Cardiol. 1994;24:1725–31.
37. McKenney ML, Schultz KA, Boyd JH, Byrd JP, Alloosh M, Teague SD, et al. Epicardial adipose excision slows the progression of porcine coronary atherosclerosis. J Cardiothorac Surg. 2014;9:2.
38. Corradi D. The ventricular epicardial fat is related to the myocardial mass in normal, ischemic and hypertrophic hearts. Cardiovasc Pathol. 2004;13:313–6.

2 Physiology and Cardioprotection of the Epicardial Adipose Tissue

Gianluca Iacobellis

Key Points

- Epicardial adipose tissue (EAT) has physiological and cardioprotective properties.
- EAT expresses genes encoding for adipokines, such as adiponectin, adrenomedullin, and omentin, and other pathways with potential cardioprotective functions.
- EAT serves as a buffer protecting the heart against high fatty acid levels, as source of energy feeding the myocardium with fatty acids, as brown fat defending the myocardium against hypothermia, and as pad protecting abnormal curvature of the coronary arteries.

Introduction

Epicardial adipose tissue (EAT) is a peculiar visceral fat depot with a dichotomous role, either physiological or pathological. EAT has cardioprotective properties and functions. The mechanisms that regulate the balance between protective and harmful effects of EAT are not clearly understood. Most of the physiological properties of the EAT are well preserved in healthy individuals. The thermogenic functions of the EAT rapidly decreased in the first months or years of life, but they remain potentially active. The equilibrium between the detrimental and beneficial effects is delicate and under the influence of several hemodynamic and metabolic factors. EAT expresses potential cardioprotective gene pathways that are downregulated by unfavorable local and systemic conditions. Otherwise, EAT can upregulate protective genes in response to chronic or acute damages. Certainly, the physiological role of EAT within the heart is complex and not completely explored. However, the EAT functions can be grossly distinguished in nutritional, regulatory, metabolic, thermogenic, and mechanical (Table 2.1). Because of its anatomical proximity to the heart and the absence of fascial boundaries, EAT interacts and modulates the myocardium and coronary arteries through the local and direct secretion of bioactive molecules (Fig. 2.1).

G. Iacobellis (✉)
Division of Endocrinology, Diabetes and Metabolism, Department of Medicine, University of Miami, Miller School of Medicine, Miami, FL, USA
e-mail: giacobellis@med.miami.edu

G. Iacobellis (ed.), *Epicardial Adipose Tissue*, Contemporary Cardiology,
https://doi.org/10.1007/978-3-030-40570-0_2

Table 2.1 Cardioprotective properties of epicardial fat

Nutritional
Mobilizable energy store for the myocardium; local energy source by channeling fatty acids to the myocardium; highest free fatty acid synthesis, incorporation, and breakdown; high lipolysis and insulin-induced lipogenesis; buffering high fatty acid levels to protect the heart
Metabolic
Adiponectin effects: anti-inflammatory, decreased expression of adhesion molecules, suppression of cytokine production and lipid accumulation in macrophages, increase myocardial fatty acid combustion
Adrenomedullin effects: vasodilation, antioxidative, angiogenic, anti-apoptotic, and anti-inflammatory
Omentin effects: vasodilation, improved insulin sensitivity
Expression of glucagon-like peptide-1 receptor (GLP-1R), and sodium-glucose cotransporter 2 (SGLT2)
Thermogenic
Brown fatlike activity via expression of uncoupling protein 1 (UCP-1) and other markers of BAT: defend the myocardium against hypothermia, white-to-beige adipocyte transformation; improve mitochondrial signaling genes; regulation of myocardial lipid and glucose metabolism; UCP-1-mediated reduced inflammation and oxidative stress
Regulatory
Regulation of potassium channel activity, mesoderm development, regulation of body fluid levels, wound healing, ER nuclear signaling pathway, membrane organization, and biogenesis
Mechanical
Mechanical protection against abnormal curvature of the coronary arteries

Epicardial Fat Nutrifying the Myocardium

EAT is actively involved in lipid and energy homeostasis, serving as both lipid storage and local source of energy by channeling free fatty acids (FFAs) to the myocardium [1]. EAT displays the greatest capacity for free fatty acid release and uptake and lower rate of glucose utilization, among any other visceral fat depots. In fact, free fatty acid synthesis, rate of incorporation and breakdown, rates of lipolysis, and insulin-induced lipogenesis are higher in EAT than in other visceral fat depots [1]. Insulin increases the rate of lipogenesis but not that of fatty acid incorporation in EAT [1]. Myocardium uses and metabolizes free fatty acids from the coronary arterial blood, and free fatty acid oxidation is responsible for about 70% of the energy production of the heart. Physiologically EAT works as a buffer, absorbing free fatty acids and protecting the heart against the toxic effect of excessively high fatty acid levels. The high basal rates of fatty acid incorporation and lipogenesis of EAT serve as a rapidly mobilizable energy store for the myocardium. Given the proximity to the heart, due to the absence of muscle fascia that separates the two tissues, FFAs are transported from the EAT directly into the myocardium. Free fatty acids can diffuse bidirectionally in interstitial fluid across concentration gradients. EAT

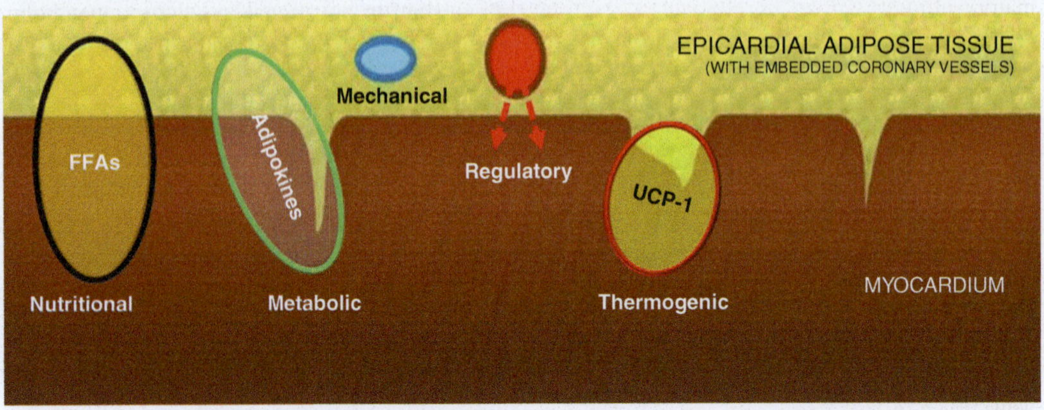

Fig. 2.1 Graphic depicting how epicardial adipose tissue (EAT) modulates the proximal and underlying myocardium through the local and direct secretion of bioactive molecules that exert nutritional, regulatory, metabolic, thermogenic, and mechanical functions

also secretes vasoactive factors that regulate coronary arterial tone and so facilitate the FFA influx. Fatty-acid-binding protein 4, highly expressed in EAT, participates in the intracellular transport of FFAs from epicardial fat into the myocardium [2]. Compared to subcutaneous adipose tissue, human EAT is rich in saturated fatty acids [3], such as myristic acid (14:0), palmitic acid (16:0), and stearic acid (18:0), whereas unsaturated fatty acids are lower. This profound difference in fatty acid composition accounts for the different rate of mobilization, deposition, and synthesis of FFAs between epicardial and subcutaneous fat.

Epicardial Fat Cardioprotective Adipokines

EAT can be considered an endocrine organ. It is a metabolically active organ and a source of several bioactive molecules that can influence the myocardium and coronary arteries [4–6]. EAT expresses and secretes a number of cytokines, pro- and anti-inflammatory adipokines, vasoactive factors, and growth factors [4–6]. Two major mechanisms of interaction between the myocardium and the epicardial fat, i.e., paracrine and vasocrine, have been suggested [7, 8]. Paracrine release of cytokines from periadventitial EAT could traverse the coronary wall by diffusion from outside to inside. Given the dense inflammatory infiltrate within the human EAT and its complex cellularity, it seems reasonable to suspect that cytokines are secreted by different cells. Adipokines secreted from epicardial adipocytes and stromal and vascular cells may diffuse in interstitial fluid across the adventitia, media, and intima and then interact respectively with vasa vasorum and endothelial and vascular smooth muscle cells of the coronary arteries. Alternatively, adipokines and free fatty acids might be released from epicardial tissue directly into vasa vasorum and be transported downstream into the arterial wall, in a vasocrine signaling mechanism [7, 8]. EAT is enriched in genes coding for cardioprotective adipokines such as adiponectin and adrenomedullin, both with potential anti-inflammatory and anti-atherogenic properties [9–11]. It is unclear how the expression and secretion of these adipokines is regulated [12]. EAT might exert its cardioprotective effect through adiponectin and adrenomedullin secretion in response to local or systemic metabolic or mechanical insults. Alternatively, it has been suggested that EAT cardioprotective adipokine gene and protein expression is higher in individuals with lower risk of cardiovascular, hypothesizing therefore a protective transcriptome reducing the risk of major cardiovascular events. However, it is plausible to hypothesize that both mechanisms may coexist.

Adiponectin

Adiponectin, a serum protein of 30 kDa, a member of the complement factor C1q family, is produced and secreted exclusively by adipose tissue. Adiponectin may have anti-inflammatory and anti-atherogenic properties, and hypoadiponectinemia can play a role in the pathogenesis of coronary artery disease [9–11]. Human EAT expresses adiponectin, as first discovered by Iacobellis et al. [13]. Adiponectin protein expression was studied in EAT in vivo both in patients with severe coronary artery disease and in subjects without normal coronary arteries. Given the anatomical proximity, epicardial fat could exert its favorable effects on the adjacent coronary artery through increased adiponectin production. Adiponectin can decrease the expression of adhesion molecules in the endothelial cells in response to local inflammation and suppress cytokine production and lipid accumulation in macrophages. EAT secreted adiponectin which contributes to myocardial fatty acid combustion. Unfortunately, adiponectin gene and protein expression in patients with coronary artery disease is downregulated (Fig. 2.2) [13, 14]. The lower EAT adiponectin expression can therefore contribute to favor free fatty acid myocardial accumulation over combustion. However, is EAT adiponectin secreted directly into the intracoronary circulation? Given the absence of anatomical barriers separating the fat from the underlying coronary

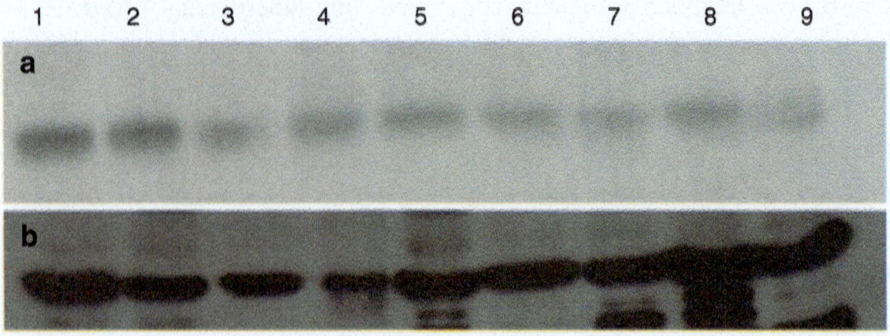

Fig. 2.2 (**a**) Western blot showing higher epicardial adipose tissue (EAT) adiponectin expression in patients without coronary artery disease (CAD), lanes 1–2, as compared to that in patients CAD lanes from 3 to 9. Total proteins were extracted from frozen EAT collected in patients who underwent cardiac surgery. (**b**) Monoclonal antibody for adiponectin (dilution 1:2500) that recognizes the C-terminal globular domain of human adiponectin. (© Georg Thieme Verlag KG. From Iacobellis et al. [14], with permission)

arteries, this could be assumed. To address whether EAT secretosome can be directly transported into the coronary lumen, plasma levels of adiponectin were measured in peripheral vein circulation and in left coronary artery during coronary angiography [14]. EAT for adiponectin protein extraction was obtained from the same subjects with or without coronary artery disease who underwent elective cardiac surgery. Remarkably, intracoronary plasma adiponectin levels significantly correlated with epicardial fat adiponectin protein expression ($r = 0.68$, $p = 0.02$) in all subjects. The intracoronary adiponectin levels were predicted by both peripheral adiponectin levels and EAT adiponectin protein expression. It is interesting to note that intracoronary adiponectin levels rapidly and significantly increased after coronary revascularization [15]. Although these studies could not demonstrate an independent correlation, EAT could contribute, at least partially, to adiponectin levels in the coronary circulation.

Adrenomedullin

Adrenomedullin has been indicated to have cardioprotective effects, as well as adiponectin. Adrenomedullin is a peptide with vasodilating, antioxidative, angiogenic, anti-apoptotic, and anti-inflammatory properties [16–18]. However, the role of adrenomedullin in cardiovascular diseases is not completely understood and results are contradictory. Some studies found higher whereas others lower adrenomedullin circulating levels in subjects with coronary artery disease [18–21]. Circulating plasma adrenomedullin levels are upregulated after an acute myocardial infarction suggesting an adaptive response to modulate myocardial tolerance to ischemia-reperfusion injury [18–20]. Whether EAT expresses adrenomedullin and plays a protective role on the coronary arteries mediated by this adipokine was evaluated. Adrenomedullin and its receptors are expressed and secreted by the EAT [22]. Adrenomedullin proteins were present in blood vessel walls and in the stromal fraction of EAT. Adrenomedullin could originate from epicardial adipocytes and macrophages infiltrating the fat depot [22]. Interestingly it has been suggested that adrenomedullin can increase epicardial adipocyte sizes by inhibiting the catecholamine-induced lipolysis [22]. EAT adrenomedullin was investigated in different cardiovascular conditions, such as heart failure and coronary artery disease. Findings of these studies seem to be contradictory, although explanatory mechanisms may clarify the apparent discordance. Adrenomedullin is related to 11beta-HSD-1 expression and its expression in EAT was higher in subjects with chronic coronary artery disease [22]. Higher expression of mRNA encoding for adrenomedullin was observed also in the epicardial fat of patients with systolic heart failure [20]. On the contrary, intracoronary adrenomedullin concentrations were significantly lower in subjects with coronary ischemic disease than in those without [24]. This study failed to demonstrate that EAT independently contributes to intracoronary adrenomedullin levels [24]. Coronary sinus adrenomedullin levels were not statistically different than those in left coronary artery suggesting that adrenomedullin was not secreted from EAT into the coronary artery lumen [24]. If adrenomedullin was secreted transmurally from epicardial fat into the coronary artery lumen, adrenomedullin levels in coronary sinus should have been higher than those in arterial blood. EAT adrenomedullin expression can be upregulated in response to acute hypoxemia, such as in myocardial infarction or acute heart failure [18–20, 23]. By the contrast, the chronic hypoxic insult can progressively downregulate epicardial fat adrenomedullin secretion and so explain the lower plasma concentration in advanced stages of coronary artery disease [21, 24]. Undoubtedly, EAT is a source of adrenomedullin under pathological conditions. However, epicardial fat adrenomedullin secretion is regulated by coronary status and other hemodynamic factors that can differently affect its circulating levels.

Omentin

Omentin-1, another adipocytokine mainly expressed in visceral adipose tissue, displays also cardioprotective functions by inhibiting the inflammatory response and improving insulin resistance. Omentin is closely associated with adiponectin. Remarkably, omentin treatment increases adipogenesis-induced adiponectin levels on stromal cells of epicardial fat [25]. EAT expresses omentin-1 gene but the mRNA levels are lower in patients with coronary artery disease [26]. Interestingly EAT omentin-1 expression was lower in fat depot adjacent to coronary stenotic segments than in that proximal to nonstenotic segments [26]. However, results are not univocal. In fact, omentin expression in the EAT was found higher in nonobese patients with coronary artery disease [27] and affected by type 2 diabetes [28].

Epicardial as Brown Fat

Brown adipose tissue generates heat, nonshivering thermogenesis, in response to cold temperatures and activation of the autonomic nervous system. Brown fat dissipates energy through uncoupling protein (UCP)-1-mediated heat production. Brown fat is also a secretagogue depot. Brown fat secretosome can locally and systemically influence fuel and energy metabolism. However, the role of brown fat in humans is unclear. Activation of brown fat can increase energy expenditure, reduce adiposity, and improve insulin sensitivity, glucose, and lipid metabolism. Brown fat activation would be the ideal fat burner and therefore weight loss mediator, but unfortunately most of the brown fat is lost in the transition from infancy to adult life in humans. Brown fat was first identified in hibernating animals and newborns. More recent studies found brown fat or brown fatlike, also called beige, adipocytes also in adult humans. Brown adipose tissue could be further categorized as visceral and subcutaneous [29, 30]. Visceral brown fat is represented around the heart and the vessels. Visceral brown fat can be located around the aorta, common carotid artery, brachiocephalic artery, and anterior mediastinum internal mammary artery. Clinically, a significant uptake of 18F-fluorodeoxyglucose (18F-FDG) by the heart suggested that brown adipose tissue may lie close to the heart or directly within the myocardial tissue [31]. Brown fat can be visualized also around the kidneys, adrenals, liver, and pancreas. It is of interest to report that the mRNA expression of adiponectin was found significantly higher in brown adipose tissue than in white adipose tissue surrounding pheochromocytoma and that catecholamine and serum adiponectin levels significantly correlated with brown fat markers and adiponectin mRNA levels [32]. Subcutaneous brown fat includes depots located between the anterior neck muscles, in the supraclavicular fossa posterior to the brachial plexus, under the clavicles, in the axilla, and in the inguinal area [29, 30].

Human EAT also displays brown fat features and properties, as recently discovered by

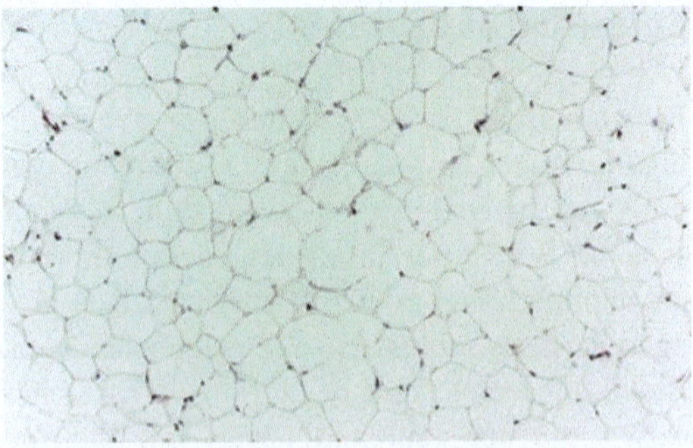

Fig. 2.3 Epicardial histology section from patient showing the small and unilocular epicardial adipocytes. (From Sacks et al. [35], with permission from Oxford University Press)

Sacks and colleagues [33–35]. Histologically, EAT should better defined as beige fat [35]. In fact, small unilocular adipocytes without UCP-1 immunostaining are described in EAT (Fig. 2.3). Hence, epicardial adipocytes display histological similarities with in vitro in beige lineage adipocytes [35]. Brown fat-specific gene UCP-1 and other brown fat regulatory genes, such as brown adipocyte differentiation transcription factors PR-domain-missing 16 (PRDM16) and peroxisome proliferator-activated receptor gamma coactivator-1 alpha (PGC-1α), were all highly expressed in human EAT [34]. PRDM16 and PGC-1α regulate the transformation of brown adipocyte precursors into their mature cellular forms containing UCP-1 in humans. UCP-1 was found significantly higher in human EAT as compared to other fat depots and basically undetectable in subcutaneous fat [34]. EAT UCP-1 expression increased with body mass index and was similar in women and men, whereas it was not influenced by statin or thiazolidinedione therapy [34]. In cases of hypothermia, chronic exposure to cold promotes EAT PGC-1α activation, a key mediator of the white-to-beige adipocyte transformation [34].

While age seems to have only a minimal or no effect on EAT volume or thickness in humans, the brown fat activity of EAT changes and decreases with aging [35]. The structure and architecture of EAT differs among the neonate, infant, and child, with profound regulatory effects on UCP-1, as nicely described by Ojha et al. [36]. In their study, the authors noted that epicardial fat can maintain a good number of UCP1-positive cells into childhood. Autoptic studies confirmed histological evidence of brown fat in the pericardium and EAT in human infants and children under 10 years [29, 30]. The proportion of brown adipocytes decreases in favor of more unilocular white adipocytes in subjects older than 25 years. This suggests the transition from brown to beige fat features of EAT in adult life. To evaluate the loss of brown adipocytes with age and maturation, the presence of UCP1 was analyzed within the EAT and other adipose tissues in young sheep during the first month of life [37]. The authors found that UCP1 abundance was reduced by 28 days of age, although UCP1 signal remained in the EAT as compared to the other fat depots [37].

All together, these findings suggest that under physiological conditions EAT displays brown fat like activity to protect the myocardium against hypothermia. However, the role of EAT to serve as brown fat to the myocardium is still unclear. EAT is thought to provide direct heating to the myocardium and protect the heart during a drop in core body temperature or during unfavorable hemodynamic conditions, such as ischemia or hypoxia.

If this is correct, brown fatlike activity of EAT would be either up- or downregulated in advanced coronary artery disease. Upregulation would be anticipated as compensatory response to the chronic hypoxic insult whereas downregulation would be expected as consequences of the fibrotic and apoptotic involution that EAT may suffer in end-stage organ disease, as suggested by McAninch et al. [38]. Nevertheless results are controversial and not yet conclusive. In fact, UCP-1 expression was similar in patients without and with severe coronary atherosclerosis in a single study [34]. However, an alternative pathway has been recently proposed. Singh et al., using a genetic approach and heatmap, identified other possible cardioprotective pathway genes involving PGC-1α for evaluation of their effects to attenuate heart failure in both mice and humans. Interestingly, the authors suggested a role of the epicardial fat heme oxygenase-1 (HO1) PGC-1α in modulating the inflammation, mitochondrial activity, and left ventricle function [39]. PGC-1α and PRDM16 are the major inducers of adipocyte browning and thermogenic activation of brown fat. This study highlights the role that EAT PGC-1α and HO-1 can play in mitochondrial function and biogenesis. Singh et al. have shown that humans with heart diseases have a reduction of HO-1 PGC-1α and PRDM16 in EAT compared to visceral controls, with reciprocal increases in pro-inflammatory cytokines. Remarkably, the increase in brown fat and mitochondrial signaling genes was associated with a decrease in inflammatory adipokines in EAT and an improvement in left ventricular function in obese mice. Of note, EAT was highly enriched with *KCNK17*, overexpressed in human brown fat in comparison to white fat [40].

Interestingly, potential UCP-1-mediated cardioprotective function of EAT may be not only related to the myocardial thermoregulation. In fact, recent transcriptomic analysis of different fat depots confirmed that EAT has a unique UCP-1 signature profile and the higher *UCP1* expression in EAT was associated with a downregulation of T cell-related immune pathways, such as T cell receptor signaling, iCOS-iCOSL signaling in T helper cells, Th2 pathway, T helper cell differentiation, calcium-induced T lymphocyte apoptosis, and B cell receptor [41]. Upregulation of *UCP1* in EAT was also associated with a downregulation of TNFα and reactive oxygen species [41].

So it is plausible to think that epicardial fat may function like brown fat to defend the heart against hypothermia and possibly again inflammation and oxidative stress. While EAT turns into a beige fat depot in adult life, it retains the genetic and cellular potential to switch on its early brown fat activity. In fact, UCP-1 expression was present and abundant in epicardial of adult humans [34]. EAT may adapt itself to different metabolic circumstances and function as brown-like or beige fat depot as needed. However, this fascinating hypothesis requires further investigations.

Epicardial Fat Regulatory Transcriptome

Microarray study showed the human EAT is also highly enriched in genes encoding for factors and proteins that play a regulatory function of the heart morphology and structure [38]. Epicardial and subcutaneous fat samples were obtained from patients undergoing cardiac surgery and evaluated using Genechip Human Gene 2.0 ST arrays (Affymetrix, Santa Clara, CA, USA). EAT was highly enriched in gene coding for potassium channel activity, mesoderm development, regulation of body fluid levels, wound healing, ER nuclear signaling pathway, membrane organization, and biogenesis as compared to subcutaneous adipose tissue collected from the same subject. *ADORA1* coding for receptor implicated in cardioprotection in the face of ischemia was also upregulated in human EAT [38, 42].

Epicardial Fat Mechanical Cardioprotection

In addition to its important metabolic and thermos-energetic properties, EAT has the mechanical function of protecting the coronary artery against the torsion induced by the arterial pulse wave and cardiac contraction [43]. Positive vessel remodeling was evaluated in 147 patients by using intravascular ultrasound (IVUS). IVUS identification of septal branches, which emerge on the side of the vessel opposite the pericardium, can be used to divide the plaque into a myocardial and pericardial surface. As they are unimpaired by myocardial extravascular resistance, lesions facing the pericardium undergo a vessel expansion that is also favored by the permissive role of EAT. There is a possibility that a rim of fat tissue separates the proximal left anterior coronary artery from the underlying myocardium. This is an anatomical variant but it is unlikely to contrast the splinting effect of the myocardium during systole.

Effect of Aging and Gender on Epicardial Fat Cardioprotection

As physiological process, aging may also influence the function of EAT. This seems to occur more in female than in male, as recently suggested. A study showed decrease in EAT-secreted both pro- and anti-inflammatory cytokines in older female rather than in older male rats [44]. Another study in rats found profound changes in the expression profile of obesity-related genes in EAT with aging in female, but not in male [45]. These changes could be attributed to differences in hormonal control, adipocyte remodeling, endothelium changes, or macrophage infiltration between female and male rats [46]. A very recent study confirmed the transition from brown to white fat at 2 weeks of age in EAT of fetus lambs and showed the effect of maternal cortisol on epicardial fat maturation [6].

In humans, the effect of aging on EAT has been not well investigated, but it could affect its thermogenic properties, as previously discussed. If these results would be confirmed in humans, the detrimental effect of aging on female EAT may contribute to the higher cardiovascular risk in postmenopausal women.

References

1. Marchington JM, Pond CM. Site-specific properties of pericardial and epicardial adipose tissue: the effects of insulin and high-fat feeding on lipogenesis and the incorporation of fatty acids in vitro. Int J Obes. 1990;14:1013–22.
2. Vural B, Atalar F, Ciftci C, Demirkan A, Susleyici-Duman B, Gunay D. Presence of fatty-acid-binding protein 4 expression in human epicardial adipose tissue in metabolic syndrome. Cardiovasc Pathol. 2008;17:392–8.
3. Pezeshkian M, Mahtabipour MR. Epicardial and subcutaneous adipose tissue fatty acids profiles in diabetic and non-diabetic patients candidate for coronary artery bypass graft. Bioimpacts. 2013;3:83–9.
4. Marchington JM, Mattacks CA, Pond CM. Adipose tissue in the mammalian heart and pericardium; structure, foetal development and biochemical properties. Comp Biochem Physiol. 1989;94B:225–32.
5. Iacobellis G, Bianco AC. Epicardial adipose tissue: emerging physiological, pathophysiological and clinical features. Trends Endocrinol Metab. 2011;22:450–7.
6. Iacobellis G, Corradi D, Sharma AM. Epicardial adipose tissue: anatomic, biomolecular and clinical relationships with the heart. Nat Clin Pract Cardiovasc Med. 2005;2:536–43.
7. Judkin JS, Eringa E, Stehouwer CD. "Vasocrine signalling" from perivascular fat: a mechanism linking insulin resistance to vascular disease. Lancet. 2005;365:1817–20.
8. Mazurek T, Zhang L, Zalewski A, Mannion JD, Diehl JT, Arafat H. Human epicardial adipose tissue is a source of inflammatory mediators. Circulation. 2003;108:2460–6.
9. Matsuzawa Y, Funahashi T, Kihara S, Shimomura I. Adiponectin and metabolic syndrome. Arterioscler Thromb Vasc Biol. 2004;24:29–33. Review.
10. Yatagai T, Nagasaka S, Taniguchi A, Fukushima M, Nakamura T, Kuroe A, et al. Hypoadiponectinemia is associated with visceral fat accumulation and insulin resistance in Japanese men with type 2 diabetes mellitus. Metabolism. 2003;52:1274–8.
11. Staiger H, Tschritter O, Machann J, Thamer C, Fritsche A, Maerker E, et al. Relationship of serum adiponectin and leptin concentrations with body fat distribution in humans. Obes Res. 2003;11:368–72.
12. Iacobellis G, Barbaro G. The double role of epicardial adipose tissue as pro- and anti-inflammatory organ. Horm Metab Res. 2008;40:442–5.
13. Iacobellis G, Pistilli D, Gucciardo M, Leonetti F, Miraldi F, Brancaccio G, et al. Adiponectin expression in human epicardial adipose tissue in vivo is lower in patients with CAD. Cytokine. 2005;29:251–5.
14. Iacobellis G, di Gioia CR, Cotesta D, Petramala L, Travaglini C, De Santis V, et al. Epicardial adipose tissue adiponectin expression is related to intracoronary adiponectin levels. Horm Metab Res. 2009;41:227–31.
15. Iacobellis G, Cotesta D, Petramala L, De Santis V, Vitale D, Tritapepe L, Letizia C. Intracoronary adiponectin levels rapidly and significantly increase after coronary revascularization. Int J Cardiol. 2010;144:160–3.
16. Ishimitsu T, Ono H, Minami J, Matsuoka H. Pathophysiologic and therapeutic implications of adrenomedullin in cardiovascular disorders. Pharmacol Ther. 2006;111:909–27.
17. Bunton DC, Petrie MC, Hillier C, Johnston F, McMurray JJV. The clinical relevance of adrenomedullin: a promising profile? Pharmacol Ther. 2004;103:179–201.
18. Yasu T, Nishikimi T, Kobayashi N, Ikeda N, Ueba H, Nakamura T, et al. Up-regulated synthesis of mature-type adrenomedullin in coronary circulation immediately after reperfusion in patients with anterior acute myocardial infarction. Regul Pept. 2005;129(1–3):161–6.
19. Kobayashi K, Kitamura K, Hirayama N, Date H, Kashiwagi T, Ikushima I, et al. Increased plasma adrenomedullin in acute myocardial infarction. Am Heart J. 1996;131:676–80.

20. Hamid SA, Baxter GF. A critical cytoprotective role of endogenous adrenomedullin in acute myocardial infarction. J Mol Cell Cardiol. 2006;41:360–3.
21. Hojo Y, Uichi I, Katsuki T, Shimada K. Decreased adrenomedullin production in the coronary circulation of patients with coronary artery disease. Heart. 2000;84(1):88.
22. Silaghi A, Achard V, Paulmyer-Lacroix O, Scridon T, Tassistro V, Duncea I, et al. Expression of adrenomedullin in human epicardial adipose tissue: role of coronary status. Am J Physiol Endocrinol Metab. 2007;293:E1443–50.
23. Fosshaug LE, Dahl CP, Risnes I, Bohov P, Berge RK, Nymo S, et al. Altered levels of fatty acids and inflammatory and metabolic mediators in epicardial adipose tissue in patients with systolic heart failure. J Card Fail. 2015;21:916–23.
24. Iacobellis G, di Goia CR, Di Vito M, Petramala L, Cotesta D, De Santis V, et al. Epicardial adipose tissue and intracoronary adrenomedullin levels in coronary artery disease. Horm Metab Res. 2009;41:855–60.
25. Fernández-Trasancos Á, Agra RM, García-Acuña JM, Fernández ÁL, González-Juanatey JR, Eiras S. Omentin treatment of epicardial fat improves its anti-inflammatory activity and paracrine benefit on smooth muscle cells. Obesity (Silver Spring). 2017;25:1042–9.
26. Du Y, Ji Q, Cai L, Huang F, Lai Y, Liu Y, et al. Association between omentin-1 expression in human epicardial adipose tissue and coronary atherosclerosis. Cardiovasc Diabetol. 2016;15:90.
27. Harada K, Shibata R, Ouchi N, Tokuda Y, Funakubo H, Suzuki M, et al. Increased expression of the adipocytokine omentin in the epicardial adipose tissue of coronary artery disease patients. Atherosclerosis. 2016;251:299–304.
28. Matloch Z, Kratochvílová H, Cinkajzlová A, Lipš M, Kopecký P, Pořízka M, et al. Changes in omentin levels and its mRNA expression in epicardial adipose tissue in patients undergoing elective cardiac surgery: the influence of type 2 diabetes and coronary heart disease. Physiol Res. 2018;67:881–90.
29. Nedergaard J, Bengtsson T, Cannon B. Unexpected evidence for active brown adipose tissue in adult humans. Am J Physiol Endocrinol Metab. 2007;293:E444–52.
30. Heaton JM. The distribution of brown adipose tissue in the human. J Anat. 1972;112:35–9.
31. Cypess AM, Lehman S, Williams G, Tal I, Rodman D, Goldfine AB, et al. Identification and importance of brown adipose tissue in adult humans. N Engl J Med. 2009;360:1509–17.
32. Iacobellis G, Di Gioia C, Petramala L, Chiappetta C, Serra V, Zinnamosca L, et al. Brown fat expresses adiponectin in humans. Int J Endocrinol. 2013;2013:126751.
33. Sacks HS, Fain JN. Human epicardial adipose tissue: a review. Am Heart J. 2007;153:907–17.
34. Sacks HS, Fain JN, Holman B, Cheema P, Chary A, Parks F. Uncoupling protein-1 and related mRNAs in human epicardial and other adipose tissues: epicardial fat functioning as brown fat. J Clin Endocrinol Metab. 2009;94:3611–5.
35. Sacks HS, Fain JN, Bahouth SW, Ojha S, Frontini A, Budge H, et al. Human epicardial fat exhibits beige features. J Clin Endocrinol Metab. 2013;98:E1448–55.
36. Ojha S, Fainberg HP, Wilson V, Pelella G, Castellanos M, May ST, et al. Gene pathway development in human epicardial adipose tissue during early life. JCI Insight. 2016;1:e87460.
37. Fainberg HP, Birtwistle M, Alagal R, Alhaddad A, Pope M, Davies G, et al. Transcriptional analysis of adipose tissue during development reveals depot-specific responsiveness to maternal dietary supplementation. Sci Rep. 2018;8:9628.
38. McAninch EA, Fonseca TL, Poggioli R, Panos AL, Salerno TA, Deng Y, et al. Epicardial adipose tissue has a unique transcriptome modified in severe coronary artery disease. Obesity. 2015;23:1267–78.
39. Singh SP, McClung JA, Thompson E, Glick Y, Greenberg M, Acosta-Baez G, et al. Cardioprotective effect of heme oxygenase-1-PGC-1α signaling in epicardial fat attenuates cardiovascular risk in humans as in obese mice. Obesity (Silver Spring). 2019;27:1634–43.
40. Svensson PA, Jernas M, Sjoholm K, Hoffmann JM, Nilsson BE, Hansson M, et al. Gene expression in human brown adipose tissue. Int J Mol Med. 2011;27:227–32.
41. Chechi K, Vijay J, Voisine P, Mathieu P, Bossé Y, Tchernof A, et al. UCP1 expression-associated gene signatures of human epicardial adipose tissue. JCI Insight. 2019;4:e123618.
42. Regan SE, Broad M, Byford AM, Lankford AR, Cerniway RJ, Mayo MW, et al. A1 adenosine receptor overexpression attenuates ischemia-reperfusion-induced apoptosis and caspase 3 activity. Am J Physiol Heart Circ Physiol. 2003;284:H859–66.
43. Prati F, Arbustini E, Labellarte A, Sommariva L, Pawlowski T, Manzoli A, et al. Eccentric atherosclerotic plaques with positive remodelling have a pericardial distribution: a permissive role of epicardial fat? A three-dimensional intravascular ultrasound study of left anterior descending artery lesions. Eur Heart J. 2003;24:329–36.
44. Fei J, Cook C, Blough E, Santanam N. Age and sex mediated changes in epicardial fat adipokines. Atherosclerosis. 2010;212:488–94.
45. Kocher C, Christiansen M, Martin S, Adams C, Wehner P, Gress T, Santanam N. Sexual dimorphism in obesity-related genes in the epicardial fat during aging. J Physiol Biochem. 2017;73:215–24.
46. Richards EM, McElhaney E, Zeringue K, Joseph S, Keller-Wood M. Transcriptomic evidence that cortisol alters perinatal epicardial adipose tissue maturation. Am J Physiol Endocrinol Metab. 2019;317:E573–85.

3 Transcriptomic and Proteomic Analysis of the Epicardial Adipose Tissue

Vladimir Camarena, David W. Sant, Tyler C. Huff, and Gaofeng Wang

Key Points

- Epicardial adipose tissue (EAT) expresses a unique set of genes setting it apart from other human adipose tissues.
- Transcriptomic and proteomic studies show that EAT is a local source of adipokines with paracrine influence on the myocardium due to the intimate microcirculation shared by both tissues.
- EAT displays a unique pro-inflammatory and thermogenic gene signature.

V. Camarena · T. C. Huff
John P. Hussman Institute for Human Genomics, Department of Human Genetics, University of Miami Miller School of Medicine, Miami, FL, USA

D. W. Sant
Biomedical Informatics, Department of Biological Engineering, Utah State University, Salt Lake City, UT, USA

G. Wang (✉)
John P. Hussman Institute for Human Genomics, Dr. John T. Macdonald Foundation Department of Human Genetics, Sylvester Comprehensive Cancer Center, Miller School of Medicine, University of Miami, Miami, FL, USA
e-mail: gwang@med.miami.edu

Introduction

Adipose tissue is mainly composed of adipocytes. Adipocytes are specialized cells that store energy as lipids and triglycerides in a vacuole. Based on appearance in histological analysis, adipose tissues are classified as white, brown, or beige. Adipose tissues are subdivided into subcutaneous and visceral based on their anatomical location [1]. Subcutaneous and visceral fat are further subdivided according to location [1]. In the white adipocyte tissue (WAT), the adipocytes store lipids in a central vacuole that pushes the nuclei and the rest of the cytoplasm to the periphery of the cell. Depending of the size of the vacuole, these cells can increase in size from 30 to 230 microns. Based on the energy needs of the body, adipocytes can also synthesize fatty acids and release them to the bloodstream and are therefore located in close proximity to capillaries and other blood vessels. Brown adipose tissue (BAT) consists of smaller adipocytes [15–60 microns] which contain lipid droplets in multiple small vacuoles. They have larger cytoplasm, nuclei, and mitochondria that give them a distinct color. BAT is abundant in the fetus, human newborns, and hibernating animals. Production of heat by the mitochondria is considered to be the main role of BAT and can be regulated by extensive sympathetic innervation within the tissue [2]. Beige adipocytes are brown-like adipocytes that can appear in between white adipose

G. Iacobellis (ed.), *Epicardial Adipose Tissue*, Contemporary Cardiology,
https://doi.org/10.1007/978-3-030-40570-0_3

depots. These cells also have thermogenic function like BAT and can be induced in deposits of WAT by certain physiological conditions like cold temperatures or exercise [3]. Adipose depots serve as energy supply due to their ability to release fatty acids into the blood stream as needed for energy. However, adipose tissue can also serve as an insulator and give mechanical protection to the underlying tissue by acting as a cushion. Furthermore, adipose tissue serves endocrine and paracrine functions which were relatively overlooked until the discovery of adipokines (such as tumor necrosis factor α (TNF-α), leptin, adipsin, and adiponectin) that are produced and secreted by adipose tissue and modulate numerous physiological processes [3, 4]. Epicardial adipose tissue [EAT] is derived from the splanchnopleuric mesoderm that evolved during embryogenesis [5–8]. It is intimately located on the myocardium and coronary arteries without separation by a fascia. This tissue has a beige phenotype and is composed of small adipocytes, fibroblasts, immune cells, vasculature, and neural cells [6]. This heterogeneous tissue was historically viewed as a pathological fat deposit with no functional role. Recent proteomic studies and the rise of high-throughput sequencing technologies have now led to discoveries suggesting this to be far from the truth, providing great new insight into the physiological role of EAT.

Epicardial Fat Transcriptomics in Animals and Humans

Studies investigating EAT function have adopted numerous cellular and animal models. Studies of a diverse group of wild and domesticated animals have shown that EAT is present in many small mammals including guinea pigs, rabbits, monkeys, and cats, as well as in many large mammals like horses, whales, and humans [9]. The presence of EAT has also been found to be unrelated to the leanness of the animal. The best EAT animal model is the guinea pig, as they have epicardial fat next to the myocardium that increases in size with age, similar to humans. Additionally, they have a relatively low cost of maintenance in comparison to larger animals [10, 11]. Several gene expression studies have been done in larger animals such as pigs [12–15], but the cost of maintaining large animals in conjunction with their longevity can be limiting. Mouse models with all their available genetic tools would be ideal, but gene expression studies in mice are limited due to the small size or lack of EAT; therefore, genetically obese models like Zucker rats are typically used [9, 14, 16]. Mice can be induced to develop EAT by promoting the expression of the peroxisome proliferator-activated receptor-γ [PPARγ] which induces epithelial-to-mesenchymal transition, suggesting that a similar mechanism might occur for the development of EAT in humans and other mammals, but this has not been fully demonstrated [17].

The use of tissue explants or conditioned media from EAT is another approach to study the function of EAT [11, 18–23]. The disadvantage of tissue explants is that once the tissues are removed from their natural environment, their gene expression profile can change significantly. Using conditioned media from explants has been particularly useful for studying the effect of EAT on myocytes in cell culture systems. Additionally, human tissue recovered from autopsies has also been used to study EAT [24]. Unfortunately, postmortem studies are limited and difficult to interpret. The cause of death and the time of sample collection can lead to deterioration of the sample, which can yield low-quality RNA and may even cause a change in expression profiles, thus making gene expression studies difficult to execute.

The most common method to study EAT in humans is the use of biopsies collected during elective cardiovascular surgery. These biopsies are often compared with other adipose tissues collected from the same individual or between groups of differing pathologies. These approaches have been very useful to our understanding of EAT, but caution should be taken when interpreting results since healthy people do not undergo cardiovascular surgery. Moreover, factors such as the type of surgery, anesthesia, the time of biopsy collection, or the anxiety and medication used before surgery can alter EAT gene expression patterns [25–29].

Unique Gene Expression in Epicardial Fat

The initial work of the Caroline M. Pond lab at the end of the 1980s characterizing EAT suggested that this adipose tissue is different from other adipose tissues [9]. EAT has an increase in the uptake and release of fatty acids compared to other adipose tissues, and the size of adipocytes is significantly smaller [9, 30]. These phenotypic changes suggest that EAT would have a different transcriptomic profile from other adipose tissue. In 1995 the obese gene *leptin* [LEP] was found to be expressed at different levels in adipose tissues from different parts of the body [31]. By the beginning of the 2000s, it was clear that there was a regional difference in the gene expression of adipose tissue and that EAT may exhibit unique transcriptomic properties [32, 33].

The first exploration of gene expression in EAT was done at a single-gene level through qPCR. The majority of these studies investigated the expression of adipokines. One early study investigated the expression of adipokines in EAT compared to subcutaneous adipose tissue (SAT) from patients after coronary artery bypass grafting (CABG) surgery [34] (Fig. 3.1). In this study, it was found that EAT expresses IL-1β, IL-6, TNF-α, and MCP-1 at higher levels than subcutaneous fat. In 2005, adiponectin was found to be expressed in EAT and is thought to be the source of adiponectin found in coronary circulation [35, 36]. Despite the constitutive expression of adiponectin in EAT, levels are low in comparison to the levels in other adipose tissues like SAT or omental adipose tissue. The expression of adiponectin in EAT can decrease further under certain conditions like coronary artery disease (CAD) [35, 37–40]. Resistin, another adipokine, was found to be expressed in EAT along with CD45 (inflammatory cell marker) and t-PA (endothelial cell marker) [37]. Other adipokines also found to be expressed in EAT include visfatin, leptin, omentin, RANTES (the protein encoded by the *CCL5* gene), adrenomedullin, natriuretic peptide receptor, PPAR-gamma, and SFRP4 [39, 41–44]. Cellular pathways activated by adipokines are subsequently found to be upregulated in EAT. Inflammatory pathways like NF-kappa-B (NFκB) and c-Jun N-terminal kinases (NFκB, IkK, IKK-β, JNK-1 and 2) were found to be upregulated in the EAT of patients with CAD compared to the EAT of patients without CAD [45].

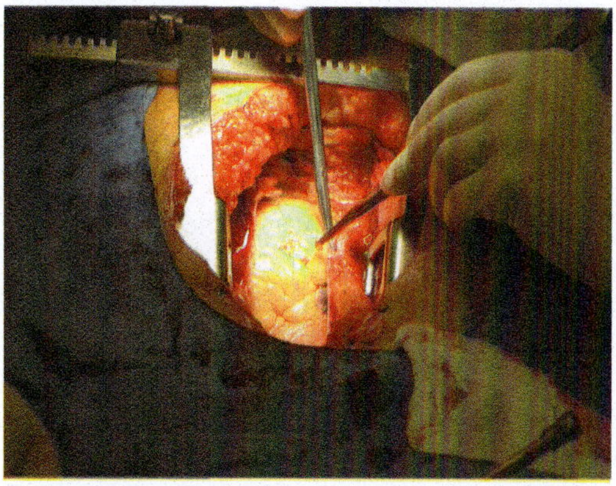

Fig. 3.1 EAT is collected (average 0.5–1 gram) during cardiothoracic surgeries. EAT samples are usually obtained near the proximal segment of the right coronary artery, deep to the visceral layer of the pericardium prior to the patients being placed on-pump. SAT samples can be obtained from the median sternotomy site. Each tissue sample is immediately frozen over dry ice and then stored at −80 °C until processing for RNA analysis. Fresh fat sample is used for flow cytometry

Proteomic approaches followed qPCR. Using these approaches, it was found that proteins involved in the oxidative stress pathway were upregulated in EAT relative to SAT [46]. It was suggested that due to its proximity to myocardium, EAT is under higher oxidative stress and this might drive its inflammatory response. Another mechanism that could explain increased oxidative stress in EAT is the AGE-RAGE pathway, which has also been shown to have higher expression in EAT compared to SAT [47]. Pathways that regulate lipid metabolism are also activated in EAT but at a lower level than in SAT [48].

EAT has been found to express uncoupling protein 1 [UCP1], a thermogenic protein also considered to be a brown adipocyte marker [49]. Further studies confirmed the high expression of UCP1 in EAT along with other thermogenic markers like Prdm16, Cpt1b, Ppargcla, and Cox4iL [23]. Other brown adipocyte markers like Zicl and Lhx8 were not detectable in EAT, while beige markers TBX1, SLC36a2, TMEM26, P2rx5, and Tnfrsf9 were expressed [23]. These markers suggests that EAT is a beige fat and gives support to the hypothesis of epicardial adipogenesis by mesenchymal transformation induced by PPAR γ activation [17, 23]. Genes involved in autophagy and unfolded protein response (UPR) were found to have high expression in EAT compared to SAT, such as GRP78, GRP94, ERN1, PERK, CEBE, mTOR, BECN1, PINK1, and BIM [50].

Several studies have investigated the secretome, or the repertoire of all secreted molecules, of adipocytes from both EAT and SAT using tissue explants. Apolipoprotein A-1, fatty acid binding protein (FABP), orosomucoid, resistin, actin A, FABP4, apolipoprotein A1, and S100A9 were found to be released from EAT [18, 19, 51–55, 56]. EAT was found to express pregnancy-associated plasma protein-A (PAPP-A) at 15 times the level of SAT. PAPP-A enhances insulin-like growth factor (IGF) action through cleavage of IGF binding-protein 4 (IGFBP4). Addition of PAPP-A to the culture of human cardiomyocyte cell lines subsequently induced IGF signaling, indicating that PAPP-A secretion from EAT can induce IGF signaling in the heart [57]. Additionally, the expression and secretion of genes involved in inflammatory response was high in EAT compared to SAT, consistent with transcription studies [22]. Moreover, a reduction in adiponectin expression after stimulation with high glucose and macrophage conditioned media was found in EAT, but not in SAT [20].

Later studies investigated large numbers of genes through the use of microarray technology. The first microarray study found 73 genes upregulated and 94 genes downregulated in EAT of patients with CAD in comparison to SAT. In the same study of CAD patients, EAT was found to have only 23 genes upregulated in comparison to mediastinal adipose tissue (MAT), an adipose tissue that displays characteristics of brown adipose tissue. This experiment indicated that the EAT expression profile is more closely related to MAT than SAT. Analysis of the biological pathways found that genes upregulated in EAT in comparison to SAT were involved in cardiotoxicity, hepatotoxicity, and nephrotoxicity. Of particular note, ADORA1 is involved in myocardial ischemia and prostaglandin D2 involved in atherosclerosis, both of which are upregulated in EAT [58].

A 2013 microarray study looked into the difference between EAT, SAT, and omental adipose tissue (OAT) in patients with CAD [59]. In EAT, 55 genes were found upregulated in the inflammatory and immune response, confirming the previous observations that found these pathways to be preferentially expressed in EAT [59]. One important finding was a high expression of serglycin (SRGN) in EAT. Using adipocyte mouse cell lines, this group further confirmed that serglycin was secreted from the adipocytes and that TNF-α can stimulate its secretion.

A microarray study in 2015 confirmed that EAT is an inflammatory tissue and that in comparison with SAT, it has high expression of gene involved in endothelial function, coagulation, immune signaling, potassium transport and apoptosis and lower expression of genes involved in protein metabolism, oxidative stress, and TGF-beta signaling [60] (Fig. 3.2).

Microarray analysis has been used to determine whether different regions of adipose depots in EAT can have differential gene expression [61]. This study assessed gene expression in the preatrial, peri-ventricular, and pericoronary EAT from a large population of 40 individuals. They found first that globally EAT when compared with SAT matches the gene expression a beige fats because of the upregulation of genes involved in cell-cell interaction, oxidative phosphorylation, and cardiac muscle contraction [61]. Genes involved in the peroxisome proliferator-activated receptor (PPAR) gamma signaling and fatty acid metabolism were downregulated [61]. Using gene ontology analysis, they also found extracellular matrix remodeling, thrombosis, and inflammatory processes to be high in all EAT compared to SAT. Additionally, they found

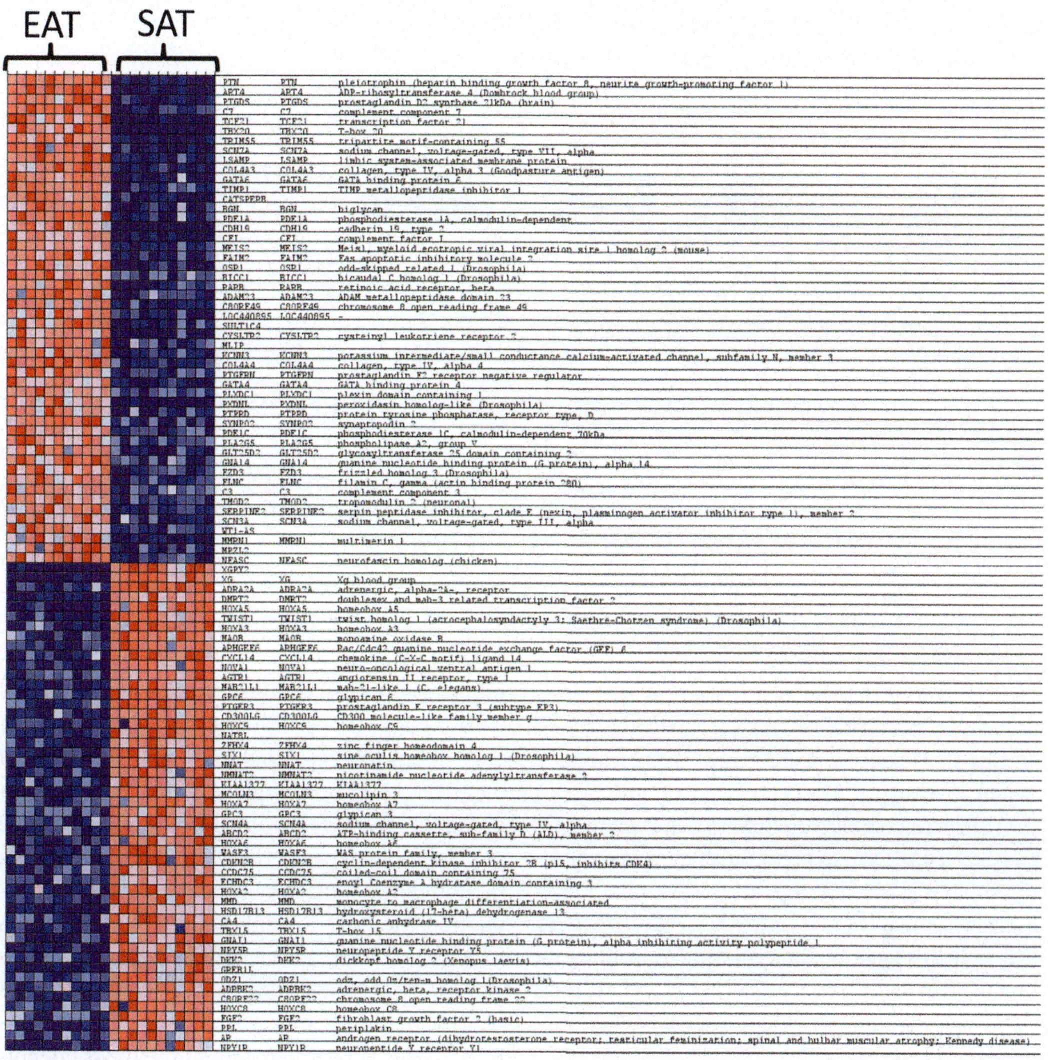

Fig. 3.2 Heat map of the 50 most enriched genes in EAT samples compared with SAT samples. Heat mapping demonstrates the unique transcriptome of EAT. Gene expression values are represented as colors (red, increased expression; blue, decreased expression) with the degree of color saturation indicating the degree of expression. As compared to SAT from the same subject, EAT is enriched with genes involved in endothelial function, coagulation, immune signaling, potassium transport, and apoptosis. Heat map generated by Broad Institute's Gene Set Enrichment Analysis. EAT, epicardial adipose tissue; SAT, subcutaneous adipose tissue. (From McAninch et al. [60], with permission from John Wiley)

a subset of genes to be enriched in EAT from each region. A total of 622 genes were preferentially expressed in peri-ventricular EAT including UCP1 and genes involved in inflammation. Peri-atrial EAT had 2571 preferentially expressed genes including genes involved in oxidative phosphorylation, cell adhesion, cardiac muscle contraction, and intracellular calcium signaling. Peri-coronary EAT had 1170 genes preferentially expressed, many involved in proliferation, O-N- glycan biosynthesis, and sphingolipid metabolism. The differences reported indicate the there is a specific signature in the transcriptome of EAT in comparison to SAT. Additionally, each fat depot within the EAT has its own specific gene expression suggesting that the role of

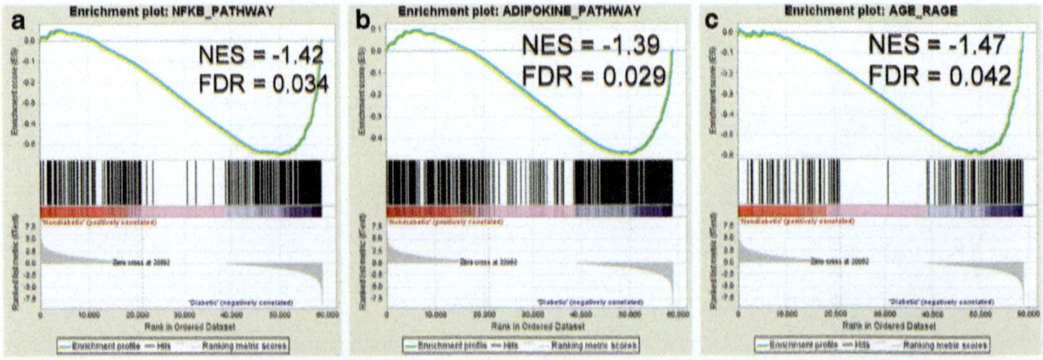

Fig. 3.3 Gene set enrichment analysis of EAT in diabetic samples. (**a**) Genes in the NF-κB pathway are significantly enriched in diabetic samples, NES = −1.42, FDR = 0.034. (**b**) Genes in the adipokine database are significantly enriched in diabetic samples. NES = −1.39, FDR = 0.029. (**c**) Genes in the AGE-RAGE database are significantly enriched in diabetic samples. NES = −1.47, FDR = 0.042. GSEA, gene set enrichment analysis; NES, normalized enrichment score; FDR, false discovery rate; NF-κB, nuclear factor-κB; AGE-RAGE, advanced glycation end-products-receptor advanced glycation end products. (From Camarena et al. [63], with permission from Elsevier)

the EAT varies depending of where it is located around the heart [61].

In 2016 a study was published using microarray to investigate the expression of miRNA in EAT [62]. In comparison to SAT, EAT was found to have a miRNA expression pattern that indicates that it is pro-inflammatory and highly metabolically active [62]. In patients with CAD, EAT was found to have an altered miRNA profile with a downregulation of genes involved in lipid metabolism, mitochondrial function, nuclear receptor transcriptional activity, and an upregulation of miRNAs involved in antigen presentation, chemokine signaling, and inflammation. For example, miR103 3p was found to be a modulator of CCL13 in EAT [62].

While microarrays have proven very useful, they are limited to only a predetermined set of probes that correspond to a selected group of genes. Whole transcriptome sequencing [RNA-seq] technology allows for unbiased quantification of transcripts expressed in tissue. In 2017, an RNA-seq study compared the transcriptomes of EAT and SAT in a small set of patients with and without type 2 diabetes mellitus (T2DM) [63]. The SAT between diabetic and nondiabetic patients had only 3 differential transcripts, indicating that T2DM did not significantly alter the transcriptome of SAT. In contrast, 592 genes were found to be differentially expressed in EAT between the diabetic and nondiabetic patients. Gene enrichment analysis found an upregulation of genes involved in many inflammation-related pathways in diabetic EAT, including inflammatory response, cytokine production, leukocyte migration, NF-κB, JAK-STAT, and AGE-RAGE (Fig. 3.3). This large change in gene expression might be explained by changes in expression of a set of transcription factors which can drive massive transcriptomic changes [63]. Fifty transcription factors were found to be differentially expressed between diabetic and nondiabetic EAT, including members of the NF-κB family (RELB, REL, NFκB1, and NFκB2) and FOS family (*FOSL1* and *FOSL2*) [63] (Fig. 3.4). Additionally, numerous adipokines and adipokine receptors were found to be upregulated. Surprisingly, there were no observed changes in genes related to oxidative stress. This study demonstrates that the transcriptome in EAT is markedly different from that in SAT, especially in pathological states such as diabetes. It also indicates that there is an increase in inflammation, innate immune response, and endothelium damage in diabetic patients (Fig. 3.5) [63].

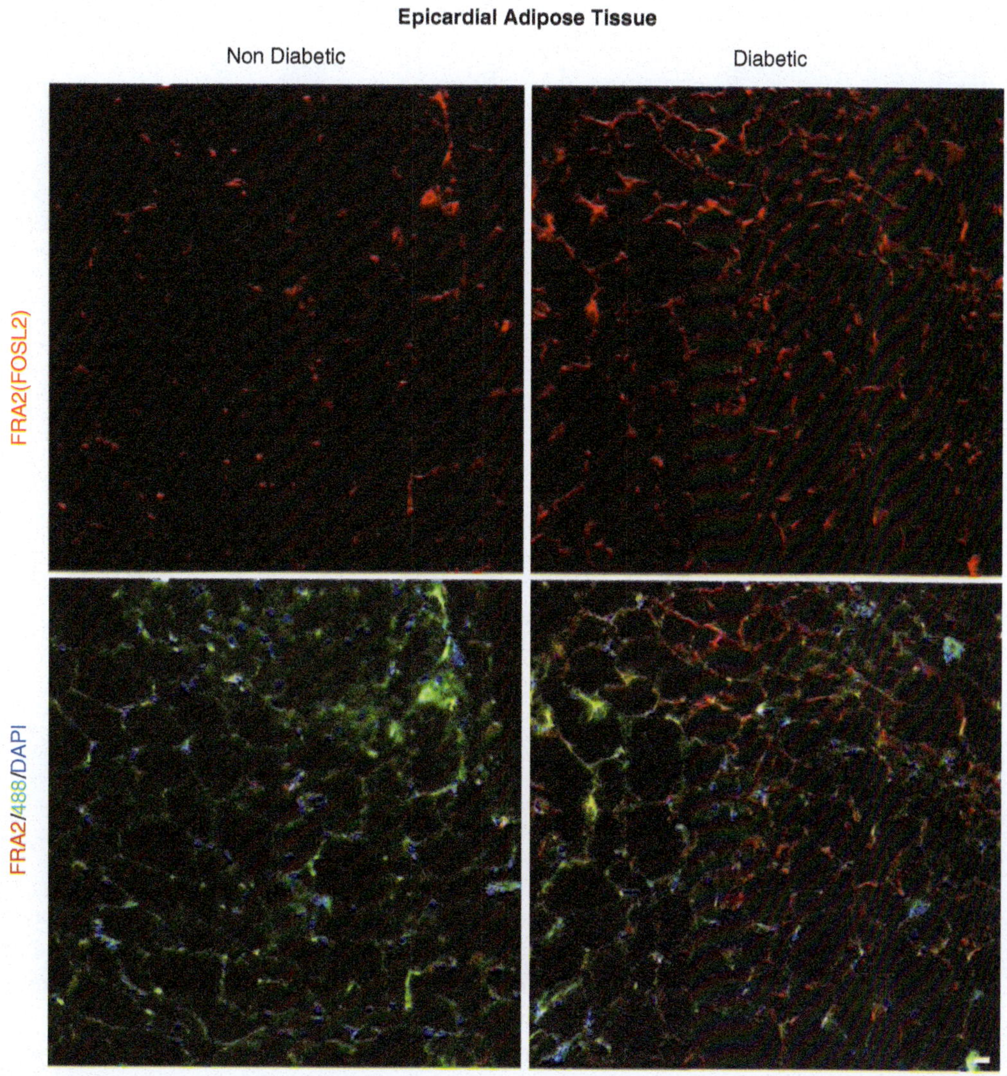

Fig. 3.4 Immunofluorescence of *FOSL2* in EAT. FRA2 (*FOSL2)* was found increased in immunofluorescence diabetic EAT compared to non-diabetic EAT (top panel). DAPI was used to label the nucleus, and autofluorescence of the tissue was collected at 488 nm excitation (*merged bottom panel*). (From Camarena et al. [63], with permission from Elsevier)

UCP1 has been reported to affect the metabolic activity of EAT. UCP1 is the gene for thermogenin, found in the mitochondria of BAT and responsible for the generation of heat. A 2019 RNA-seq study compared the transcriptome of EAT with high UCP1 expression to the transcriptome of EAT with low UCP1 expression [23, 64]. The EAT from patients with high UCP1 exhibited a low level of expression of genes in immune-related pathways [including T-cell homeostasis] and had lower production of reactive oxygen species. These results suggest a reciprocal relationship between UCP1 and adaptive immunity.

Another method for investigating differences between EAT and SAT is to study the lipid profile which is consequently influenced by the transcriptomic profile of the cell through proteins. One study used liquid chromatography–mass spectrometry to investigate the lipid

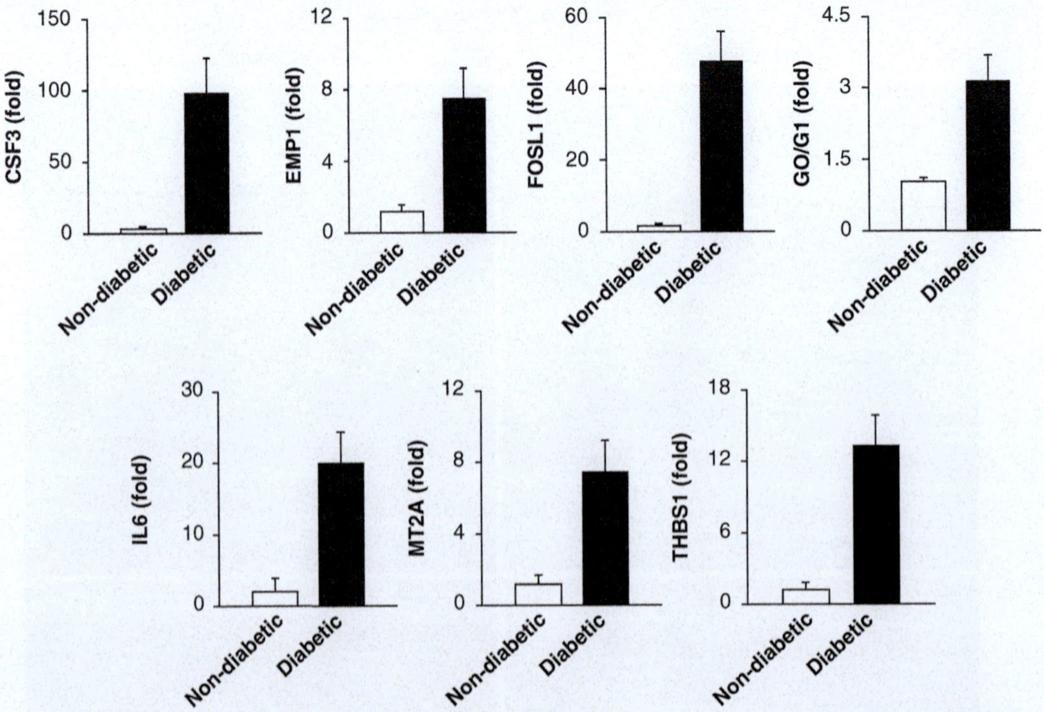

Fig. 3.5 Quantitative real-time PCR of upregulated genes in diabetes. qPCR results of selected genes encoding for inflammatory, oxidative stress, and transcription factors in diabetes. Values are relative to non-diabetic control expression. White bars represent non-diabetic EAT expression and black bars represent diabetic EAT expression. (From Camarena et al. [63], with permission from Elsevier)

profile of SAT and EAT. They found a lower content of triacylglycerols (TAGs) and glycerophosphatidylethanolamine (Pes), but a higher content of glycerophosphocholines (PCs) in EAT. These lipid types are generally found in protective adipose tissues rather than in ones that are traditionally used for energy storage. This suggests a protective function of EAT for sheltering the heart against lipid overload, whereas the SAT is thought to be a depot of energetically rich lipids [65].

In summary, EAT has a unique gene expression profile that distinguishes it from other adipose tissues. It has a beige phenotype, with small adipocytes and a stroma made of other cells including immune cells, endothelial cells, fibroblast, and nervous cells. The expression profile differs not only from other fat deposits in the body but also between different fat deposits around the heart. Newer technologies such as high-throughput sequencing allows for detailed investigation of the whole transcriptome. Furthermore, profound changes in gene and protein expression have been found to occur in disease states such as diabetes or CAD.

Epicardial Fat Paracrine/Endocrine Function

One of the unique aspects of EAT is that in addition to protecting underlying tissue and providing metabolic support for the heart, it also has unique endocrine and paracrine functions [18, 36, 42, 45, 66–69]. From the first initial investigations into EAT gene expression, it has been demonstrated that EAT is a source of adipokines, which can serve both endocrine and paracrine functions [26, 34, 35, 37–40, 70]. Paracrine, or local effects, will have a direct impact on the heart for two main reasons: (1) EAT touches the myocardium and lacks a fascia to separate the tissues as normally happens in other parts of the body, and (2) the EAT is also supported by coronary circulation that irrigates the heart [7, 9, 71, 72]. Evidence of local diffusion of adipokines has been found in studies correlating EAT gene expression with levels of adipokines found in both global plasma collected in major veins and the local plasma collected in the coronary arteries [36, 42, 43, 68, 69, 73–75].

One of the adipokines with paracrine effects is activin A, which is released from EAT. Activin A has been found to induce the expression of certain microRNAs in cardiomyocytes including miR-143, which has been found to block insulin signaling by reducing the insulin-induced AKT phosphorylation [52]. Another secreted adipokine is orosomucoid, which has been shown to increase endothelial proliferation [55]. Further release of orosomucoid can be caused by treatment with isoproterenol, suggesting that the innervation of EAT can influence the release of adipokines [55].

Some adipokines have also been shown to exhibit endocrine effects. Examples include neuromedin U, which regulates blood pressure among other functions. Chemokine ligand 5 (CCL5 or RANTES) and secreted frizzled-related protein (SFRP4) are both adipokines with endocrine function that have been found to be expressed in EAT and are both involved in metabolic syndrome [42, 44, 76]. The hormones secreted from the EAT have also been found to be important for the migration of monocytes and adhesion of those monocytes to endothelial cells [19].

The secretion of adipokines has been found to change in disease states such as diabetes and CAD. Resistin, among other proteins, was found to be secreted at higher levels from the EAT of patients with CAD [18]. Furthermore, the conditioned media from EAT explants from CAD patients was found to increase endothelial cell permeability in culture more than conditioned media from EAT explants from patients without CAD [18]. Despite having similar levels of APOA1 RNA transcripts, the EAT from patients with CAD was found to release significantly less APOA1 protein than the EAT from healthy patients [51]. APOA1 is an adipokine that affects the lipid metabolism in cells that it reaches. EAT from diabetic patients was found to express 27 adipokines and adipokine receptors at higher levels than EAT from nondiabetic patients. In particular, the adipokines that increased in expression affected pathways including NF-κB, JAK-STAT, and AGE-RAGE [63]. These diabetes-related changes in adipokine expression were not found in the SAT from the same patient cohort.

The EAT, like all adipose tissues, is composed of multiple cell types. The most abundant and distinct cells are the adipocytes, but other stromal cells are found in the EAT as well, including fibroblasts, immune cells, nervous cells, and endothelial cells. Histological analysis and correlation and gene expression indicate that the adipocytes are not the only cells secreting adipokines in the EAT [30, 43, 59, 70, 77]. Immune cells have been thought to be particularly important. Several studies have separated out the different cell types using various methods and studied the effects of each cell type [82]. Analysis of separate cell types showed that endothelial cells have a high secretion of molecules involved in inflammation and adhesion (VCAM and ICAM) compared to adipocytes [20, 23].

The non-adipocyte cells within the EAT have been shown to influence the expression patterns in adipocytes. For instance, when adipocytes from EAT are cultured with media from immune cells in culture, there is a reduction in the expression of adiponectin in the adipocytes [20]. Stromal vascular cells secrete adiponectin in EAT. This secretion of adiponectin was found to increase after treatment with omentin, which then reduced TNF-α expression in the adipocytes [58]. Furthermore, the culture media from the omentin-treated adipocytes led to less migration of smooth muscle cells than media from untreated adipocytes [78]. Mesenchymal cells collected from EAT were found to express pregnancy-associated plasma protein A [PAPP-A], while mature adipocytes from EAT did not, and the levels of PAPP-A were higher in cultures of EAT than SAT [57].

The cells within EAT not only influence other cells of the body but are influenced by cells around them. Using large numbers of EAT and myocardium samples from human patients, the paracrine effect of adiponectin on the myocardium and the feedback from this tissue was demonstrated [14]. Oxidation products released from cardiomyocytes trigger PPAR-gamma receptor activation in EAT, mediating upregulation of adiponectin [14]. The increased adiponectin helps the myocardium suppress free radical production through inhibition of nicotinamide adenine dinucleotide phosphate (NADPH) oxidases in the cardiomyocytes [14]. Polymorphism that increase ADIPOQ expression led to reduced myocardial NADPH oxidase-derived O2 [14]. These feedback mechanisms showed that increased myocardial oxidative stress elevates local EAT adiponectin expression to subsequently reduce oxidative stress in the adjacent myocardium.

Further studies with more extensive gene expression analysis like microarrays or high-throughput sequencing further elaborate upon the endocrine/paracrine function of adipose tissue. For example, prostaglandin D2 (PTGDS0, involved in atherosclerosis was upregulated in EAT [59]. Serglycin found in the serum was found to be secreted from adipocytes in culture [59]. Large sets of genes involved in secretion by the immune system were found upregulated in the EAT of CAD patients [79].

Even there is differential paracrine/endocrine activities in different EAT deposit locations. For example, in peri-ventricular EAT, there are high levels of omentin when compared with other regions [61]. Furthermore, whole genome transcriptome sequencing of patient EAT from diabetics and non-diabetics found large changes in gene expression of adipokines and their putative downstream pathways like NF-κB pathway, JAK-STAT pathway, and the AGE-RAGE pathway [63].

The secretion of proteins are not the only mechanism to regulate the endocrine/paracrine function of the EAT and miRNA are also involved. For example, miR-103-3p was found highly expressed in the EAT of CAD patients, and it could be regulating the expression of CCL13 [62]. Moreover, secretome from T2DM EAT patients reduce cardiomyocyte contractility in vitro via activation of renin angiotensin system and induction of miR-208a [34].

In summary, it is clear that gene expression profiling gives strong support to the hypothesis that EAT is an endocrine/paracrine organ. The adipokines secreted have been shown to have both endocrine and paracrine effects. These secretions do not match those of other adipose tissues. The expression and secretion of adipokines change in disease states. Stromal cells such as fibroblasts, immune cells, and endothelial cells within the EAT have been found to express adipokines and influence the expression of adipokines in adipocytes. These findings provide evidence of the unique endocrine/paracrine function occurring in EAT and its importance in cardiac function.

Epicardial Fat Immunological/ Inflammation Function

Gene expression analysis studies have shown that EAT has high expression of immune cell-specific markers as well as genes involved in immune regulation. Markedly high levels of cytokines and chemokines were noted in even the earliest gene expression studies on EAT biopsies [10, 19, 39, 43, 45, 53, 73, 75, 77, 80–83]. These findings have been repeatedly confirmed in findings from microarrays [59, 61, 79], microRNA microarrays [62], proteomics [23, 84], and whole-transcriptome sequencing [63, 64]. Interestingly, different regions of the EAT were also found to exhibit different levels of inflammatory markers. Peri-ventricular EAT was found to have higher expression of genes involved in inflammation than other regions of the EAT [61].

Experimental data show the presence of many types of immune cells and inflammation in EAT [45, 74, 77, 85]. However, the presence of many of these immune cells only occurs in EAT along with specific pathologies such as CAD, metabolic syndrome, or diabetes [86]. Surprisingly, inflammatory rheumatic disease does not result in increased EAT inflammation [86]. The immune cells found in EAT include macrophages, T cells, and dendritic cells [77, 85, 87–90].

As with other aspects of gene expression, the expression of immune-related genes changes in disease states such as diabetes and CAD. Cytokine signaling pathways such as the NF-κB and JNK pathways were found upregulated in EAT in patients with CAD compared to patients without CAD [45]. A second study confirmed the finding that a large set of genes involved in immune signaling was upregulated in the EAT of CAD patients [79]. Many genes involved in inflammatory response, particularly within the AGE-RAGE pathway, were also found upregulated in the EAT from patients with diabetes in comparison to patients without diabetes [63].

The driving force behind inflammation in healthy EAT is not well understood. Human biopsies and explant experiments have the drawback of being collected only from patients undergoing surgery, indicating that they are unhealthy. Some animal models have shown constituent inflammation in the EAT, particularly in guinea pigs [10, 12]. Chronic or acute inflammation elsewhere in the body has been suggested to possibly drive changes in expression in the EAT that lead to an inflammatory response. Surprisingly, the inflammatory response of EAT has been found to be much higher in disease states than the response in SAT and other adipose tissues [63].

An alternative explanation for inflammation in EAT is that the EAT might have an immune response due to bacterial infections. One study showed that the EAT could have bacterial DNA. Using high-throughput sequencing, DNA from 76 bacterial species were detected in the EAT of humans undergoing coronary artery bypass grafting [91]. The presence of this DNA most likely represents antigen-presenting cell translocation after engulfing bacteria in other locations of the body. Surprisingly, the most abundant species of bacteria detected was *Cyanobacteria streptophyta*, which is also known as blue-green algae and not known to colonize humans.

In summary, EAT is known to have high expression of inflammatory markers, and many different types of immune cells can be found in the EAT depending on the disease physiology. An increase of inflammation in the EAT has been shown in both CAD and diabetes. The cause of constitutive inflammation in the EAT is unknown, but some studies suggest that the EAT may simply have a much stronger inflammatory response than other adipose tissues, causing it to become inflamed more often than would be expected.

Factors That Modulate Epicardial Fat Gene Expression

Exercise

Exercise has been hypothesized to have an effect on gene expression in EAT. A study in pigs demonstrated that exercise can change the expression of inflammatory genes in EAT [12]. Specifically, the inflammatory response in the peri-myocardial EAT was decreased in guinea pigs after 16 weeks training of aerobic exercise. In the same experiment, it was found that exercise causes a decrease in adiponectin expression in visceral adipose tissue, but little changes in the inflammatory response of SAT were observed [12].

Age and Sex

Expression differences in adipose tissue due to sex have been reported [92, 93]. The most obvious difference is the preferential deposition of SAT in different locations of the body according to the sex. In EAT specifically, it has been reported that adiponectin and leptin expression were both higher in women than in men [38]. However, a later study has found only minimal differences [63]. Age has also shown to influence expression in EAT [94]. Elderly patients exhibited lower levels of adiponectin in EAT than young non-obese patients, but similar levels to young obese patients [95]. Changes in expression in the myocardium were also found in elderly patients, particularly an increase in LKB1, PP2A, PP2C, and AMPK activation [95]. The possible effect of age and sex in the EAT gene expression is still unclear and need to be further investigated.

Surgery

The difficulty of accessing a tissue that touches the heart has led to the majority of human EAT samples being collected during surgery. The process of surgery, however, is believed to impact the gene expression profile of EAT. Cardiac surgery results in an increase in cytokine production in both SAT and EAT cytokine production, which could play a role in postoperative insulin resistance [25]. Additionally, markers of many immune cell types increased in EAT, while a small number of immune cell markers increased in SAT after surgery. In the blood, it was found that resistin, leptin, IL-6, TNF-α, MCP-1, and cortisol increase in the blood after surgery while adiponectin decreases [25]. This is consistent with findings that cardiac surgery activates peripheral monocytes, which would be found throughout the body after surgery [29]. Angiotensinogen expression increased in EAT following surgery but remained unchanged in SAT [27]. Fibroblast growth factor 21 and other factors such as serum glucose, insulin, CRP, IL-6, IL-8, MCP-1, and TNF-α also increase in the EAT following cardiac surgery [28].

Overall, these findings indicate that surgery itself is an important factor that affects the gene expression profile of EAT. Researchers working with EAT cannot avoid the surgical procedure but should therefore try to minimize its effect and standardize sample collection by taking samples at the beginning of the surgical procedure.

Diseases

Due to the prevalence of surgeries related to CAD, it has been the best-studied disease for EAT expression, and several differences in expression between patients with CAD and without CAD have been reported [18, 19, 35, 37, 39, 40, 43, 45, 47, 48, 58, 68, 69, 73, 80, 87, 96–99]. However, the genetic profile of EAT has been studied in other diseases like hypertension [40, 76, 100], atrial fibrillation [13, 21, 84, 101–105], myocardial infarction [54, 79, 106, 107], heart failure [108, 109], and metabolic syndrome [11, 15, 16, 34, 42, 50, 52, 55, 63, 65, 90, 109–114], and diabetes [63]. The genetic profile of EAT in disease has numerous implications in cardiac pathology. Due to limitations of space, these effects will not be thoroughly covered here, but these changes include an increase in the expression of inflammatory markers and adipokines, as mentioned in previous sections of this chapter.

Medication

Most human samples obtained for study come from patients that are acutely or chronically medicated. Unfortunately, there is evidence that medication can alter the expression profile of EAT. For example, IL-6 levels in EAT were reduced in CABG patients treated with statin when compared to patients that did not receive treatment [37]. Metabolic syndrome is associated with an increased expression of IL1B, IL1RA, and IL-10, but this increase in expression was not found in patients treated with pioglitazone [115]. Pioglitazone was also found to reduce the presence of macrophages and lymphocytes in patients with CAD, which would affect the expression pattern in EAT [116]. Simvastatin was found to actually increase the number of inflammatory cells in CAD patients, but the cells were found to gather at the edge of the EAT and around blood vessels rather than distributed throughout the tissue [116]. Sildenafil [PDE5 inhibitor] has been found to downregulate miR-22-3p in patients with T2DM, which would affect the expression of SIRT1 in tissues including EAT [117]. Liraglutide (a glucagon-like peptide 1 analog) indicated in T2DM has an unexplained cardioprotective effect in patients with diabetic cardiomyopathy [118, 119]. This beneficial effect could be directly modulated by receptors of glucagon-like peptide 1 and 2 that were found to be expressed in EAT and that might be responsible for the liraglutide-mediated reduction of EAT in T2DM patients [119].

Concluding Remarks

The EAT does have a unique expression profile which greatly influences its effect on the heart and cardiovascular function. However, many conditions may affect the expression profile of EAT. These conditions include exercise, age, sex, surgery, disease, and medications. It is particularly important to keep this in mind regarding studies of gene expression in EAT because the majority of studies will include samples taken from patients undergoing surgery, who are more likely to be elderly, sedentary, diseased, and currently taking medication. The need for practical models that can be better controlled and manipulated will fuel the development of new approaches to study the function of EAT. Animal models like guinea pig are promising since gene expression studies showed similar findings to what was already observed in humans, though additional models are warranted. Nevertheless, the analysis of gene expression is probably the best window to offer a glimpse into the functional role of the EAT.

Acknowledgments We apologize to colleagues whose works we were not able to cite here due to space limitations. The work on the EAT transcriptome in the Wang Lab is supported by the grant R01NS089525 from the National Institutes of Health.

References

1. Zwick RK, Guerrero-Juarez CF, Horsley V, Plikus MV. Anatomical, physiological, and functional diversity of adipose tissue. Cell Metab. 2018;27:68–83.
2. Kajimura S, Spiegelman BM, Seale P. Brown and beige fat: physiological roles beyond heat generation. Cell Metab. 2015;22:546–59.
3. Gupta RK. Adipocytes. Curr Biol. 2014;24:R988–93.
4. Fasshauer M, Bluher M. Adipokines in health and disease. Trends Pharmacol Sci. 2015;36:461–70.
5. Iacobellis G, Bianco AC. Epicardial adipose tissue: emerging physiological, pathophysiological and clinical features. Trends Endocrinol Metab. 2011;22:450–7.
6. Iacobellis G, Barbaro G. Epicardial adipose tissue feeding and overfeeding the heart. Nutrition. 2019;59:1–6.
7. Iacobellis G, Willens HJ. Echocardiographic epicardial fat: a review of research and clinical applications. J Am Soc Echocardiogr. 2009;22:1311–9. quiz 1417-8
8. Talman AH, Psaltis PJ, Cameron JD, Meredith IT, Seneviratne SK, Wong DT. Epicardial adipose tissue: far more than a fat depot. Cardiovasc Diagn Ther. 2014;4:416–29.
9. Marchington JM, Mattacks CA, Pond CM. Adipose tissue in the mammalian heart and pericardium: structure, foetal development and biochemical properties. Comp Biochem Physiol B. 1989;94:225–32.
10. Swifka J, Weiss J, Addicks K, Eckel J, Rosen P. Epicardial fat from guinea pig: a model to study the paracrine network of interactions between epicardial fat and myocardium? Cardiovasc Drugs Ther. 2008;22:107–14.
11. Greulich S, de Wiza DH, Preilowski S, Ding Z, Mueller H, Langin D, et al. Secretory products of guinea pig epicardial fat induce insulin resistance and impair primary adult rat cardiomyocyte function. J Cell Mol Med. 2011;15:2399–410.
12. Company JM, Booth FW, Laughlin MH, Arce-Esquivel AA, Sacks HS, Bahouth SW, et al. Epicardial fat gene expression after aerobic exercise training in pigs with coronary atherosclerosis: relationship to visceral and subcutaneous fat. J Appl Physiol (1985). 2010;109:1904–12.
13. Chilukoti RK, Giese A, Malenke W, Homuth G, Bukowska A, Goette A, et al. Atrial fibrillation and rapid acute pacing regulate adipocyte/adipositas-related gene expression in the atria. Int J Cardiol. 2015;187:604–13.
14. Antonopoulos AS, Margaritis M, Verheule S, Recalde A, Sanna F, Herdman L, et al. Mutual regulation of epicardial adipose tissue and myocardial redox state by PPAR-gamma/adiponectin signaling. Circ Res. 2016;118(5):842–55.
15. Oclon E, Latacz A, Zubel-Lojek J, Pierzchala-Koziec K. Hyperglycemia-induced changes in miRNA expression patterns in epicardial adipose tissue of piglets. J Endocrinol. 2016;229:259–66.
16. Distel E, Penot G, Cadoudal T, Balguy I, Durant S, Benelli C. Early induction of a brown-like phenotype by rosiglitazone in the epicardial adipose tissue of fatty Zucker rats. Biochimie. 2012;94:1660–7.
17. Yamaguchi Y, Cavallero S, Patterson M, Shen H, Xu J, Kumar SR, et al. Adipogenesis and epicardial adipose tissue: a novel fate of the epicardium induced by mesenchymal transformation and PPARgamma activation. Proc Natl Acad Sci U S A. 2015; 112:2070–5.
18. Langheim S, Dreas L, Veschini L, Maisano F, Foglieni C, Ferrarello S, et al. Increased expression and secretion of resistin in epicardial adipose tissue of patients with acute coronary syndrome. Am J Physiol Heart Circ Physiol. 2010;298:H746–53.

19. Karastergiou K, Evans I, Ogston N, Miheisi N, Nair D, Kaski JC, et al. Epicardial adipokines in obesity and coronary artery disease induce atherogenic changes in monocytes and endothelial cells. Arterioscler Thromb Vasc Biol. 2010;30:1340–6.
20. Fernandez-Trasancos A, Guerola-Segura R, Paradela-Dobarro B, Alvarez E, Garcia-Acuna JM, Fernandez AL, et al. Glucose and inflammatory cells decrease adiponectin in epicardial adipose tissue cells: paracrine consequences on vascular endothelium. J Cell Physiol. 2016;231:1015–23.
21. Viviano A, Yin X, Zampetaki A, Fava M, Gallagher M, Mayr M, et al. Proteomics of the epicardial fat secretome and its role in post-operative atrial fibrillation. Europace. 2018;20:1201–8.
22. Gruzdeva OV, Akbasheva OE, Dyleva YA, Antonova LV, Matveeva VG, Uchasova EG, et al. Adipokine and cytokine profiles of epicardial and subcutaneous adipose tissue in patients with coronary heart disease. Bull Exp Biol Med. 2017;163:608–11.
23. Chechi K, Voisine P, Mathieu P, Laplante M, Bonnet S, Picard F, et al. Functional characterization of the Ucp1-associated oxidative phenotype of human epicardial adipose tissue. Sci Rep. 2017;7:15566.
24. Furuhashi M, Fuseya T, Murata M, Hoshina K, Ishimura S, Mita T, et al. Local production of fatty acid-binding protein 4 in epicardial/perivascular fat and macrophages is linked to coronary atherosclerosis. Arterioscler Thromb Vasc Biol. 2016;36:825–34.
25. Kremen J, Dolinkova M, Krajickova J, Blaha J, Anderlova K, Lacinova Z, et al. Increased subcutaneous and epicardial adipose tissue production of proinflammatory cytokines in cardiac surgery patients: possible role in postoperative insulin resistance. J Clin Endocrinol Metab. 2006;91:4620–7.
26. Silaghi A, Achard V, Paulmyer-Lacroix O, Scridon T, Tassistro V, Duncea I, et al. Expression of adrenomedullin in human epicardial adipose tissue: role of coronary status. Am J Physiol Endocrinol Metab. 2007;293:E1443–50.
27. Roubicek T, Dolinkova M, Blaha J, Haluzikova D, Bosanska L, Mraz M, et al. Increased angiotensinogen production in epicardial adipose tissue during cardiac surgery: possible role in a postoperative insulin resistance. Physiol Res. 2008;57:911–7.
28. Kotulak T, Drapalova J, Kopecky P, Lacinova Z, Kramar P, Riha H, et al. Increased circulating and epicardial adipose tissue mRNA expression of fibroblast growth factor-21 after cardiac surgery: possible role in postoperative inflammatory response and insulin resistance. Physiol Res. 2011;60:757–67.
29. Kotulak T, Drapalova J, Lips M, Lacinova Z, Kramar P, Riha H, et al. Cardiac surgery increases serum concentrations of adipocyte fatty acid-binding protein and its mRNA expression in circulating monocytes but not in adipose tissue. Physiol Res. 2014;63:83–94.
30. Eiras S, Teijeira-Fernandez E, Salgado-Somoza A, Couso E, Garcia-Caballero T, Sierra J, et al. Relationship between epicardial adipose tissue adipocyte size and MCP-1 expression. Cytokine. 2010;51:207–12.
31. Masuzaki H, Ogawa Y, Isse N, Satoh N, Okazaki T, Shigemoto M, et al. Human obese gene expression. Adipocyte-specific expression and regional differences in the adipose tissue. Diabetes. 1995;44:855–8.
32. Arner P. Regional differences in protein production by human adipose tissue. Biochem Soc Trans. 2001;29:72–5.
33. Dusserre E, Moulin P, Vidal H. Differences in mRNA expression of the proteins secreted by the adipocytes in human subcutaneous and visceral adipose tissues. Biochim Biophys Acta. 2000;1500:88–96.
34. Mazurek T, Zhang L, Zalewski A, Mannion JD, Diehl JT, Arafat H, et al. Human epicardial adipose tissue is a source of inflammatory mediators. Circulation. 2003;108:2460–6.
35. Iacobellis G, Pistilli D, Gucciardo M, Leonetti F, Miraldi F, Brancaccio G, et al. Adiponectin expression in human epicardial adipose tissue in vivo is lower in patients with coronary artery disease. Cytokine. 2005;29:251–5.
36. Date H, Imamura T, Ideguchi T, Kawagoe J, Sumi T, Masuyama H, et al. Adiponectin produced in coronary circulation regulates coronary flow reserve in nondiabetic patients with angiographically normal coronary arteries. Clin Cardiol. 2006;29:211–4.
37. Baker AR, Silva NF, Quinn DW, Harte AL, Pagano D, Bonser RS, et al. Human epicardial adipose tissue expresses a pathogenic profile of adipocytokines in patients with cardiovascular disease. Cardiovasc Diabetol. 2006;5:1.
38. Iglesias MJ, Eiras S, Pineiro R, Lopez-Otero D, Gallego R, Fernandez AL, et al. Gender differences in adiponectin and leptin expression in epicardial and subcutaneous adipose tissue. Findings in patients undergoing cardiac surgery. Rev Esp Cardiol. 2006;59:1252–60.
39. Cheng KH, Chu CS, Lee KT, Lin TH, Hsieh CC, Chiu CC, et al. Adipocytokines and proinflammatory mediators from abdominal and epicardial adipose tissue in patients with coronary artery disease. Int J Obes. 2008;32:268–74.
40. Eiras S, Teijeira-Fernandez E, Shamagian LG, Fernandez AL, Vazquez-Boquete A, Gonzalez-Juanatey JR. Extension of coronary artery disease is associated with increased IL-6 and decreased adiponectin gene expression in epicardial adipose tissue. Cytokine. 2008;43:174–80.
41. Fain JN, Sacks HS, Buehrer B, Bahouth SW, Garrett E, Wolf RY, et al. Identification of omentin mRNA in human epicardial adipose tissue: comparison to omentin in subcutaneous, internal mammary artery periadventitial and visceral abdominal depots. Int J Obes. 2008;32:810–5.
42. Madani R, Karastergiou K, Ogston NC, Miheisi N, Bhome R, Haloob N, et al. RANTES release by human adipose tissue in vivo and evidence for depot-specific differences. Am J Physiol Endocrinol Metab. 2009;296:E1262–8.

43. Shibasaki I, Nishikimi T, Mochizuki Y, Yamada Y, Yoshitatsu M, Inoue Y, et al. Greater expression of inflammatory cytokines, adrenomedullin, and natriuretic peptide receptor-C in epicardial adipose tissue in coronary artery disease. Regul Pept. 2010;165:210–7.
44. Ji Q, Zhang J, Du Y, Zhu E, Wang Z, Que B, et al. Human epicardial adipose tissue-derived and circulating secreted frizzled-related protein 4 (SFRP4) levels are increased in patients with coronary artery disease. Cardiovasc Diabetol. 2017;16:133.
45. Baker AR, Harte AL, Howell N, Pritlove DC, Ranasinghe AM, da Silva NF, et al. Epicardial adipose tissue as a source of nuclear factor-kappaB and c-Jun N-terminal kinase mediated inflammation in patients with coronary artery disease. J Clin Endocrinol Metab. 2009;94:261–7.
46. Salgado-Somoza A, Teijeira-Fernandez E, Fernandez AL, Gonzalez-Juanatey JR, Eiras S. Proteomic analysis of epicardial and subcutaneous adipose tissue reveals differences in proteins involved in oxidative stress. Am J Physiol Heart Circ Physiol. 2010;299:H202–9.
47. Rodino-Janeiro BK, Salgado-Somoza A, Teijeira-Fernandez E, Gonzalez-Juanatey JR, Alvarez E, Eiras S. Receptor for advanced glycation end-products expression in subcutaneous adipose tissue is related to coronary artery disease. Eur J Endocrinol. 2011;164:529–37.
48. Jaffer I, Riederer M, Shah P, Peters P, Quehenberger F, Wood A, et al. Expression of fat mobilizing genes in human epicardial adipose tissue. Atherosclerosis. 2012;220:122–7.
49. Chechi K, Blanchard PG, Mathieu P, Deshaies Y, Richard D. Brown fat like gene expression in the epicardial fat depot correlates with circulating HDL-cholesterol and triglycerides in patients with coronary artery disease. Int J Cardiol. 2013;167:2264–70.
50. Burgeiro A, Fonseca AC, Espinoza D, Carvalho L, Lourenco N, Antunes M, et al. Proteostasis in epicardial versus subcutaneous adipose tissue in heart failure subjects with and without diabetes. Biochim Biophys Acta Mol basis Dis. 2018;1864:2183–98.
51. Salgado-Somoza A, Teijeira-Fernandez E, Fernandez AL, Gonzalez-Juanatey JR, Eiras S. Changes in lipid transport-involved proteins of epicardial adipose tissue associated with coronary artery disease. Atherosclerosis. 2012;224:492–9.
52. Blumensatt M, Greulich S, Herzfeld de Wiza D, Mueller H, Maxhera B, Rabelink MJ, et al. Activin A impairs insulin action in cardiomyocytes via up-regulation of miR-143. Cardiovasc Res. 2013;100:201–10.
53. Agra RM, Teijeira-Fernandez E, Pascual-Figal D, Jesus SM, Fernandez-Trasancos A, Sierra J, et al. Differential behavior between S100A9 and adiponectin in coronary artery disease. Plasma or epicardial fat. Life Sci. 2014;100:147–51.
54. Rachwalik M, Zysko D, Diakowska D, Kustrzycki W. Increased content of resistin in epicardial adipose tissue of patients with advanced coronary atherosclerosis and history of myocardial infarction. Thorac Cardiovasc Surg. 2014;62:554–60.
55. Fandino-Vaquero R, Fernandez-Trasancos A, Alvarez E, Ahmad S, Batista-Oliveira AL, Adrio B, et al. Orosomucoid secretion levels by epicardial adipose tissue as possible indicator of endothelial dysfunction in diabetes mellitus or inflammation in coronary artery disease. Atherosclerosis. 2014;235:281–8.
56. Obokata M, Iso T, Ohyama Y, Sunaga H, Kawaguchi T, Matsui H, et al. Early increase in serum fatty acid binding protein 4 levels in patients with acute myocardial infarction. Eur Heart J Acute Cardiovasc Care. 2018;7:561–9.
57. Conover CA, Bale LK, Frye RL, Schaff HV. Cellular characterization of human epicardial adipose tissue: highly expressed PAPP-A regulates insulin-like growth factor I signaling in human cardiomyocytes. Physiol Rep. 2019;7:e14006.
58. Guauque-Olarte S, Gaudreault N, Piche ME, Fournier D, Mauriege P, Mathieu P, et al. The transcriptome of human epicardial, mediastinal and subcutaneous adipose tissues in men with coronary artery disease. PLoS One. 2011;6:e19908.
59. Imoto-Tsubakimoto H, Takahashi T, Ueyama T, Ogata T, Adachi A, Nakanishi N, et al. Serglycin is a novel adipocytokine highly expressed in epicardial adipose tissue. Biochem Biophys Res Commun. 2013;432:105–10.
60. McAninch EA, Fonseca TL, Poggioli R, Panos AL, Salerno TA, Deng Y, et al. Epicardial adipose tissue has a unique transcriptome modified in severe coronary artery disease. Obesity (Silver Spring). 2015;23:1267–78.
61. Gaborit B, Venteclef N, Ancel P, Pelloux V, Gariboldi V, Leprince P, et al. Human epicardial adipose tissue has a specific transcriptomic signature depending on its anatomical peri-atrial, peri-ventricular, or peri-coronary location. Cardiovasc Res. 2015; 108:62–73.
62. Vacca M, Di Eusanio M, Cariello M, Graziano G, D'Amore S, Petridis FD, et al. Integrative miRNA and whole-genome analyses of epicardial adipose tissue in patients with coronary atherosclerosis. Cardiovasc Res. 2016;109:228–39.
63. Camarena V, Sant D, Mohseni M, Salerno T, Zaleski ML, Wang G, et al. Novel atherogenic pathways from the differential transcriptome analysis of diabetic epicardial adipose tissue. Nutr Metab Cardiovasc Dis. 2017;27:739–50.
64. Chechi K, Vijay J, Voisine P, Mathieu P, Bosse Y, Tchernof A, et al. UCP1 expression-associated gene signatures of human epicardial adipose tissue. JCI Insight. 2019;4. https://doi.org/10.1172/jci.insight.123618.
65. Tomasova P, Cermakova M, Pelantova H, Vecka M, Kratochvilova H, Lips M, et al. Minor lipids profiling in subcutaneous and epicardial fat tissue using LC/MS with an optimized preanalytical phase. J

Chromatogr B Analyt Technol Biomed Life Sci. 2019;1113:50–9.
66. Chaldakov GN, Fiore M, Stankulov IS, Manni L, Hristova MG, Antonelli A, et al. Neurotrophin presence in human coronary atherosclerosis and metabolic syndrome: a role for NGF and BDNF in cardiovascular disease? Prog Brain Res. 2004;146:279–89.
67. Iacobellis G, di Gioia CR, Cotesta D, Petramala L, Travaglini C, De Santis V, et al. Epicardial adipose tissue adiponectin expression is related to intracoronary adiponectin levels. Horm Metab Res. 2009;41:227–31.
68. Iacobellis G, di Gioia CR, Di Vito M, Petramala L, Cotesta D, De Santis V, et al. Epicardial adipose tissue and intracoronary adrenomedullin levels in coronary artery disease. Horm Metab Res. 2009;41:855–60.
69. Spiroglou SG, Kostopoulos CG, Varakis JN, Papadaki HH. Adipokines in periaortic and epicardial adipose tissue: differential expression and relation to atherosclerosis. J Atheroscler Thromb. 2010;17:115–30.
70. Iacobellis G. Epicardial and pericardial fat: close, but very different. Obesity (Silver Spring). 2009;17:625; author reply 626–7.
71. Iacobellis G, Corradi D, Sharma AM. Epicardial adipose tissue: anatomic, biomolecular and clinical relationships with the heart. Nat Clin Pract Cardiovasc Med. 2005;2:536–43.
72. Gao X, Mi S, Zhang F, Gong F, Lai Y, Gao F, et al. Association of chemerin mRNA expression in human epicardial adipose tissue with coronary atherosclerosis. Cardiovasc Diabetol. 2011;10:87.
73. Shimabukuro M, Hirata Y, Tabata M, Dagvasumberel M, Sato H, Kurobe H, et al. Epicardial adipose tissue volume and adipocytokine imbalance are strongly linked to human coronary atherosclerosis. Arterioscler Thromb Vasc Biol. 2013;33:1077–84.
74. Dozio E, Malavazos AE, Vianello E, Briganti S, Dogliotti G, Bandera F, et al. Interleukin-15 and soluble interleukin-15 receptor alpha in coronary artery disease patients: association with epicardial fat and indices of adipose tissue distribution. PLoS One. 2014;9:e90960.
75. Mitchell JD, Maguire JJ, Kuc RE, Davenport AP. Expression and vasoconstrictor function of anorexigenic peptides neuromedin U-25 and S in the human cardiovascular system. Cardiovasc Res. 2009;81:353–61.
76. Zhou Y, Wei Y, Wang L, Wang X, Du X, Sun Z, et al. Decreased adiponectin and increased inflammation expression in epicardial adipose tissue in coronary artery disease. Cardiovasc Diabetol. 2011;10:2.
77. Fernandez-Trasancos A, Fandino-Vaquero R, Agra RM, Fernandez AL, Vinuela JE, Gonzalez-Juanatey JR, et al. Impaired adipogenesis and insulin resistance in epicardial fat-mesenchymal cells from patients with cardiovascular disease. J Cell Physiol. 2014;229:1722–30.
78. Fernandez-Trasancos A, Agra RM, Garcia-Acuna JM, Fernandez AL, Gonzalez-Juanatey JR, Eiras S. Omentin treatment of epicardial fat improves its anti-inflammatory activity and paracrine benefit on smooth muscle cells. Obesity (Silver Spring). 2017;25:1042–9.
79. Blumensatt M, Fahlbusch P, Hilgers R, Bekaert M, Herzfeld de Wiza D, Akhyari P, et al. Secretory products from epicardial adipose tissue from patients with type 2 diabetes impair mitochondrial beta-oxidation in cardiomyocytes via activation of the cardiac renin-angiotensin system and induction of miR-208a. Basic Res Cardiol. 2017;112:2.
80. Malavazos AE, Ermetici F, Coman C, Corsi MM, Morricone L, Ambrosi B. Influence of epicardial adipose tissue and adipocytokine levels on cardiac abnormalities in visceral obesity. Int J Cardiol. 2007;121:132–4.
81. Dozio E, Dogliotti G, Malavazos AE, Bandera F, Cassetti G, Vianello E, et al. IL-18 level in patients undergoing coronary artery bypass grafting surgery or valve replacement: which link with epicardial fat depot? Int J Immunopathol Pharmacol. 2012;25:1011–20.
82. Wang Q, Shen H, Min J, Gao Y, Liu K, Xi W, et al. YKL-40 is highly expressed in the epicardial adipose tissue of patients with atrial fibrillation and associated with atrial fibrosis. J Transl Med. 2018;16:229.
83. Jiang DS, Zeng HL, Li R, Huo B, Su YS, Fang J, et al. Aberrant epicardial adipose tissue extracellular matrix remodeling in patients with severe ischemic cardiomyopathy: insight from comparative quantitative proteomics. Sci Rep. 2017;7:43787.
84. Vianello E, Dozio E, Arnaboldi F, Marazzi MG, Martinelli C, Lamont J, et al. Epicardial adipocyte hypertrophy: association with M1-polarization and toll-like receptor pathways in coronary artery disease patients. Nutr Metab Cardiovasc Dis. 2016;26:246–53.
85. Andersen JK, Oma I, Prayson RA, Kvelstad IL, Almdahl SM, Fagerland MW, et al. Inflammatory cell infiltrates in the heart of patients with coronary artery disease with and without inflammatory rheumatic disease: a biopsy study. Arthritis Res Ther. 2016;18:232.
86. Hirata Y, Kurobe H, Akaike M, Chikugo F, Hori T, Bando Y, et al. Enhanced inflammation in epicardial fat in patients with coronary artery disease. Int Heart J. 2011;52:139–42.
87. Gurses KM, Ozmen F, Kocyigit D, Yersal N, Bilgic E, Kaya E, et al. Netrin-1 is associated with macrophage infiltration and polarization in human epicardial adipose tissue in coronary artery disease. J Cardiol. 2017;69:851–8.
88. Miksztowicz V, Morales C, Barchuk M, Lopez G, Poveda R, Gelpi R, et al. Metalloproteinase 2 and 9 activity increase in epicardial adipose tissue of patients with coronary artery disease. Curr Vasc Pharmacol. 2017;15:135–43.

89. Mraz M, Cinkajzlova A, Klouckova J, Lacinova Z, Kratochvilova H, Lips M, et al. Dendritic cells in subcutaneous and epicardial adipose tissue of subjects with type 2 diabetes, obesity, and coronary artery disease. Mediat Inflamm. 2019;2019:5481725.
90. Pedicino D, Severino A, Ucci S, Bugli F, Flego D, Giglio AF, et al. Epicardial adipose tissue microbial colonization and inflammasome activation in acute coronary syndrome. Int J Cardiol. 2017;236:95–9.
91. White UA, Tchoukalova YD. Sex dimorphism and depot differences in adipose tissue function. Biochim Biophys Acta. 2014;1842:377–92.
92. Chang E, Varghese M, Singer K. Gender and sex differences in adipose tissue. Curr Diab Rep. 2018;18:69.
93. Palmer AK, Kirkland JL. Aging and adipose tissue: potential interventions for diabetes and regenerative medicine. Exp Gerontol. 2016;86:97–105.
94. Niemann B, Pan R, Teschner M, Boening A, Silber RE, Rohrbach S. Age and obesity-associated changes in the expression and activation of components of the AMPK signaling pathway in human right atrial tissue. Exp Gerontol. 2013;48:55–63.
95. Dutour A, Achard V, Sell H, Naour N, Collart F, Gaborit B, et al. Secretory type II phospholipase A2 is produced and secreted by epicardial adipose tissue and overexpressed in patients with coronary artery disease. J Clin Endocrinol Metab. 2010;95:963–7.
96. Salgado-Somoza A, Teijeira-Fernandez E, Rubio J, Couso E, Gonzalez-Juanatey JR, Eiras S. Coronary artery disease is associated with higher epicardial retinol-binding protein 4 (RBP4) and lower glucose transporter (GLUT) 4 levels in epicardial and subcutaneous adipose tissue. Clin Endocrinol. 2012;76:51–8.
97. Silaghi A, Silaghi H, Scridon T, Pais R, Achard V. Glucocorticoid receptors in human epicardial adipose tissue: role of coronary status. J Endocrinol Investig. 2012;35:649–54.
98. Cappellano G, Uberti F, Caimmi PP, Pietronave S, Mary DA, Dianzani C, et al. Different expression and function of the endocannabinoid system in human epicardial adipose tissue in relation to heart disease. Can J Cardiol. 2013;29:499–509.
99. Teijeira-Fernandez E, Eiras S, Grigorian-Shamagian L, Fernandez A, Adrio B, Gonzalez-Juanatey JR. Epicardial adipose tissue expression of adiponectin is lower in patients with hypertension. J Hum Hypertens. 2008;22:856–63.
100. Kourliouros A, Karastergiou K, Nowell J, Gukop P, Tavakkoli Hosseini M, Valencia O, et al. Protective effect of epicardial adiponectin on atrial fibrillation following cardiac surgery. Eur J Cardiothorac Surg. 2011;39:228–32.
101. Suffee N, Moore-Morris T, Farahmand P, Rucker-Martin C, Dilanian G, Fradet M, et al. Atrial natriuretic peptide regulates adipose tissue accumulation in adult atria. Proc Natl Acad Sci U S A. 2017;114:E771–80.
102. Wang Q, Xi W, Yin L, Wang J, Shen H, Gao Y, et al. Human epicardial adipose tissue cTGF expression is an independent risk factor for atrial fibrillation and highly associated with atrial fibrosis. Sci Rep. 2018;8:3585.
103. Wang Q, Min J, Jia L, Xi W, Gao Y, Diao Z, et al. Human Epicardial adipose tissue activin a expression predicts occurrence of postoperative atrial fibrillation in patients receiving cardiac surgery. Heart Lung Circ. 2019;28:1697–705.
104. Couselo-Seijas M, Lopez-Canoa JN, Agra-Bermejo RM, Diaz-Rodriguez E, Fernandez AL, Martinez-Cereijo JM, et al. Cholinergic activity regulates the secretome of epicardial adipose tissue: association with atrial fibrillation. J Cell Physiol. 2019;234:10512–22.
105. Zangi L, Oliveira MS, Ye LY, Ma Q, Sultana N, Hadas Y, et al. Insulin-like growth factor 1 receptor-dependent pathway drives epicardial adipose tissue formation after myocardial injury. Circulation. 2017;135:59–72.
106. Agra RM, Teijeira-Fernandez E, Pascual-Figal D, Sanchez-Mas J, Fernandez-Trasancos A, Gonzalez-Juanatey JR, et al. Adiponectin and p53 mRNA in epicardial and subcutaneous fat from heart failure patients. Eur J Clin Investig. 2014;44:29–37.
107. Perez-Belmonte LM, Moreno-Santos I, Gomez-Doblas JJ, Garcia-Pinilla JM, Morcillo-Hidalgo L, Garrido-Sanchez L, et al. Expression of epicardial adipose tissue thermogenic genes in patients with reduced and preserved ejection fraction heart failure. Int J Med Sci. 2017;14:891–5.
108. Teijeira-Fernandez E, Eiras S, Grigorian-Shamagian L, Salgado-Somoza A, Martinez-Comendador JM, Gonzalez-Juanatey JR. Diabetic and nondiabetic patients express similar adipose tissue adiponectin and leptin levels. Int J Obes. 2010;34:1200–8.
109. Gormez S, Demirkan A, Atalar F, Caynak B, Erdim R, Sozer V, et al. Adipose tissue gene expression of adiponectin, tumor necrosis factor-alpha and leptin in metabolic syndrome patients with coronary artery disease. Intern Med. 2011;50:805–10.
110. Castro RB, Longui CA, Faria CD, Silva TS, Richeti F, Rocha MN, et al. Tissue-specific adaptive levels of glucocorticoid receptor alpha mRNA and their relationship with insulin resistance. Genet Mol Res. 2012;11:3975–87.
111. Agra RM, Fernandez-Trasancos A, Sierra J, Gonzalez-Juanatey JR, Eiras S. Differential association of S100A9, an inflammatory marker, and p53, a cell cycle marker, expression with epicardial adipocyte size in patients with cardiovascular disease. Inflammation. 2014;37:1504–12.
112. Moreno-Santos I, Perez-Belmonte LM, Macias-Gonzalez M, Mataro MJ, Castellano D, Lopez-Garrido M, et al. Type 2 diabetes is associated with decreased PGC1alpha expression in epicardial adipose tissue of patients with coronary artery disease. J Transl Med. 2016;14:243.

113. Liu Y, Fu W, Lu M, Huai S, Song Y, Wei Y. Role of miRNAs in epicardial adipose tissue in CAD patients with T2DM. Biomed Res Int. 2016;2016: 1629236.
114. Sacks HS, Fain JN, Cheema P, Bahouth SW, Garrett E, Wolf RY, et al. Inflammatory genes in epicardial fat contiguous with coronary atherosclerosis in the metabolic syndrome and type 2 diabetes: changes associated with pioglitazone. Diabetes Care. 2011;34:730–3.
115. Grosso AF, de Oliveira SF, Higuchi Mde L, Favarato D, Dallan LA, da Luz PL. Synergistic anti-inflammatory effect: simvastatin and pioglitazone reduce inflammatory markers of plasma and epicardial adipose tissue of coronary patients with metabolic syndrome. Diabetol Metab Syndr. 2014;6:47.
116. Fiore D, Gianfrilli D, Giannetta E, Galea N, Panio G, di Dato C, et al. PDE5 inhibition ameliorates visceral adiposity targeting the miR-22/SIRT1 pathway: evidence from the CECSID trial. J Clin Endocrinol Metab. 2016;101:1525–34.
117. Iacobellis G, Mohseni M, Bianco SD, Banga PK. Liraglutide causes large and rapid epicardial fat reduction. Obesity (Silver Spring). 2017;25:311–6.
118. Marso SP, Daniels GH, Brown-Frandsen K, Kristensen P, Mann JF, Nauck MA, et al. Liraglutide and cardiovascular outcomes in type 2 diabetes. N Engl J Med. 2016;375:311–22.
119. Iacobellis G, Camarena V, Sant DW, Wang G. Human epicardial fat expresses glucagon-like peptide 1 and 2 receptors genes. Horm Metab Res. 2017;49:625–30.

Pathology and Cardiotoxicity of the Epicardial Adipose Tissue

4

Gianluca Iacobellis

Key Points

- Myocardial lipid content increases with the degree of visceral adiposity and may contribute to cause cardiomyocytes apoptosis and adverse structural and functional cardiac changes.
- Large and abnormal epicardial fat accumulation can increase myocardial triglyceride content and cause morphological changes of the heart, such as left ventricular hypertrophy and atrial myopathy.
- Excessive epicardial fat can affect both diastolic filling and relaxation, in some cases the systolic function.

Visceral Adiposity and Cardiovascular Risk

Historically obese individuals have been considered at higher cardiovascular risk than individuals with normal body weight. However, there is an almost univocal consensus in considering the visceral fat a stronger independent cardio-metabolic risk factor than overall obesity. Subjects with visceral fat accumulation are considered at higher cardiovascular risk than individuals with prevalent peripheral adiposity. The exact mechanisms that lead to a different anatomical fat accumulation in humans are still unclear. Different visceral fat depots seem to have different physiological and pathological properties.

Human body fat is functionally heterogeneous and not equally distributed. Local fat accumulation seems to be more important than overall body fat. Indeed, more attention was recently focused on the visceral and intra-organ fat and their local pathological effects and clinical implications. If increased visceral fat is considered a major determinant of a poor cardio-metabolic profile, the excessive intra-organ fat is recently thought to play a key role in the obesity-related organ damages. Intracellular ectopic fat infiltration seems to be even more important than general obesity or intra-abdominal visceral adiposity. Intra-organ fatty infiltration is associated with end-organ damages and increased cardiovascular risk [1–3]. Ectopic fat deposition occurs also within the heart and may cause a metabolic cardiomyopathy [1–3]. EAT can exert cardiotoxic effects through different and complex mechanisms which are discussed in this chapter and summarized in Table 4.1.

G. Iacobellis (✉)
Division of Endocrinology, Diabetes and Metabolism, Department of Medicine, University of Miami, Miller School of Medicine, Miami, FL, USA
e-mail: giacobellis@med.miami.edu

G. Iacobellis (ed.), *Epicardial Adipose Tissue*, Contemporary Cardiology,
https://doi.org/10.1007/978-3-030-40570-0_4

Table 4.1 Mechanisms of epicardial fat cardiotoxicity

Imbalance between myocardial uptake and oxidation of nonesterified fatty acids
Increased rate of fatty acid incorporation and infiltration within the cardiomyocytes
Accumulation of fatty acid intermediates in the cytoplasm
Cardiomyocytes steatosis
Cardiomyocytes fibrosis
Cardiomyocytes apoptosis
Dense inflammatory cell infiltrate
Fibrotic changes within epicardial fat ganglia
Electromechanical changes in atrial tissue due to higher free fatty acids infiltration

Myocardial Lipotoxicity of Epicardial Fat

Obesity leads not only to increased fat depots in classical adipose tissue locations but also to significant lipid accumulation and infiltration within and around other tissues and internal organs. Ectopic fat deposition may occur within the heart and affect cardiovascular function. EAT can be considered ectopic fat accumulation of the heart.

EAT is higher in high-fat-diet-fed experimental animals and in obese subjects, particularly in those presenting with excessive abdominal adiposity [4, 5]. Excessive epicardial adipose tissue can produce lipotoxic effects throughout an abnormal lipid deposition and fatty infiltration in the myocardium [6–9]. As cardiomyocytes fat storage capacity is very limited, high levels of plasma lipids cause cardiac steatosis, dysfunction, and ultimately failure, as observed in morbid obesity and uncontrolled diabetes [6]. High-fat feeding increases the rate of fatty acid incorporation in all adipose depots [10]. An imbalance between myocardial uptake and oxidation of nonesterified fatty acids has been proposed as a possible causative mechanism of this relation [8]. Nonadipocytes and cardiac cells have a very limited capacity to store excess fat. If they are exposed to high levels of plasma lipids, as usually occurs in obesity, triglycerides can accumulate and increase within cardiomyocytes. Although much of this excess lipid may be stored in a relatively neutral form such as triglycerides, some fatty acids that enter the cell may contribute to apoptosis by lipotoxicity [1, 2]. An imbalanced diet can affect gut microbiome and consequently influence adipose tissue metabolism, including EAT. Pericardial and epicardial adipose tissue respond similarly to high-fat feeding, but the magnitude of the response is greater in the EAT depot [10]. The increased myocardial triglyceride content can be considered as result of the free fatty acids overload and saturation of the physiological free fatty acids oxidative capacity by the heart. Intra-myocardial free fatty acids undergo peroxidation and saturation, leading to the accumulation of fatty acid intermediates in the cytoplasm and functional damage to the heart.

Myocardial lipid content increases with the degree of adiposity and may contribute to the adverse structural and functional cardiac adaptations seen in obese persons. The detrimental accumulation of high triglycerides levels in cardiomyocytes affects left ventricle and promotes cardiac fibrosis and apoptosis in obese rats and in high-fat-fed rabbits. Postmortem studies showed excessive triglycerides accumulation within the cytosol in morbid obese subjects and that the infiltration of EAT between myocardial fibers occurred especially in the right ventricular wall.

The term myocardial apoptosis implies cardiomyocyte loss that occurs through apoptosis or programmed cell death [1, 2]. Myocardial apoptosis has been reported in heart failure and cardiomyopathies. When lipids over-accumulate in nonadipose tissues during overnutrition, fatty acids enter deleterious pathways such as ceramide production, which, through increased nitric oxide formation, causes apoptosis of lipid-laden cells, such as beta cells and cardiomyocytes. Long-chain saturated fatty acids induce apoptosis through a mechanism involving the generation of reactive intermediates. In human cardiomyopathies, lipid accumulation that results from downregulation of fatty acid metabolism may also trigger apoptotic cell death.

Remarkably, EAT is highly enriched in genes coding for cell apoptosis, as described in a microarray analysis in patients with coronary artery diseases [11]. The same study showed that EAT inflammatory transcriptome was downregulated in subjects with advanced disease, whereas the pro-fibrotic genes were actually upregulated. It could be speculated that the apoptotic activity of the EAT led to fibrotic changes within the adipocytes and contiguous cardiomyocytes.

Excessive release of free fatty acids from the EAT into the cardiomyocytes has been recently evoked as contributory to the development and progression of atrial fibrillation [12, 13]. Free fatty acids can be transported from the peri-atrial EAT to the left atrium and lead to electromechanical changes in atrial tissue, favoring electrical impulses breakthrough and reentry. Increased EAT could also influence the intrinsic autonomic system, increasing the propensity for atrial fibrillation.

Magnetic resonance spectroscopy studies described that EAT in humans and myocardial fat in animals were both positively associated with the mass of the left ventricle and let ventricular hypertrophy [14–18]. Hydrogen-1 MR (1H-MR) spectroscopy was used to determine myocardial fat content. Magnetic proton spectroscopy was validated for the evaluation of myocardial fat content in humans by showing similar accuracy of direct biochemical measurements in lean and obese Zucker rats [14–18]. 1H-MR spectroscopic myocardial fat content is expressed as a percentage of triglycerides content compared to water content. An independent and significant relation of EAT, as measured with echocardiography, and myocardial triglycerides content, as measured by proton magnetic resonance spectroscopy, has been described by Iacobellis's group [19]. Multivariate linear regression analysis showed EAT thickness as the most significant independent correlate of myocardial fat ($p < 0.001$). Kankaanpaa found an important and concurrent threefold and twofold elevation in myocardial and EAT in obese individuals [8]. The independent correlation of epicardial, visceral fat depot, and lipid content within the cardiac cells further suggests the occurrence of a direct crosstalk between the epicardial adipocytes and the cardiomyocytes. This is allowed by the absence of anatomical barriers between the EAT and the myocardium. Additionally this underlines the difference between epicardial and pericardial fat, external to the myocardium.

Myocardial fat has been previously associated with increased visceral and hepatic fat and more generally with obesity and diabetes mellitus. Intrahepatic fat accumulation is a major determinant of the hepatic insulin resistance causing hyperglycemia. The accumulation of triglyceride in and around the myocardium leads to peripheral vascular resistance and left ventricular hypertrophy in obese individuals [8]. Obesity and insulin resistance are associated with an increased myocardial uptake and oxidation of fatty acids. This leads to increased oxygen requirements and decreased cardiac efficiency. This also causes a mismatch between free fatty acid uptake and oxidation that eventually increases the production of fatty acid intermediates, free radicals, and excess storage in myocardial triglycerides, causing cardiomyocyte apoptosis, increased oxidative stress, and impairment in cardiac function.

However, the role of intramyocardial triglyceride accumulation in the pathogenesis of left ventricular dysfunction is not fully elucidated. Myocardial triglycerides content may present a separate entity that is influenced by factors beyond visceral adiposity. The correlation between EAT and intra-myocardial lipid content was not univocally described [20]. One study found myocardial triglycerides as the only parameter independently associated with EAT volume [21]. Myocardial triglycerides content decreased and epicardial and pericardial fat depots increased in non-diabetic subjects with dilated cardiomyopathy. Myocardial triglycerides could play a specific role in the myocardial energy metabolism in congestive heart failure [22].

Epicardial Fat and Heart Chambers

Microscopic Changes

The presence of subepicardial adipose tissue and adiposity *cordis* have been described in the early

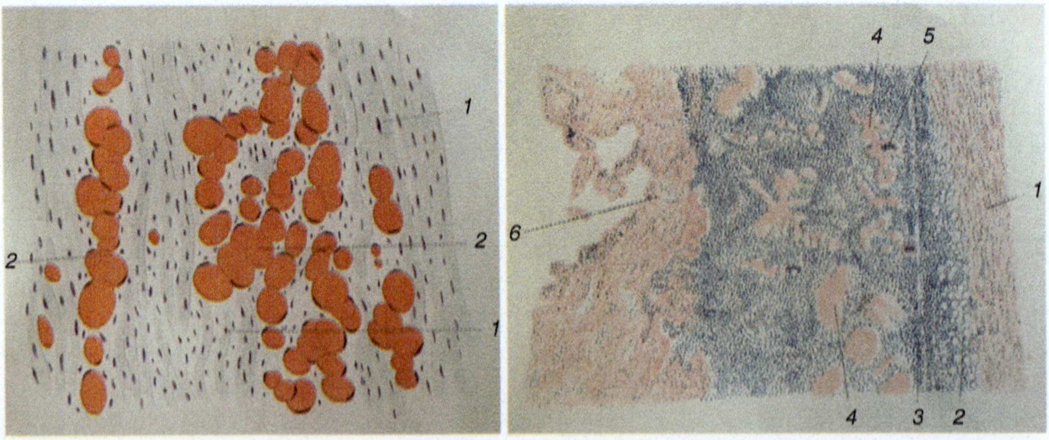

Fig. 4.1 Example of adiposity cordis with presence of fat cells (*indicated by number* 2) within the myocardium (indicated by number 1) (*left panel*). Subepicardial adipose tissue (*indicated by number* 2) in a case of acute turberculosis pericarditis (*right panel*). (Microanatomical lithograph from Anst v. F. Reichhold. München, 1899. From author's own collection)

nineteenth century as depicted in Fig. 4.1. Epicardial adipocytes display an intrinsic pro-inflammatory and atherogenic profile. A dense inflammatory infiltrate, mainly represented by macrophages, is commonly detected in EAT of subjects with coronary artery disease [10, 23]. Compared with subcutaneous fat, EAT showed thickened connective tissue septa with dense inflammatory cell infiltrates that extended to the periseptal areas of the fat lobules (Fig. 4.2) [24]. Microvessels of EAT contained variable degrees of leukocyte accumulation, whereas no sign of cellular retention was observed in subcutaneous fat. When specific inflammatory cell markers were used, epicardial adipose tissue demonstrated presence of T lymphocytes (CD3+), macrophages (CD68+), and mast cells (Fig. 4.3). Interestingly, the ratio of EAT pro-inflammatory M1 macrophages and anti-inflammatory M2 macrophages is unbalanced in patients with coronary artery disease [24, 25]. The presence of macrophages and mast cells in epicardial adipose tissue could also be reactive to underlying plaque rupture and instability. The number of CD8+ T cells is significantly higher in patients with coronary artery disease as compared to control, whereas CD4+ cells were not detected in the EAT. The cardiac ganglionated plexus in EAT incorporates the autonomic innervation (both sympathetic and parasympathetic) of the heart. Fibrotic changes within EAT ganglia can affect atrial function and contribute to the development of atrial fibrillation [26].

Macroscopic Changes

Excessive local fat accumulation can affect the heart through both biochemical and physical mechanisms. Due to its anatomical and functional vicinity to the myocardium, EAT has been reported to have an impact on all the heart chambers and influence their morphology and function, as discussed in detail below and summarized in Table 4.2.

Epicardial Fat and Ventricles

In the 1950s, Reiner et al. studied epicardial adipose tissue in normal, hypertensive and ischemic hearts [27, 28]. In a later autoptic study of human hearts, Corradi et al. investigated the relationship between ventricular myocardial and EAT in normal hearts and those that were ischemic, hypertrophic, or both [29]. Left, right, and total ventricular fat weights were significantly greater in hypertrophic hearts, but there was no

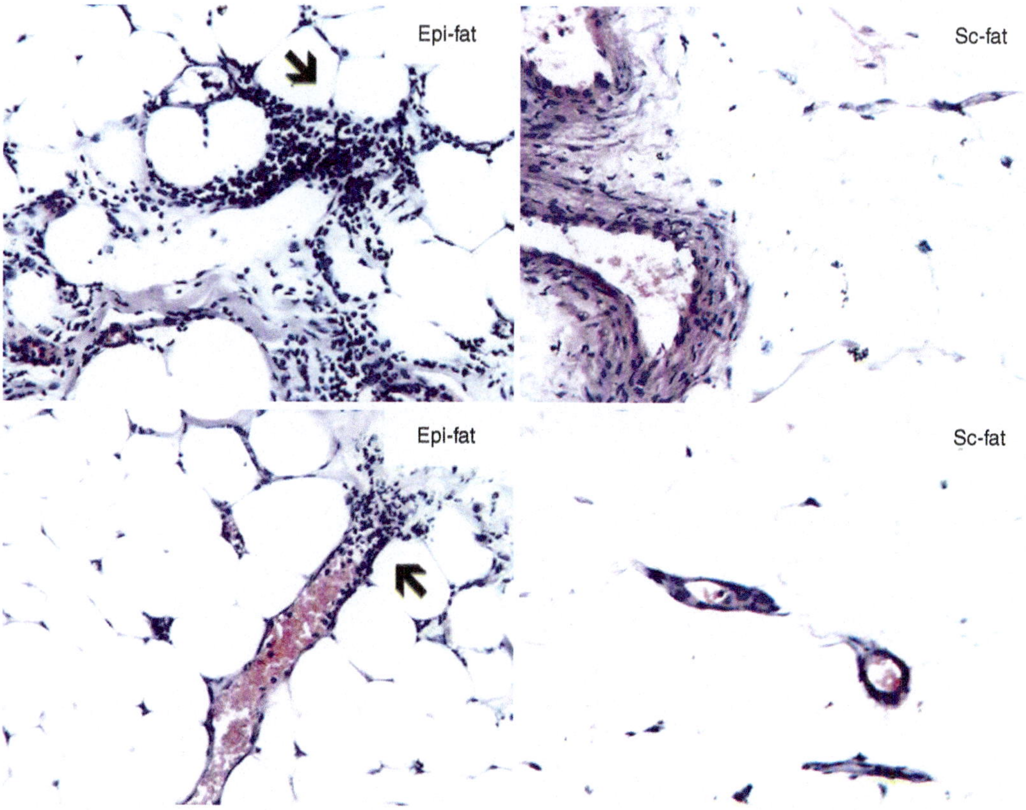

Fig. 4.2 Histopathological features of epicardial and subcutaneous adipose tissues. On the left, epicardial adipose tissue (*Epi-fat*) shows dense inflammatory infiltrates (*arrow*) involving mostly septa. On the right, subcutaneous adipose tissue (*Sc-fat*) from the same patient shows absence of inflammatory cells. Hematoxylin and eosin stain; magnification ×10. (From Mazurek et al. [24], with permission https://www.ahajournals.org/doi/10.1161/01.CIR.0000099542.57313.C5)

relationship to ischemia. EAT located over both ventricles accounted for around 20% of the total ventricular mass in all groups. When hypertrophied, EAT occupies the space between the ventricle, sometimes even covering the whole surface of the epicardium [29, 30].

Although left ventricular mass far exceeds that of the right ventricle, the absolute amount of fat tissue was similar in the right and left ventricles. As a result, the ratio of fat to myocardium weight for the right side of the heart was more than three times that of the left side: the mean weight of fat per 1 g muscle mass in the right ventricle was 0.61 g in women and 0.48 g in men, while the values in the left ventricle were 0.17 and 0.15 g, respectively. Although in non-hypertrophied hearts there was a significant correlation between body mass index and the total EAT weight ($p < 0.05$), this was not the case in hypertrophied hearts. Corradi et al. thus concluded that a constant ratio of fat to muscle exists in each ventricle, which is not influenced by ischemia or hypertrophy [29]. In the hypertrophic heart, the hypertrophy is mainly on the right-hand side and the adipose tissue also fills the epicardial spaces between these sites (Fig. 4.4) [30].

The effect of EAT on the ventricles has been evaluated in clinical studies. Increased EAT has been largely associated with increased left ventricular mass and abnormal geometry [31–35]. A recent meta-analysis reviewed the clinical studies measuring EAT with either computed

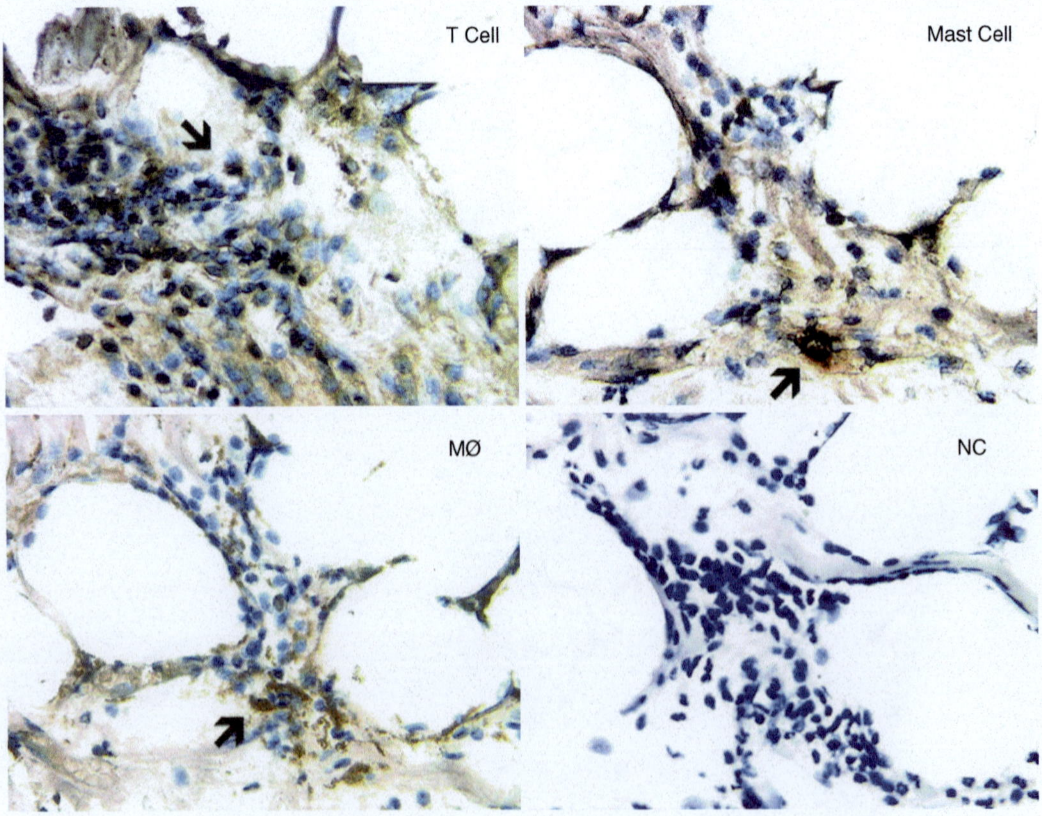

Fig. 4.3 Immunohistochemistry of cellular infiltrates in epicardial adipose tissue shows T cells (CD3+), macrophages (MØ; CD68+), and mast cells (tryptase +) that are depicted by arrows. NC indicates negative control. Magnification ×40. (From Mazurek et al. [24], with permission)

Table 4.2 Epicardial fat-related heart abnormalities

Epicardial fat-related heart abnormalities
Increased left ventricular mass
Left ventricular hypertrophy
Left ventricular remodeling
Right ventricle hypertrophy
Atrial dilation
Impaired diastolic relaxation
Impaired diastolic filling
Reduced systolic function

tomography (CT) or magnetic resonance imaging (MRI) and its relationship with left ventricular mass and geometry [36]. This meta-analysis considered only EAT volume whereas did not include linear, echocardiographic, measurement of EAT thickness. Most of the studies agreed that EAT can independently affect left ventricular mass, although one study suggests this effect could be limited to not obese subjects, due to the concurrent influential roles of obesity by itself [37]. EAT volume is correlated with left ventricular mas and left ventricular remodeling index (ratio of mass/end-diastolic volume) [33], although the effect of EAT on left ventricular geometry is controversial [31]. Multiple factors, such as obesity, hypertension, and coronary artery disease, can influence left ventricle geometry. Higher EAT volume was associated with higher left ventricular mass in obese participants in the Framingham Heart study, although the association was attenuated after adjustment for other adiposity [38]. However, this study measured the overall fat depot located within the pericardial sac, with no distinction between epicardial and pericardial fat. Interestingly studies in metabolically healthy, yet severe obese subjects, showed that the uncomplicated obesity was associated with adapted and appropriate changes in

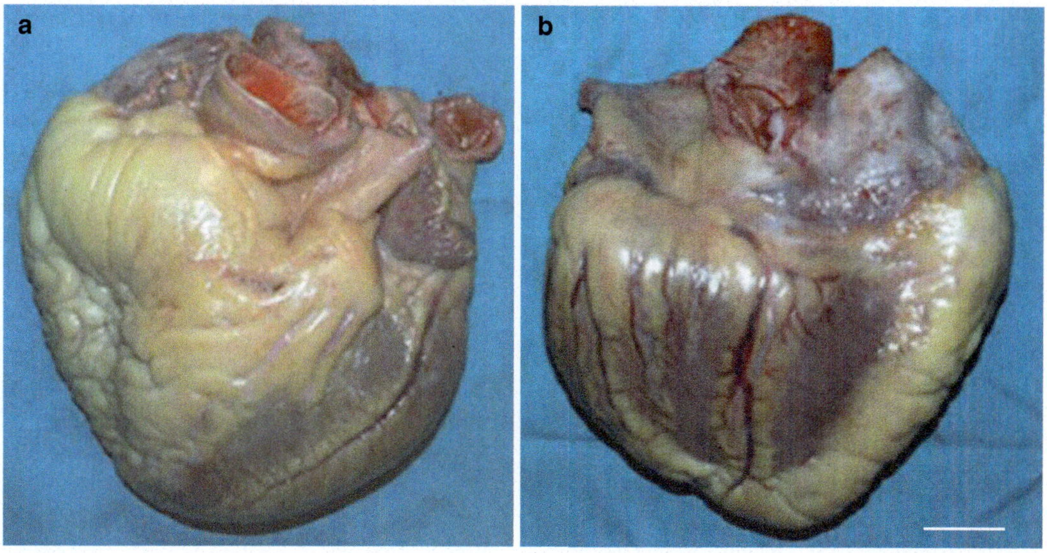

Fig. 4.4 Macroscopic appearance of epicardial fat in pathology. (**a**) Anterior view of a hypertrophic (900 g) heart. (**b**) Posterior view of a hypertrophic (900 g) heart. In the hypertrophic heart – the hypertrophy is mainly on the right hand. (From Iacobellis et al. [30], with permission)

left ventricle structure and function [39, 40]. Metabolically healthy obese are likely to present with more peripheral, subcutaneous fat accumulation, rather than with visceral, abdominal, or truncal fat phenotype. The peripheral adiposity phenotype, not well described by the body mass index, is associated with lower EAT. This can likely explain the appropriateness of the left ventricular changes in obese subjects with lower EAT accumulation.

The positive relationship between the amount of EAT and ventricular myocardial mass was also reported in echocardiographic studies. EAT thickness was related to indexed left ventricular mass, independently of body mass index, fat mas, and age in healthy individuals with a wide range of adiposity [31]. Echocardiographic findings are therefore in agreement with postmortem and CT or MRI studies. It can be assumed that EAT has an impact on left ventricular mass, regardless if it is calculated as linear or volumetric measure. Autopsy and imaging findings strongly suggest, therefore, that an increase in myocardial mass during cardiac hypertrophy is associated with a consensual and proportional increase in epicardial adipose mass. Mechanical and biomolecular mechanisms have been evoked to explain these correlations. Increased EAT by adding to the mass of the ventricles may increase the work of pumping. Increased left ventricle mass in morbidly obese subjects could be due to a direct effect of excess EAT. Higher EAT can increase left ventricle afterload and subsequent increased the output, ultimately leading to left ventricular remodeling in central obese subjects.

The physiological and pathological accumulation of EAT of the right ventricle has been also investigated in both autoptic and clinical studies in humans [40–43]. Schejbal found that the highest epicardial fat layer thickness was along the sharp heart edge – the ventrolateral edge of the right ventricle – decreasing from the heart bases to the apex [40]. Interestingly, the thickness of the EAT on the surface of the right ventricle in the histological slides was concordant with the echocardiographic values described by Iacobellis and others [43]. As the EAT mass increases, the weight of the ventricle wall increases, and in some cases the whole heart weight may be positively affected. Interestingly, a decompensated right ventricle is associated with thinning of the EAT layer. Autoptic studies in humans found age not to be a major factor of EAT morphology and thickness.

Epicardial Fat and Atria

As EAT is ubiquitously distributed around the heart chambers, it is likely to affect the atria, as well. EAT can be found in the free walls of the atria and around the two appendages. The detrimental effect of abnormal EAT on atrial morphology and function has been investigated. A very recent quantitative meta-analysis showed that CT measured EAT volume was associated with left atrial dilation (pooled B-coefficient: 0.12 mm; 95% confidence interval [CI] 0.08 to 0.17; I2: 97%) [44]. Increase in ultrasound-measured EAT thickness is significantly correlated with enlarged atria in morbidly obese subjects [45]. EAT thickness in morbidly obese subjects was significantly related to left atrium($r = 0.65$, $p = 0.02$) and right atrium ($r = 0.63$, $p = 0.02$) diameter [45]. The amount and the fibro-fatty changes of epicardial adipose tissue that accumulates around the atria are associated with the risk, persistence, and severity of atrial fibrillation [46]. Fibro-fatty infiltrations of the subepicardium could also contribute to the functional disorganization of the atrial myocardium. Given its contiguity, EAT is thought to contribute to fibrosis of the neighboring atrial myocardium by secreting inflammatory cytokines such as interleukins (ILs), tumor necrosis factor (TNF)-alpha, and profibrotic factors such as matrix metalloproteinases (MMPs) and activin A [13].

Epicardial Fat and Diastole

Obesity and conditions with excessive visceral adiposity, such type 2 diabetes, have been commonly associated with diastolic dysfunction [47]. However, due to its anatomical and functional contiguity to the atria, EAT may directly affect the diastole. Obese subjects, particularly those with abdominal and truncal fat accumulation, tend to have higher EAT. Both EAT volume and thickness effects on diastolic function were evaluated. CT EAT volume was associated with higher E/E′ ratio (pooled B-coefficient: 0.28 cm/s; 95% CI 0.08 to 0.49; I2: 67%), lower E′ velocity (pooled B-coefficient: −0.16 cm/s; 95% CI −0.22 to −0.09; I2: 43%), and E/A ratio (pooled B-coefficient: −0.01; 95% CI −0.02 to −0.001; I2: 70%), independently of body mass index, from a recent meta-analysis of 19 studies [44]. Increase in EAT thickness is significantly correlated with enlarged atria and impaired right and left ventricular diastolic filling in morbidly obese subjects [45]. EAT thickness in morbidly obese subjects was significantly related to both mitral ($r = 0.40$, $p = 0.04$) and tricuspidal ($r = 0.41$, $p = 0.04$) E/A ratio. Correlations were essentially unchanged when echocardiographic variables were adjusted for BMI, age, and sex [45].

The effects of epicardial adipose tissue can be mediated by both biochemical and mechanical pathways. The local release of EAT adipokines can affect diastolic function and impair diastolic relaxation through fibrosis, inflammation, and collagen turnover [48, 49]. The lower expression of the cardioprotective adiponectin can also modify diastolic function [50–52]. EAT may directly contribute to impair diastolic function in subjects with increased visceral adiposity. A direct mechanical obstacle and compression of the excessive EAT pad can affect the diastolic filling. The association of EAT with aortic stiffness has been proposed as another mechanism affecting diastolic filling [53]. Increased pressure in late systole can also affect diastolic dysfunction.

A recent meta-analysis showed that CT- or MRI-measured EAT volume has an independent effect on diastolic function parameters over adiposity markers [36]. However, the cause-effect relation between the fat and the diastole can be confounded by the effects of age, obesity-related changes, normal systolic function, and the U-shaped relationship of E/A ratio with diastolic function that makes it difficult to assess without taking into consideration additional covariates [54]. Obese subjects may present with adaptive changes in both filling and relaxation. However, it is important to underline that some of the studies have also included pericardial fat that misses the direct contiguity with the myocardial atria. This could explain the lack of independent correlation with E/A ratio. Hence, causality cannot be fully proved; some of these findings should be interpreted with caution. As noted for the left ventricular mass, the methodology used to measure EAT, either CT or echocardiography, seems not to be so relevant in determining the association between the fat and the diastolic dysfunction.

Epicardial Fat and Systole

The role of EAT in affecting the systole has been studied. Nevertheless, if there is almost a consensus about the effects of the fat on left ventricle morphology and diastole, not all of the studies found a similar correlation with the systolic function. Two recent meta-analyses concluded there was no or weak association between epicardial and left ventricular systolic function [36, 44]. There were weak and inconsistent associations of CT measured EAT volume and systolic parameters. However, one study found a strong and independent association between EAT and longitudinal strain as a marker of subclinical myocardial dysfunction [55]. EAT volume was also independently associated with impaired myocardial systolic function despite preserved left ventricular ejection fraction and absence of severe coronary artery disease, in nonobese and obese subjects [55, 56]. EAT seems to inversely correlate with systolic parameters in conditions of preserved ejection fraction. The correlation with EAT and systolic function can actually be linear rather than inverse, in the setting of heart failure. In fact, a stepwise decrease in CT or ultrasound measured EAT volume in patients with impaired cardiac function and congestive heart failure was reported [35, 57]. Subjects with reduced ejection fraction tend to have less EAT as compared to controls or those with normal ejection fraction. The mechanism causing a decreased EAT in patients with impaired systolic function is unclear. Several mechanisms have been evoked to explain this finding. As myocardial function deteriorates, EAT may suffer fibrotic changes and turn up apoptotic mechanisms contributing to EAT mass reduction. However, the relation and role of EAT with systolic function is still not completely understood.

References

1. Unger RH, Orci L. Lipoapoptosis: its mechanism and its diseases. Biochim Biophys Acta. 2002;1585:202–12.
2. Unger RH. Lipotoxic diseases. Annu Rev Med. 2002;53:319–36.
3. Iozzo P. Myocardial, perivascular, and epicardial fat. Diabetes Care. 2011;34(Suppl 2):S371–9.
4. Marchington JM, Pond CM. Site-specific properties of pericardial and epicardial adipose tissue. The effects of insulin and high-fat feeding on lipogenesis and the incorporation of fatty acids in vitro. Int J Obes. 1990;14:1013–22.
5. Vural B, Atalar F, Ciftci C, Demirkan A, Susleyici-Duman B, Gunay D. Presence of fatty-acid-binding protein 4 expression in human epicardial adipose tissue in metabolic syndrome. Cardiovasc Pathol. 2008;17:392–8.
6. Zhou YT, Grayburn P, Karim A, Shimabukuro M, Higa M, Baetens D, Orci L, Unger RH. Lipotoxic heart disease in obese rats: implications for human obesity. Proc Natl Acad Sci U S A. 2000;97:1784–9.
7. Granér M, Nyman K, Siren R, Pentikäinen MO, Lundbom J, Hakkarainen A, et al. Ectopic fat depots and left ventricular function in nondiabetic men with nonalcoholic fatty liver disease. Circ Cardiovasc Imaging. 2014;8(1):e001979.
8. Kankaanpää M, Lehto HR, Pärkkä JP, Komu M, Viljanen A, Ferrannini E, et al. Myocardial triglyceride content and epicardial fat mass in human obesity: relationship to left ventricular function and serum free fatty acid levels. J Clin Endocrinol Metab. 2006;91:4689–95.
9. Pezeshkian M, Mahtabipour MR. Epicardial and subcutaneous adipose tissue fatty acids profiles in diabetic and non-diabetic patients candidate for coronary artery bypass graft. Bioimpacts. 2013;3:83–9.
10. Marchington JM, Mattacks CA, Pond CM. Adipose tissue in the mammalian heart and pericardium; structure, foetal development and biochemical properties. Comp Biochem Physiol. 1989;94B:225–32.
11. McAninch EA, Fonseca TL, Poggioli R, Panos AL, Salerno TA, Deng Y, et al. Epicardial adipose tissue has a unique transcriptome modified in severe coronary artery disease. Obesity. 2015;23:1267–78.
12. Hatem SN, Redheuil A, Gandjbakhch E. Cardiac adipose tissue and atrial fibrillation: the perils of adiposity. Cardiovasc Res. 2016;109:502–9.
13. Venteclef N, Guglielmi V, Balse E, Gaborit B, Cotillard A, Atassi F, et al. Human epicardial adipose tissue induces fibrosis of the atrial myocardium through the secretion of adipo-fibrokines. Eur Heart J. 2015;36:795–805a.
14. McGavock JM, Lingvay I, Zib I, Tillery T, Salas N, Unger R, et al. Cardiac steatosis in diabetes mellitus: a 1H-magnetic resonance spectroscopy study. Circulation. 2007;116:1170–5.

15. Szczepaniak LS, Dobbins RL, Metzger GJ, Sartoni-D'Ambrosia G, Arbique D, Vongpatanasin W. Myocardial triglycerides and systolic function in humans: in vivo evaluation by localized proton spectroscopy and cardiac imaging. Magn Reson Med. 2003;49:417–23.
16. Felblinger J, Jung B, Slotboom J, Boesch C, Kreis R. Methods and reproducibility of cardiac/respiratory double-triggered 1H-MR spectroscopy of the human heart. Magn Reson Med. 1999;42:903–10.
17. den Hollander JA, Evanochko WT, Pohost GM. Observation of cardiac lipids in humans by localized 1H magnetic resonance spectroscopic imaging. Magn Reson Med. 1994;32:175–80.
18. Reingold JS, McGavock JM, Kaka S, Tillery T, Victor RG, Szczepaniak LS. Determination of triglyceride in the human myocardium by magnetic resonance spectroscopy: reproducibility and sensitivity of the method. Am J Physiol Endocrinol Metab. 2005;289:E935–9.
19. Malavazos AE, Di Leo G, Secchi F, Lupo EN, Dogliotti G, Coman C, et al. Relation of echocardiographic epicardial fat thickness and myocardial fat. Am J Cardiol. 2010;105:1831–5.
20. Granér M, Siren R, Nyman K, Lundbom J, Hakkarainen A, Pentikäinen MO, et al. Cardiac steatosis associates with visceral obesity in nondiabetic obese men. J Clin Endocrinol Metab. 2013;98:1189–97.
21. Gaborit B, Kober F, Jacquier A, Moro PJ, Cuisset T, Boullu S, et al. Assessment of epicardial fat volume and myocardial triglyceride content in severely obese subjects: relationship to metabolic profile, cardiac function and visceral fat. Int J Obes. 2012;36:422–30.
22. Granér M, Pentikäinen MO, Nyman K, Siren R, Lundbom J, Hakkarainen A, et al. Cardiac steatosis in patients with dilated cardiomyopathy. Heart. 2014;100:1107–12.
23. Bambace C, Telesca M, Zoico E, Sepe A, Olioso D, Rossi A, et al. Adiponectin gene expression and adipocyte diameter: a comparison between epicardial and subcutaneous adipose tissue in men. Cardiovasc Pathol. 2011;20:e153–6.
24. Mazurek T, Zhang L, Zalewski A, Mannion JD, Diehl JT, Arafat H. Human epicardial adipose tissue is a source of inflammatory mediators. Circulation. 2003;108:2460–6. https://www.ahajournals.org/doi/10.1161/01.CIR.0000099542.57313.C5.
25. Hirata Y, Tabata M, Kurobe H, Motoki T, Akaike M, Nishio C, et al. Coronary atherosclerosis is associated with macrophage polarization in epicardial adipose tissue. J Am Coll Cardiol. 2011;58:248–55.
26. Zhou Q, Zhang L, Wang K, Xu X, Ji M, Zhang F. Effect of interconnection between cervical vagus trunk, epicardial fat pad on sinus node function, and atrial fibrillation. Pacing Clin Electrophysiol. 2014;37:356–63.
27. Reiner L. Statistical analysis of the epicardial fat weight in human hearts. AMA Arch Pathol. 1995;60:369–73.
28. Reiner L. The weight of the human heart, II. Hypertensive cases. Arch Pathol. 1961;71:180–201.
29. Corradi D. The ventricular epicardial fat is related to the myocardial mass in normal, ischemic and hypertrophic hearts. Cardiovasc Pathol. 2004;13:313–6.
30. Iacobellis G, Corradi D, Sharma AM. Epicardial adipose tissue: anatomic, biomolecular and clinical relationships with the heart. Nat Clin Pract Cardiovasc Med. 2005;2:536–43.
31. Iacobellis G, Ribaudo MC, Zappaterreno A, Iannucci CV, Leonetti F. Relation between epicardial adipose tissue and left ventricular mass. Am J Cardiol. 2004;94:1084–7.
32. Iacobellis G, Pond CM, Sharma AM. Different "weight" of cardiac and general adiposity in predicting left ventricle morphology. Obesity (Silver Spring). 2006;14:1679–84.
33. Doesch C, Haghi D, Fluchter S, Suselbeck T, Schoenberg SO, Michaely H, Borggrefe M, Papavassiliu T. Epicardial adipose tissue in patients with heart failure. J Cardiovasc Magn Reson. 2010;12:40.
34. Doesch C, Haghi D, Suselbeck T, Schoenberg SO, Borggrefe M, Papavassiliu T. Impact of functional, morphological and clinical parameters on epicardial adipose tissue in patients with coronary artery disease. Circ J. 2012;76:2426–34.
35. Doesch C, Streitner F, Bellm S, Suselbeck T, Haghi D, Heggemann F, et al. Epicardial adipose tissue assessed by cardiac magnetic resonance imaging in patients with heart failure due to dilated cardiomyopathy. Obesity (Silver Spring). 2013;21:E253–61.
36. Nerlekar N, Muthalaly RG, Wong N, Thakur U, Wong DT, Brown AJ, Marwick TH. Association of volumetric epicardial adipose tissue quantification and cardiac structure and function. J Am Heart Assoc. 2018;7:e009975.
37. Bakkum MJ, Danad I, Romijn MA, Stuijfzand WJ, Leonora RM, Tulevski II, et al. The impact of obesity on the relationship between epicardial adipose tissue, left ventricular mass and coronary microvascular function. Eur J Nucl Med Mol Imaging. 2015;42:1562–73.
38. Fox CS, Gona P, Hoffmann U, Porter SA, Salton CJ, Massaro JM, et al. Pericardial fat, intrathoracic fat, and measures of left ventricular structure and function: the Framingham Heart Study. Circulation. 2009;119:1586–91.
39. Iacobellis G. True uncomplicated obesity is not related to increased left ventricular mass and systolic dysfunction. J Am Coll Cardiol. 2004;44:225.
40. Iacobellis G, Ribaudo MC, Zappaterreno A, Iannucci CV, Di Mario U, Leonetti F. Adapted changes in left ventricular structure and function in severe uncomplicated obesity. Obes Res. 2004;12:1616–21.
41. Tansey DK. Fat in the right ventricle of the normal heart. Histopathology. 2005;46:98–104.
42. Schejbal V. Epicardial fatty tissue of the right ventricle morphology, morphometry and functional significance. Pneumologie. 1989;43:490–9.

43. Iacobellis G. Relation of epicardial fat thickness to right ventricular cavity size in obese subjects. Am J Cardiol. 2009;104:1601–2.
44. Mancio J, Azevedo D, Fragao-Marques M, Falcao-Pires I, Leite-Moreira A, Lunet N, et al. Meta-analysis of relation of epicardial adipose tissue volume to left atrial dilation and to left ventricular hypertrophy and functions. Am J Cardiol. 2019;123:523–31.
45. Iacobellis G, Leonetti F, Singh N, M Sharma A. Relationship of epicardial adipose tissue with atrial dimensions and diastolic function in morbidly obese subjects. Int J Cardiol. 2007;115:272–3.
46. Iacobellis G. Is obesity a risk factor for atrial fibrillation? Nat Clin Pract Cardiovasc Med. 2005;2:134–5.
47. Dorbala S, Crugnale S, Yang D, Di Carli MF. Effect of body mass index on left ventricular cavity size and ejection fraction. Am J Cardiol. 2006;97:725–9.
48. Mak GJ, Ledwidge MT, Watson CJ, Phelan DM, Dawkins IR, Murphy NF, et al. Natural history of markers of collagen turnover in patients with early diastolic dysfunction and impact of eplerenone. J Am Coll Cardiol. 2009;54:1674–82.
49. Silberman GA, Fan TH, Liu H, Jiao Z, Xiao HD, Lovelock JD, et al. Uncoupled cardiac nitric oxide synthase mediates diastolic dysfunction. Circulation. 2010;121:519–28.
50. Greenstein AS, Khavandi K, Withers SB, Sonoyama K, Clancy O, Jeziorska M, et al. Local inflammation and hypoxia abolish the protective anticontractile properties of perivascular fat in obese patients. Circulation. 2009;119:1661–70.
51. Iacobellis G, Pistilli D, Gucciardo M, Leonetti F, Miraldi F, Brancaccio G, et al. Adiponectin expression in human epicardial adipose tissue in vivo is lower in patients with coronary artery disease. Cytokine. 2005;29:251–5.
52. Iacobellis G, Cotesta D, Petramala L, De Santis V, Vitale D, Tritapepe L, Letizia C. Intracoronary adiponectin levels rapidly and significantly increase after coronary revascularization. Int J Cardiol. 2010;144:160–3.
53. Hachiya K, Fukuta H, Wakami K, Goto T, Tani T, Ohte N. Relation of epicardial fat to central aortic pressure and left ventricular diastolic function in patients with known or suspected coronary artery disease. Int J Cardiovasc Imaging. 2014;30:1393–8.
54. Nagueh SF, Smiseth OA, Appleton CP, Byrd BF III, Dokainish H, Edvardsen T, et al. Recommendations for the evaluation of left ventricular diastolic function by echocardiography: an update from the American Society of Echocardiography and the European Association of Cardiovascular Imaging. J Am Soc Echocardiogr. 2016;29:277–314.
55. Ng AC, Goo SY, Roche N, van der Geest RJ, Wang WY. Epicardial adipose tissue volume and left ventricular myocardial function using 3-dimensional speckle tracking echocardiography. Can J Cardiol. 2016;32:1485–92.
56. Homsi R, Yuecel S, Schlesinger-Irsch U, Meier-Schroers M, Kuetting D, Luetkens J, et al. Epicardial fat, left ventricular strain, and T1-relaxation times in obese individuals with a normal ejection fraction. Acta Radiol. 2019;60:1251–7.
57. Iacobellis G, Zaki MC, Garcia D, Willens HJ. Epicardial fat in atrial fibrillation and heart failure. Horm Metab Res. 2014;46:587–9.

5 Echocardiographic Imaging of the Epicardial Adipose Tissue

Gianluca Iacobellis

Key Points

- Epicardial fat can be visualized and measured using standard two-dimensional echocardiography.
- Epicardial fat thickness is generally identified as the echo-free space between the outer wall of the myocardium and the visceral layer of pericardium and is measured perpendicularly on the free wall of the right ventricle at end-systole.
- Echocardiographic epicardial fat measurement has several advantages, including its low cost, easy accessibility, rapid applicability, and good reproducibility.

Introduction

Excessive visceral adiposity is a well-established risk factor for cardiovascular diseases. The measurement of visceral fat can help with the stratification of the cardiovascular risk [1, 2]. In a clinical setting, visceral fat can be measured by surrogate markers, such as waist circumference alone or the ratio of waist circumference to hip circumference. However, these markers are not precise and greatly operator dependent. More direct measurements of visceral fat, including magnetic resonance imaging (MRI) and/or computed tomography (CT), are certainly precise, but they are expensive and cumbersome. There is therefore a compelling need and growing interest in less expensive and more reliable imaging markers of visceral adiposity [3]. Although much attention has been focused on the measurement of intra-abdominal fat, interest in nontraditional visceral fat depots, such as EAT, is relatively recent. Iacobellis et al. first developed a method to measure EAT thickness by using standard transthoracic echocardiography [4, 5]. Echocardiographic assessment of EAT thickness meets the criteria of specificity, not invasivity and easy availability, although there are advantages and limitations, summarized in Table 5.1.

Table 5.1 Advantages and limitations of echocardiographic epicardial fat thickness

Advantages	Limitations
Direct measure of visceral fat	High variability
Consistency with autopsy finding	Operator dependent
Noninvasive, simple, and inexpensive	No volumetric assessment
Correlation with myocardial fat content	No regional epicardial fat measurement
Concurrent assessment of cardiac function	Inaccurate estimate of the total amount of fat
Reproducible during interventions	No direct assessment of myocardial fat content

G. Iacobellis (✉)
Division of Endocrinology, Diabetes and Metabolism, Department of Medicine, University of Miami, Miller School of Medicine, Miami, FL, USA
e-mail: giacobellis@med.miami.edu

G. Iacobellis (ed.), *Epicardial Adipose Tissue*, Contemporary Cardiology,
https://doi.org/10.1007/978-3-030-40570-0_5

Methodology

EAT thickness can be visualized and measured with two-dimensional (2D) echocardiography using commercially available echocardiographic equipment, as first invented and validated by Iacobellis et al. [3–5].

Standard parasternal long-axis and short-axis views from 2D images permit the most accurate measurement of EAT thickness on the right ventricle with optimal cursor beam orientation in each view. The measurement of EAT on top of the right ventricle is consistent with anatomical findings. In fact, autopsy showed large EAT accumulation on the right ventricle [6]. EAT is commonly identified as the relatively echo-free space between the outer wall of the myocardium and the visceral layer of pericardium; its thickness is measured perpendicularly on the free wall of the right ventricle at end-systole in three cardiac cycles (Fig. 5.1). Because it is compressed during diastole, EAT thickness is best measured at end-systole at the point on the free wall of the right ventricle at which the ultrasound beam is oriented in a perpendicular manner, using the aortic annulus as an anatomic landmark. EAT thickness can also appear as hyperechoic space, if in large amount (>15 mm). Maximum EAT thickness is measured from 2D parasternal long-axis images at the point on the free wall of the right ventricle along the midline of the ultrasound beam, perpendicular to the aortic annulus, used as an anatomic landmark for this view. For mid-ventricular parasternal short-axis assessment, maximum EAT thickness is measured from 2D images on the right ventricular free wall along the midline of the ultrasound beam perpendicular to the interventricular septum at midchordal and tip of the papillary muscle level, as anatomic landmarks. The average value of three cardiac cycles from each echocardiographic view is determined. The majority of population-based clinical studies have reported excellent interobserver and intraobserver agreement for EAT thickness measurement [7–10]. Intraclass correlation coefficients have ranged from 0.90 to 0.98 and from 0.93 to 0.98, respectively, indicating good reproducibility and reliability. Concordance of long-axis and short-axis average EAT thickness measurement was also excellent at 0.98 (95% confidence interval, 0.97–0.98) [5].

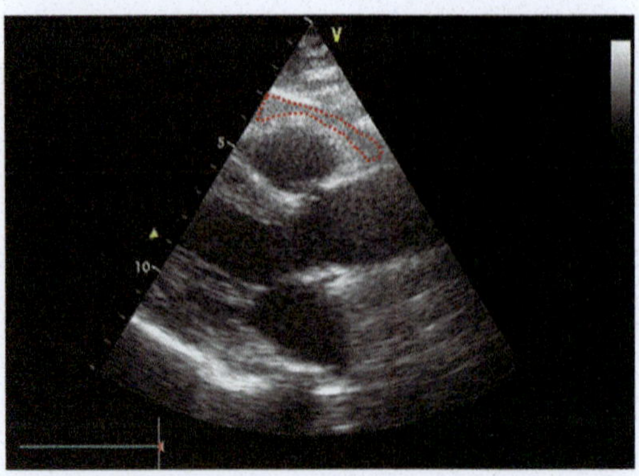

Fig. 5.1 Epicardial fat thickness (*within red dashed shape*) is identified as the echo-free space between the outer wall of the myocardium and the visceral layer of pericardium in the parasternal long-axis view. Epicardial fat thickness is measured during end-systole at the point on the free wall of the right ventricle along the midline of the ultrasound beam, with the best effort to be perpendicular to the aortic annulus, used as an anatomic landmark. (From Iacobellis et al. [3], with permission from Elsevier)

Epicardial Versus Pericardial Fat Thickness

Epicardial and pericardial fat are two embryologically, anatomically, and clinically distinct depots. This is not a matter of terminology. Ultrasound-measured EAT can be distinguished from pericardial fat. Pericardial fat thickness can be identified as the hypoechoic space anterior to the EAT and parietal pericardium (Fig. 5.2). Pericardial fat usually does not deform substantially with cardiac cycles and does not appear hyperechoic. However, fat thickness deformation is not a good way of distinguishing between the two depots.

Epicardial Fat Thickness Range

Echocardiographic EAT thickness varies from a minimum of 1 mm to a maximum measured value of almost 25 mm [5]. The wide range of EAT thicknesses likely reflects the substantial

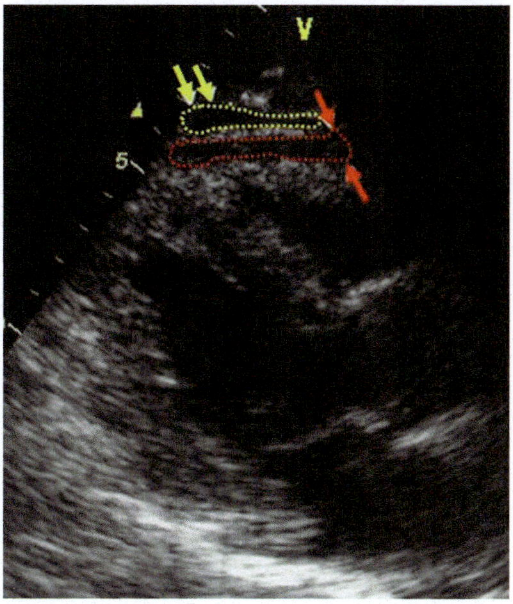

Fig. 5.2 Pericardial fat (*within yellow arrows and yellow dashed shape*) can be identified as the hypoechoic space anterior to the epicardial fat (*within red arrows and red dashed shape*). Pericardial fat usually does not deform substantially with cardiac cycles and does not appear as hyperechoic space. Modified parasternal long-axis view. (From Iacobellis et al. [3], with permission from Elsevier)

variation in abdominal visceral fat distribution. Iacobellis et al. found median EAT thicknesses of 7 mm in men and 6.5 mm in women in a large population of patients who underwent transthoracic echocardiography for standard clinical indications [5]. Jeong et al. reported a mean EAT thickness of 6.3 mm in more than 200 subjects who underwent coronary angiography [8]. Natale et al. set the normal upper limit to 7 mm, on the basis of the mean value and distribution of EAT thickness in 50 normal volunteers [9].

Echocardiographic Epicardial Fat Is a Marker of Visceral Fat

EAT thickness is a marker of visceral fat. Echocardiographic EAT strongly reflects the intra-abdominal accumulation of visceral fat as measured on MRI and does so better than waist circumference [9]. Correlation between echocardiographic EAT thickness and EAT volume, assessed by MR imaging, was excellent ($r = 0.90$, $p < 0.01$). Bland-Altman test confirmed the agreement between MR imaging of EAT volume and echocardiographic EAT thickness [4]. Subjects with higher waist circumferences have higher EAT thickness. Echocardiographic EAT thickness is therefore an independent predictor of visceral adiposity and weakly reflects the degree of obesity as defined by body mass index [11].

Advantages of Echocardiographic Epicardial Fat Thickness

Echocardiographic EAT measurement may have some advantages as an index of high cardiometabolic risk:

(a) It is a direct measure of visceral fat rather than an anthropometric measure, such as waist circumference, that includes muscle and skin layers. The echocardiographic measurement of EAT provides a more sensitive and specific measure of true visceral fat content, avoiding the possible confounding effect of increased subcutaneous abdominal fat.
(b) The location of the EAT measurement is consistent with autopsy describing a large accumulation at the ventrolateral edge of the right ventricle.
(c) It is an objective, noninvasive, simple, and certainly less expensive measure of visceral fat than MRI or CT.
(d) Echocardiographic EAT is a direct measure of ectopic fat deposition, whereas anthropometric measures can be associated only with ectopic fat deposition.
(e) It can be measured even from echocardiograms that were not specifically performed to optimize the measurement of EAT. It can be quantified with other echocardiographic parameters, such LV mass and ejection fraction, traditionally associated with cardiovascular risk.
(f) Echocardiographic EAT could be a more reliable quantitative therapeutic marker during interventions modulating and reducing visceral adiposity.

Limitations of Echocardiographic Epicardial Fat Thickness

Echocardiography may be not the optimal technique for the quantification of EAT. Although the majority of studies have shown excellent coefficients of interobserver and intraobserver variability, a single study raised some concerns on the dispersion and variability in the measurement of EAT thickness [12]. A moderate concordance in echocardiographic EAT measurement and a relatively poor agreement with measurement on multidetector computed tomography (MDCT) were reported in this study. Given the small number of patients with interpretable results on MDCT and the use of end-diastolic EAT thickness in the study, the actual variability of this measurement is still in question. However, if the echocardiographic quantification of EAT is performed for cardiometabolic risk stratification, the reproducibility of this measurement is undoubtedly a critical issue.

Echocardiographic EAT thickness is a linear measurement at a single location and therefore may not reflect the variability of fat thickness or total EAT volume. Although the anterior layer of EAT is the one commonly measured by echocardiography, this region may have the most variability in fat content as measured using MRI and MDCT. EAT thickness is usually smaller in the vicinity of the mid right ventricular free wall and greater in the distal portion of the right ventricular free wall. MRI or CT measurements of EAT thickness in the atrioventricular groove or interventricular groove areas may give a more accurate assessment of EAT amount. MDCT is more sensitive and specific than echocardiography for measuring fat thickness in deeper EAT layers as well as the thickest part of the EAT in the atrioventricular grooves [13–15]. EAT has a conspicuous distribution around the heart, and 2D echocardiographic assessment may not be a completely accurate estimate of the total amount of fat. Three-dimensional echocardiography could provide a noninvasive and more accurate volumetric assessment of EAT thickness. EAT volume, rather than its thickness, may in fact be the most consistent measure of risk [16].

The variability of echocardiographic measurement techniques has also resulted in inconsistencies among studies. EAT thickness when measured just to the right of the aortic annular plane may increase in size abruptly compared with thickness measured either at or just to the left of the aortic annular plane (Fig. 5.3). This abrupt increase in end-systolic EAT thickness is due to the steep downward turn of the free wall of the right ventricle as it approaches the proximal ascending aorta. In such cases, we recommend measuring the largest EAT thickness to the left of the annular plane. During which cardiac cycle echocardiographic EAT should be measured has also been a subject of debate. Some echocardiographic studies have measured EAT thickness at end-diastole rather than end-systole. We recommend that maximum EAT thickness is better measured at end-systole, as highlighted before [3]. When scrolling through the cardiac cycle, in some cases, the largest EAT thickness may fail to correspond to true end-systole or end-diastole. Also in these cases, we recommend measuring EAT thickness at end-systole.

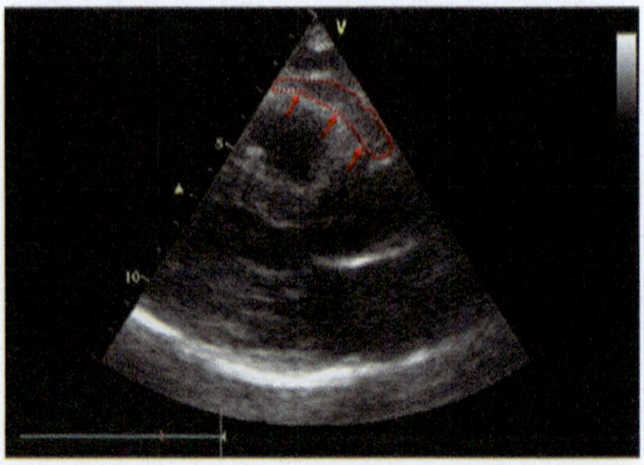

Fig. 5.3 Large echocardiographic epicardial fat thickness. Large epicardial fat thickness (*within red arrows and red dashed shape*) when measured just to the right of the aortic annular plane may abruptly increase in size. This abrupt increase in end-systolic epicardial fat thickness is due to the steep downward turn of the free wall of the right ventricle as it approaches the proximal ascending aorta. In these cases, it is recommended to measure the largest epicardial fat thickness to the left of the annular plane. (From Iacobellis et al. [3], with permission from Elsevier)

Potential limitations of echocardiography also include difficulties in differentiating between EAT thickness and pericardial fat, as well as changes in the velocity of sound in adipose tissue. Although there are no current data on how and whether the latter might affect the accuracy of EAT thickness measurement using echocardiography, it would be of interest to evaluate whether it is necessary to correct for this confounding factor when determining the amount of EAT.

References

1. Yusuf S, Hawken S, Ounpuu S, Dans T, Avezum A, Lanas F, INTERHEART Study Investigators, et al. Effect of potentially modifiable risk factors associated with myocardial infarction in 52 countries (the INTERHEART study): case-control study. Lancet. 2004;364:937–52.
2. Fox CS, Massaro JM, Hoffmann U, Pou KM, Maurovich-Horvat P, Liu CY, et al. Abdominal visceral and subcutaneous adipose tissue compartments: association with metabolic risk factors in the Framingham Heart Study. Circulation. 2007;116:39–48.
3. Iacobellis G, Willens HJ. Echocardiographic epicardial fat: a review of research and clinical applications. J Am Soc Echocardiogr. 2009;22:1311–9.
4. Iacobellis G, Assael F, Ribaudo MC, Zappaterreno A, Alessi G, Di Mario U, et al. Epicardial fat from echocardiography: a new method for visceral adipose tissue prediction. Obes Res. 2003;11:304–10.
5. Iacobellis G, Willens HJ, Barbaro G, Sharma AM. Threshold values of high risk echocardiographic epicardial fat thickness. Obesity (Silver Spring). 2008;16:887–92.
6. Schejbal V. Epicardial fatty tissue of the right ventricle–morphology, morphometry and functional significance. Pneumologie. 1989;43:490–9.
7. Sade LE, Eroglu S, Bozbasx H, Özbiçer S, Hayran M, Haberal A, et al. Relation between epicardial fat thickness and coronary flow reserve in women with chest pain and angiographically normal coronary arteries. Atherosclerosis. 2009;204:580–5.
8. Jeong JW, Jeong MH, Yun KH, Oh SK, Park EM, Kim YK. Echocardiographic epicardial fat thickness and coronary artery disease. Circ J. 2007;71:536–9.
9. Natale F, Tedesco MA, Mocerino R, de Simone V, Di Marco GM, Aronne L, et al. Visceral adiposity and arterial stiffness: echocardiographic epicardial fat thickness reflects, better than waist circumference, carotid arterial stiffness in a large population of hypertensives. Eur J Echocardiogr. 2009;10: 549–55.
10. Iacobellis G, Ribaudo MC, Assael F, Vecci E, Tiberti C, Zappaterreno A, et al. Echocardiographic epicardial adipose tissue is related to anthropometric and clinical parameters of metabolic syndrome: a new indicator of cardiovascular risk. J Clin Endocrinol Metab. 2003;88:5163–8.
11. Iacobellis G. Imaging of visceral adipose tissue: an emerging diagnostic tool and therapeutic target. Curr Drug Targets Cardiovasc Haematol Disord. 2005;5:345–53.
12. Saura D, Oliva MJ, Rodríguez D, Pascual-Figal DA, Hurtado JA, Pinar E, et al. Reproducibility of echocardiographic measurements of epicardial fat thickness. Int J Cardiol. 2010;141:311–3.
13. Wang TD, Lee WJ, Shih FY, Huang CH, Chang YC, Chen WJ, et al. Relations of epicardial adipose tissue measured by multidetector computed tomography to components of the metabolic syndrome are region-specific and independent of anthropometric indexes and intraabdominal visceral fat. J Clin Endocrinol Metab. 2009;94:662–9.
14. Sarin S, Wenger C, Marwaha A, Qureshi A, Go BD, Woomert CA, et al. Clinical significance of epicardial fat measured using cardiac multislice computed tomography. J Cardiol. 2008;102:767–71.
15. Abbara S, Desai JC, Cury RC, Butler J, Nieman K, Reddy V. Mapping epicardial fat with multi-detector computed tomography to facilitate percutaneous transepicardial arrhythmia ablation. Eur J Radiol. 2006;57:417–22.
16. Greif M, Becker A, von Ziegler F, Lebherz C, Lehrke M, Broedl UC, et al. Pericardial adipose tissue determined by dual source CT is a risk factor for coronary atherosclerosis. Arterioscler Thromb Vasc Biol. 2009;29:781–6.

Computed Tomography Imaging of Epicardial Adipose Tissue

6

Bastian Balcer, Tienush Rassaf, and Amir Abbas Mahabadi

Key Points

- Computed tomography (CT) is the gold standard for quantification of epicardial adipose tissue volume, as it allows for a three-dimensional assessment, based on a semiautomated Hounsfield unit-based measurement.
- Once non-contrast- or contrast-enhanced cardiac CT imaging is performed, information on epicardial adipose tissue volume and attenuation is readily available. In addition to overall epicardial adipose tissue assessment, cardiac CT allows for quantification of local fat components such as pericoronary fat or peri-atrial fat.
- While CT-derived epicardial adipose tissue volume is strongly associated with cardiovascular risk factors, markers of subclinical atherosclerosis, as well as prevalent and incident cardiovascular disease manifestation, also fat attenuation may allow for enhanced risk prediction.

B. Balcer · T. Rassaf · A. A. Mahabadi (✉)
Department of Cardiology and Vascular Medicine, West German Heart and Vascular Center Essen, University Hospital Essen, Essen, Germany
e-mail: amir-abbas.mahabadi@uk-essen.de

Imaging Tools as Part of Primary and Secondary Prevention

Key for guiding the appropriate treatment strategy for cardiovascular disease is accurate assessment of the cardiovascular risk of an individual patient. The link between conventional risk factors for cardiovascular disease and extent of atherosclerosis manifestation can vary substantially between individual patients. Since Framingham Heart Study investigators first confirmed the existence and importance of cardiovascular risk factors in 1961 [1], scientists and clinicians have been seeking to refine the prediction of risk for cardiovascular disease. As atherosclerosis begins at a young age but is clinically silent for many years and, in addition, delaying or prevention of systemic clinical manifestations is possible during this latent period, identifying patients at risk is of major interest in daily clinical practice [2, 3]. Therefore, clinical risk stratification tools like the Framingham Risk Score (FRS) or the pooled risk equation (ASCVD score) were developed to help clinicians to assess the risk of their patients.

These algorithms usually estimate the 10-year risk for cardiovascular disease events according to the patient's age, gender, ethnicity, and traditional risk factors such as total-, low-, and high-density cholesterol levels, smoking status, diabetes, and blood pressure [4]. According to these characteristics, patients are divided into

G. Iacobellis (ed.), *Epicardial Adipose Tissue*, Contemporary Cardiology,
https://doi.org/10.1007/978-3-030-40570-0_6

risk groups for cardiovascular disease events. While patients in the high-risk group qualify for aggressive medical treatment, treatment for intermediate- and low-risk patients remains controversial [4].

In addition, several studies have outlined limitations of the risk scoring algorithms to distinguish the risk for cardiovascular disease [5–7]. In a retrospective analysis of subjects below the age of 55 in males and below 65 in females, sustaining their first myocardial infarction, Akosah et al. estimated the risk profile based on traditional risk factors. In this young collective, 88% of the MI patients would have been considered to be at low or intermediate risk immediately before the event [6]. Likewise, Brindle et al. found that 63% of MI occurred in a group of subjects of <15% of FRS in a prospective population-based study in 6643 British men [7]. Möhlenkamp et al. looking at asymptomatic marathon runners suggested that traditional risk factors underestimate the risk in master athletes [8]. Likewise, for the ASCVD score, an overestimation of risk has been described in European populations [9]. Due to this inherent limitation of the risk scoring algorithms and the uncertainties of treatment of subjects with an intermediate risk of cardiovascular events, further risk factors and risk stratification tools are needed.

Over the last three decades, the use of imaging tools has gained interest for further risk stratification. In the classification of an individual's cardiovascular risk and in the primary prevention stage, the use of different imaging modalities can be beneficial. Hence, in line with clinical guidelines appropriate use and implementation of these different imaging techniques for risk assessment purposes can influence the outcomes of cardiovascular disease prevention [10, 11]. These include cardiac computed tomography imaging that allows for detection and quantification of coronary artery calcium as a marker of underlying cardiovascular disease. Coronary artery calcium has incremental value for risk prediction and, according to the 2018 update of the American Heart Association and American College of Cardiology guidelines, is recommended for as decision aid in patients with elevated risk for future cardiovascular events [11–15]. Coronary artery calcium can be obtained noninvasively from every ECG-gated non-contrast computed tomography exam of the heart with comparable low radiation dose [16, 17]. Once non-contrast ECG-gated CT imaging of the heart and major parts of the thorax is performed, information on cardiac and vascular structures other than the coronary arteries as well as thoracic fat tissues can be obtained from the same examination without any further radiation exposure or contrast administration. The quantification of other anatomic markers than coronary artery calcium then may help to further improve the risk assessment of asymptomatic patients and therefore may increase the prognostic value of this imaging tool.

In addition to non-contrast cardiac CT, magnetic resonance imaging [MRI] of the heart and contrast-enhanced coronary CT angiography have gained more influence on cardiovascular risk stratification, especially to define structural cardiac abnormalities and robust imaging of the coronary arteries [18]. Broad availability and technical improvements of MRI and CT scanners have led to a regular use of both diagnostic methods in clinical setup. Contrast-enhanced cardiac CT is predominantly used in symptomatic patient cohorts for evaluation of suspected coronary artery disease and can reliably be used for exclusion of disease because of its high negative predictive value in clinical routine [18].

As for non-contrast-enhanced cardiac CT, also coronary CT angiography allows for evaluation of other structures, providing information on EAT volume and attenuation without the need for addition radiation exposure or contrast media to the patient. Methods and potential consequences of fat quantification from cardiac CT will be discussed in this chapter.

CT Imaging for Quantification of Fat Depots

With advances in imaging modalities, regional fat depots including visceral abdominal fat and EAT have been identified as novel markers with implications for potential risk prediction. Several studies have highlighted EAT and visceral abdominal fat as unique, pathogenic fat depots [19–23]. Abdominal visceral abdominal fat is the largest visceral fat depot in the human body with more than ten times the volume of EAT [24]. It is significantly correlated to cardiovascular disease risk factors, the metabolic syndrome [24], and systemic markers of inflammation [25]. Therefore, visceral abdominal fat is hypothesized to have a systemic effect on atherosclerosis.

Within the thorax, the pericardial sac is the anatomical border between the epicardial and the extrapericardial adipose tissues. The potential impact of a variety of fat depots on cardiovascular disease manifestation has been described and investigated. While EAT is commonly defined as fat within the pericardial sac, extrapericardial adipose tissues are defined as fat outside the pericardial sac. For pericardial adipose tissue, various definitions are used in the literature. While some authors define it as fat inside the pericardial sac [equal to EAT], others also include fat adjacent to the outer layer of the pericardial fat [26, 27]. In addition, total thoracic adipose tissue is defined as all fat within the thorax [usually only from the pulmonary artery bifurcation to the apex], which includes epicardial and extrapericardial fat but also fat surrounding the aorta and other mediastinal structures.

In addition, more selective adipose tissues within the thorax have been described from CT imaging of the thorax. This includes periaortic fat, peri-coronary fat, peri-atrial fat, and others [28–30].

Requirements for CT Imaging

Generally, the requirements regarding CT imaging that allow for fat quantification are low. A large amount of available data arises from CT exams that were acquired from electron beam CT scanners [31–33]. Similarly, other population-based studies used such as the Framingham Heart Study or the Multi-Ethnic Study of Atherosclerosis used four-slice or eight-slice multi-detector CT scanners for assessment of EAT [34–36].

Non-contrast CT scans of the heart are predominantly performed for quantification of coronary artery calcification using the Agatston method [16]. As this requires a fixed tube voltage of 120 kV, this is found in the vast majority of publications using non-contrast CT. As for coronary CT angiography, tube voltage frequently varies by scanner type, the patient's habitus, and institutional preferences. Differences in tube voltage and likewise tube current affect CT attenuation of tissue including fat tissues. This does not relevantly affect EAT volume but has to be taken into account, when fixed thresholds for fat attenuation are used. In these cases, scanning parameters are commonly included as confounders into multivariable regression analyses [37].

Methods for Assessment of EAT from CT Imaging

Most available data are based on semiautomated quantification of EAT. Fat volume and attenuation is usually quantified offline from using a dedicated workstation [38, 39]. EAT volume can be assessed by manual tracing of the pericardial sac as outer border in axial planes from the right pulmonary artery to the apex of the heart as region of interest [38, 39] (Fig. 6.1). Some investigations additionally define upper and lower limits of the pericardial sac as the bifurcation of the pulmonary trunk and the slice caudal to the posterior descending artery [40].

Within the manually traced region of interest, pixels accounted as fat (based on a predefined Hounsfield unit window) are summed for assessment of three-dimensional volume. The Hounsfield unit window used as definition of fat slightly varies in the literature. Generally, for non-contrast CT a slightly lower Hounsfield unit window is used. Table 6.1 [26, 31, 34, 37, 38, 41–44] gives an overview over selective studies and Hounsfield unit window used for definition of fat.

Another key advantage of CT-based quantification of three-dimensional quantification of thoracic fat depots is its very high reproducibility. An intraclass correlation coefficient of >0.9 was

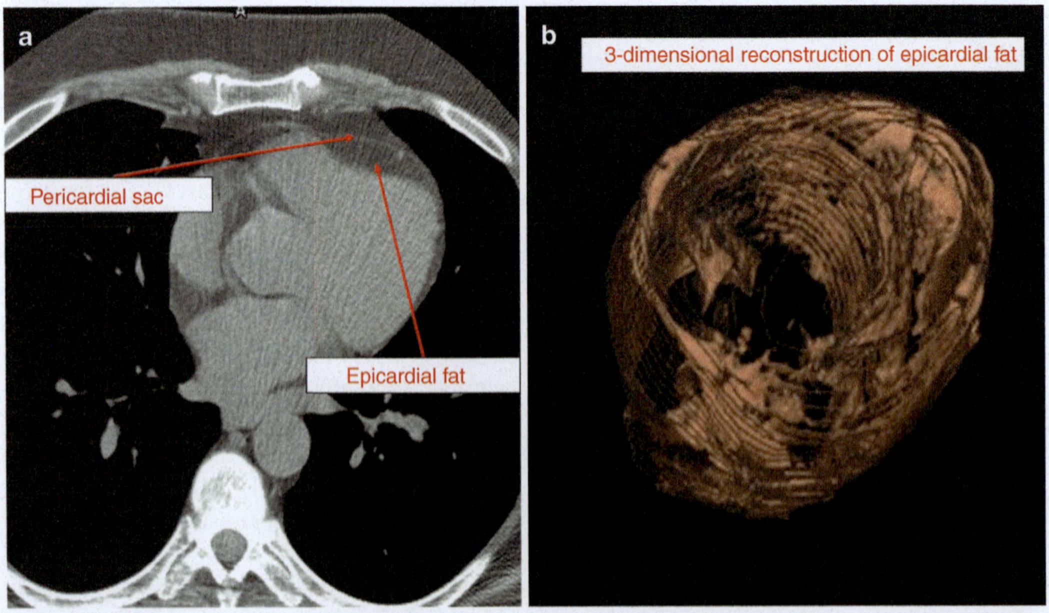

Fig. 6.1 Epicardial fat quantification from cardiac CT examination from non-contrast cardiac CT. (**a**) The pericardial sac is usually manual traced in axial images as region of interest. Within this region of interest, pixels according to a predefined Hounsfield unit range are accounted as fat. After three-dimensional reconstruction, epicardial adipose tissue volume is calculated by summation of all pixels accounted as fat. (**b**) Three-dimensional reconstruction of epicardial fat by summation of all pixels within the region of interest, accounted as fat [38, 39]. Quantification of epicardial fat from contrast-enhanced cardiac CT can be performed in similar fashion

Table 6.1 Hounsfield unit window for definition of fat in CT imaging of the heart

Study	CT imaging	HU window	Fat depot
Rosito et al. [26]	Non-contrast	−195 to −45	Pericardial fat
Ding et al. [34]	Non-contrast	−190 to −30	Pericardial fat
Mahabadi et al. [31]	Non-contrast	−195 to −45	Epicardial fat
Nichols et al. [41]	Contrast enhanced	−190 to −30	Pericardial fat
Hell et al. [42]	Contrast enhanced	−190 to −30	Epicardial fat
Schlett et al. [43]	Contrast enhanced	−190 to −30	Periaortic fat
Balcer et al. [38]	Non-contrast	−195 to −45	Peri-coronary fat
Oikonomou et al. [37]	Contrast enhanced	−190 to −30	Peri-coronary fat
Maurovich-Horvat et al. [44]	Contrast enhanced	−149 to −30	Epicardial, peri-coronary, and periaortic fat

reported in different cohorts, independent of adipose tissue evaluated and scanning characteristics [e.g., contrast enhanced vs. non-contrast]. This very low variability makes CT-derived assessment of thoracic fat depot robust and reliable measures in research and clinical practice. In addition, quantification of EAT volume from cardiac CT is less dependent of image quality as, for example, coronary anatomy. Therefore, only very few exclusion criteria apply for assessment of EAT in most studies, with previous open-heart surgery being the most commonly reason for exclusion.

In addition to semiautomated measures of epicardial and thoracic adipose tissue volumes by manual delineation of the pericardial sac in axial images, also fully automated measures have been described. Using a deep learning algorithm, Commandeur and colleagues found that automated assessment of EAT volume and attenuation is feasible within seconds using on a standard personal computer with good agreement to manual measures [45]. Further studies are needed to link these measures with predictive models.

With the use of CT imaging, radiation exposure is frequently of concern. However, with modern scanners, effective doses of 1 mSv and below can routinely be achieved, which is similar to the dose of a clinical mammogram [46]. Modern dose reduction protocols have the ability to further relevantly reduce radiation exposure of CAC scoring scans, which may ultimately relativize this concern [47].

Reference Values for CT-Derived EAT

Investigators from the Framingham Heart Study defined reference values for epicardial and extrapericardial fat in a healthy reference sample of the Offspring and Third Generation cohort [48]. They found that men had slightly higher EAT volume as compared to women, while extrapericardial fat volume was relevantly higher in men as compared to women. In addition, both fat depots relevantly increased with increasing age group, independent of gender. The investigators defined a fat volume >90th age- and gender-specific percentile in the healthy reference sample as high fat volume. In the overall cohort, 25–35% had a fat volume above this threshold, which was associated with higher body mass index and higher prevalence of metabolic syndrome [48]. However, the reference values for thoracic fat depots as described by Framingham investigators may not apply for other cohorts. With a mean EAT volume of >100 ml, they observed higher values as, e.g., for the European population-based Heinz Nixdorf Recall study cohort, for which a mean EAT volume of 85.9 ml has been observed [31]. While ethnical differences may impact overall amount of EAT volume, investigators from the Multi-Ethnic Study of Atherosclerosis found that its relationship with coronary atherosclerosis did not differ by ethnicity [35].

CT-Derived EAT and Cardiovascular Risk Factors

In the well-defined cohort of the Framingham Heart Study, investigators evaluated the association of CT-derived EAT and total thoracic volume with traditional risk factors [26]. They found that both fat depots were associated with other measures of obesity, including body mass index and waist circumference. For visceral adipose tissue volume, a strong correlation of epicardial and total thoracic fat was observed. In addition, EAT was positively linked to systolic blood pressure, blood glucose levels, and triglycerides, while a negative correlation was found with HDL cholesterol. Overall, associations were found to be stronger for women as compared to men. Within each tertile of visceral adipose tissue, the tertile of EAT further stratified the incidence of hypertension and impaired fasting glucose in women as well as metabolic syndrome in men [26]. In the European Heinz Nixdorf Recall study, CT-derived EAT was found to be significantly associated with age, gender, waist circumference, antihypertensive medication use, LDL and HDL cholesterol, diabetes, and smoking status in multivariable regression analysis [31]. Of all investigated traditional cardiovascular risk factors, systolic blood pressure and lipid-lowering therapy were the only factors without significant association in multivariable regression analysis. Unlike in the Framingham Heart Study, in this population-based cohort no relevant interaction with gender was observed. Interestingly, despite the lack in association between lipid-lowering therapy and EAT, investigators from the randomized controlled BELLES trial found that intensified as compared to moderate lipid-lowering therapy [atorvastatin 80 mg vs. pravastatin 40 mg] was associated with EAT volume regression. The effect of therapy regime on change in fat volume was present irrespective of changes in LDL cholesterol [49].

CT-Derived EAT and Markers of Subclinical Atherosclerosis

Multiple studies evaluated the link of epicardial and extrapericardial fat depots with markers of atherosclerosis. In the Offspring cohort of the Framingham Heart Study, Rosito and colleagues observed a link of epicardial and total thoracic fat volume with both coronary and aortic calcification when controlling for age and gender [26]. Interestingly, this effect was further strengthened when ancillary adjusting for visceral adipose tissue volume. In contrast, when only adjusting for traditional risk factors, no significant association of both thoracic fat depots with coronary and aortic calcification was observed. But again, the effect sizes were strengthened upon ancillary adjustment for visceral adipose tissue, observing a significant association of EAT volume with coronary artery calcification as well as a significant association of total thoracic fat volume with aortic calcification [26]. This observation supported the hypothesis of a local role of visceral adipose tissues on atherosclerosis development in the underlying vasculature. In a subset of the Multi-Ethnic Study of Atherosclerosis (MESA), one standard deviation increase in pericardial fat was associated with nearly twofold odds of calcified coronary plaque [35]. The significant association remained upon further adjustment of other cardiovascular factors and did not differ by gender and ethnicity. On the other hand, body mass index and height-adjusted waist circumference were not associated with calcified coronary plaque, suggesting that local EAT volume is a stronger predictor of coronary atherosclerosis than general measures of adiposity [35]. In the European Heinz Nixdorf Recall study, the association of CT-derived EAT volume with coronary artery calcification was no longer present when adjusting for traditional risk factors, suggesting that the link of EAT with calcified coronary plaques is ultimately explained by shared risk factors [31]. In a cross-sectional analysis of 120 patients undergoing contrast-enhanced CT angiography, pericardial fat volume was found to be associated with overall plaque burden [50]. Interestingly, pericardial fat volume was comparable in patients with predominantly calcified and with predominantly noncalcified plaque burden. In this study, addition of pericardial fat volume to Framingham risk score relevantly improved the prediction of coronary plaque. In the prospectively enrolled ROMICAT study of patients undergoing CT angiography for acute chest pain, EAT volume was not only higher in patients with plaque burden as compared to patients without detection of coronary plaque. In patients with high-risk plaque characteristics [defined as >50 luminal narrowing and positive remodeling, low attenuation plaque, or spotty calcification], even higher EAT volumes were observed [43]. In longitudinal analysis with serial non-contrast CT imaging, EAT volume was found to be significantly associated with progression of coronary artery calcification [33]. This effect was more pronounced in subjects <55 years of age and in subjects with low calcium scores at baseline examination, suggesting that the impact of EAT on plaque development is more pronounced in the early phase of atherosclerosis. Likewise, EAT was only relevantly associated with onset of calcification (coronary artery calcification score of zero at baseline and greater zero after 5 years) in the age group of <55 years [33].

CT-Derived EAT Volume and Atherosclerotic Disease Manifestation

Patient-based studies with cross-sectional design provided the first reports of an association between EAT and prevalent cardiovascular disease. In 2001, Taguchi et al. described an increased EAT volume determined by cardiac computed tomography in subjects with coronary artery disease compared to those without coronary disease in a Japanese patient cohort [51]. These results were confirmed in a population-based sample when investigators from the Framingham Heart Study described increased EAT volumes in subjects with prevalent coronary artery disease in a cross-sectional analysis in 1267 subjects from the Offspring cohort. In contrast to EAT, intrathoracic fat, as fat depot inside the thorax but outside the pericardial sac, showed no association with cardiac events. In this study, the association with coronary artery disease was independent of age and gender as well as body mass index and waist circumference, but no longer reached statistical significance when further adjusting for traditional cardiovascular risk factors [27]. Interestingly, a more pronounced link of EAT with coronary heart disease and myocardial infarction was observed, while only visceral abdominal adipose tissue volume as largest visceral fat depot of the human body was associated with stroke. This finding further supported the hypothesis of a local effect of EAT on coronary artery disease development, which ultimately overruled the systemic effect of visceral abdominal fat in this analysis. In a case-controlled subset of the Multi-Ethnic Study of Atherosclerosis, one standard deviation increase in pericardial fat was associated with 30% higher odds of developing incident coronary heart disease, while no relevant link was observed with body mass index [34]. Effect sizes for pericardial fat remained stable upon adjustment for traditional risk factors. In a population-based cohort study, Mahabadi et al. first investigated the association of CT-derived EAT volume with incident myocardial infarction with more than 32.000 patient years of follow-up [31]. In this analysis, incidence of myocardial infarction increased fivefold from 1st to 4th quartile of EAT volume. In log transformed Cox regression analysis, doubling of EAT volume was associated with 50% increased risk of incident myocardial infarction. Effect sizes were stronger for women as compared to men, which was in major parts explained by a more pronounced effect in subjects with less coronary artery calcium score (<100). This finding suggested that EAT may impact coronary artery disease development in early stages and its assessment may be of greatest value in patients with only low detection of subclinical atherosclerosis. In an observational study of 843 consecutive HIV-infected patients receiving antiretroviral therapy for at least 6 months, Raggi and colleagues investigated the complemental value of EAT and coronary artery calcification score for prediction of myocardial infarction and all-cause mortality [52]. They found that both CT-derived measures [EAT within upper tertile and coronary artery calcification score >100] independently predicted a combined endpoint of myocardial infarction and death. Likewise, in an Asian cohort of patients without known coronary artery disease undergoing coronary CT angiography, Kunita and colleagues found that the combination of EAT volume above the median and coronary artery calcification score >100 together significantly improved prediction in Cox regression analysis [53]. When investigating the link of EAT volume for prediction of coronary events with other noncoronary measures derived from non-contrast cardiac CT, EAT volume in the model together with left ventricular and left atrial axial area index, ascending and descending aortic diameters, as well as aortic valve, mitral ring, and thoracic aortic calcification remained independently associated with a combined endpoint of myocardial infarction, stroke, and cardiovascular death [32]. Of all included noncoronary measures, only left atrial size index, EAT volume, and thoracic aortic calcification from non-contrast-enhanced cardiac CT improve the prediction of incident hard cardiovascular events above CAC and established risk factors, indicating that quantification of these noncoronary measures may improve the prognostic value of this imaging technology.

However, despite the overwhelming evidence of a strong association of CT-derived EAT volume with prevalent and incident coronary artery disease manifestation, its assessment is not included into daily clinical routine. Further studies are needed to investigate how assessment of EAT directly impacts patient outcome and can alter patient management.

CT-Derived EAT and Non-atherosclerotic Cardiac Diseases

Besides the association of thoracic adipose tissues with coronary atherosclerosis, also a link of CT-derived EAT with noncoronary heart disease has been described in many studies. For development of atrial fibrillation, a role of EAT was described, which was suggested to be mediated by the inflammatory effects of EAT. Al Chekakie et al. reported higher EAT volume in subjects with atrial fibrillation compared to subjects with sinus rhythm [30]. In this study, subjects with persistent atrial fibrillation had even higher fat volume than subjects with paroxysmal atrial fibrillation. As a local effect of adipose tissue on atrial fibrillation was suggested, Wong et al. quantified peri-atrial, periventricular, and total EAT volume in 110 patients undergoing first-time ablation of atrial fibrillation compared to 20 controls in sinus rhythm [54]. They found a significant association between overall EAT volume as well as peri-atrial and periventricular fat with left atrial volumes, the presence and severity of atrial fibrillation, and poorer outcome after ablation. When comparing total EAT volume with peri-atrial fat volume, similar effects were described for atrial fibrillation burden and chronicity. Framingham investigators also reported an association of EAT with atrial fibrillation, independent of age, gender, hypertension, and body mass index in over 3000 subjects in cross-sectional analysis [55]. Furthermore, a significant correlation between EAT and left atrial dimension is described, which by itself is a strong predictor of atrial fibrillation [36]. In the Heinz Nixdorf Recall study, the link between EAT and atrial fibrillation was ultimately attenuated, when left atrial size was added to the model, whereas the association of left atrial size with atrial fibrillation was independent of the amount of fat [56]. However, longitudinal analyses are needed to establish a pathophysiological mechanism of EAT and incidence of atrial fibrillation.

Moreover, a link of EAT with left ventricular function via a lipotoxic mechanism has been suggested in the literature [57]. However, an analysis based on participants from the Framingham Heart Study could not confirm a correlation of EAT volume with left ventricular structure or function, independent of effects from general adiposity [36]. In a study on 110 patients from a health screening program without known coronary artery disease, Cavalcante et al. described a significant correlation of EAT with e′ and E/e′ as well as to left atrial size, suggesting that EAT may be associated with diastolic dysfunction [58]. These results confirm data from Iacobellis et al., showing that increase in EAT thickness is significantly correlated with atrial enlargement and impairment in diastolic filling in morbidly obese subjects [59]. Likewise, a strong association of EAT thickness with aortic valve stenosis was recently described, again suggesting a local role via promotion of inflammation [60]. Further studies are needed to confirm these results and to establish potential mechanisms for the link of EAT with measures of left ventricular size and function.

CT-Derived EAT Attenuation: A Novel and Complemental Risk Marker?

In addition to volume, CT-derived fat attenuation is suggested to reflect unfavorable metabolic activity, as it increases with vascularization, reflects higher concentration of mitochondria, and is correlated with local and systemic inflammatory markers [61–63].

Mahabadi et al. evaluated the additive value of EAT volume and attenuation in a cohort of patients with myocardial infarction. In patients with any myocardial infarction compared to stable coronary artery disease, epicardial volume was slightly higher. In addition, EAT attenuation was significantly different between both groups. Likewise, patients with type-I myocardial infarction had higher EAT attenuation and a tendency toward higher fat volume than subjects without type-I myocardial infarction. In logistic regression analysis, they observed positive associations of EAT volume with any myocardial infarction and type-I myocardial infarction in varying adjustment sets. However, despite stable effect sizes, no significant associations were observed in fully adjusted models. Likewise, also EAT attenuation was positively associated with any and type-I myocardial infarction, independently of EAT volume. In contrast to EAT volume. For fat attenuation, association with any and type-I myocardial infarction remained stable and statistically significant upon adjustment for risk factors. Interestingly, both EAT volume and attenuation were associated with myocardial infarction when adjusting for each other. To further evaluate the potential complementary value of EAT volume and attenuation, they assessed the frequencies of acute coronary syndromes in the investigated cohort stratified by EAT volume and attenuation below vs. above the median. Lowest frequencies of myocardial infarctions were observed for patients with EAT volume and attenuation below their median. Patients with diverse EAT profiles showed comparable frequencies of myocardial infarction. The highest frequencies of myocardial infarction were observed for patients with both EAT volume and attenuation above their median [39]. In the population of the EISNER study, Goeller et al. investigated the association of EAT volume and density, assessed by non-contrast-enhanced cardiac CT, with coronary artery calcification, markers of systemic inflammation, and major adverse cardiac events in asymptomatic patients [64]. They found that EAT volume was higher and fat attenuation was lower in patients with coronary atherosclerosis detection. Likewise, fat volume was positively linked with levels of PAI-1 and MCP-1 and inversely related to adiponectin and HDL cholesterol. In contrast, EAT density was inversely related to PAI-1 and LDL cholesterol and positively associated to adiponectin, sICAM-1, and HDL cholesterol. While both EAT volume and density were associated with major adverse cardiovascular events in univariate analysis, in multivariate analysis only for fat density a statistically significant association remained.

However, when EAT attenuation is assessed, methods of CT imaging have to be taken into account as scanning parameters including tube current and tube voltage and most importantly the use of contrast media relevantly impact the fat attenuation. Therefore, comparability between studies may be limited due to differences in scanning protocols.

CT-Derived Perivascular Fat Assessment and Its Implications

Following the hypothesis of a local influence of visceral adipose tissue with atherosclerosis development in the underlying vasculature, researchers started investigating the link of local peri-coronary fat depots with disease manifestation in the underlying segment. In this context, peri-coronary adipose tissue as part of the overall EATs is defined as any fat located within the pericardial sac directly surrounding the coronary arteries without any further anatomical landmarks or borders. In the literature, several anatomical definitions of peri-coronary fat have been used, including any fat until the myocardium, pericardial sac, or other coronary arteries, a radial distance from the outer vessel wall equal to the diameter of the vessel, or a maximum radius of 3 mm from the coronary artery [65–67]. Evaluating the link between the amount of local peri-coronary fat volume with the presence of plaque burden in the underlying coronary artery segment, Mahabadi et al. evaluated 311 coronary segments from contrast-enhanced coronary CT angiography [67]. They observed that per each doubling of peri-coronary fat volume, the odds for presence of plaque in the underlying coronary segment was 2.5. Associations remained statistically significant with stable effect sizes after adjustment for traditional cardiovascular risk factors and when additionally accounting for overall EAT volume. Interestingly, the effect did not differ by coronary artery segment and was not related to type of plaque [calcified or noncalcified].

In a post hoc analysis of the randomized controlled BELLES trial, the investigators found that statin therapy was associated with a decrease in peri-coronary fat attenuation [68]. The change of fat attenuation was independent of total cholesterol, low-density lipoprotein cholesterol, coronary artery calcium, and EAT volume. In contrast to EAT, the attenuation of subcutaneous fat was not impacted by statin therapy [68].

In a subset of a population-based cohort of more than 4000 subjects, Mahabadi et al. evaluated the CT-derived peri-coronary fat area of patients developing incident nonfatal myocardial infarction during 8 years of follow-up. They found that coronary arteries that developed a culprit lesion during follow-up causing a coronary event had significantly higher peri-coronary fat area at baseline as compared to coronary arteries without consecutive culprit lesion in the same patient [31].

Overall, the assessment of regional peri-coronary adipose tissue volume and attenuation can be performed differently and different methods have been described in the literature. For instance, the evaluation of Balcer et al. was based on manual delineation of regions of interest of a coronary segmentation model divided in seven coronary segments in axial planes according to the Society of Coronary Computed Tomography (SCCT): left main = 5 mm

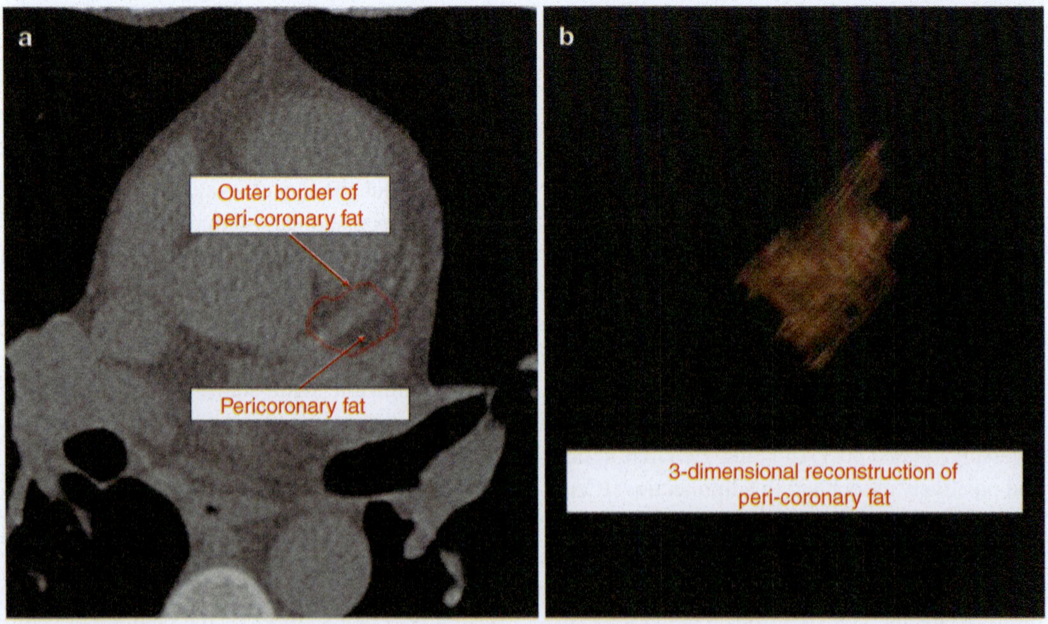

Fig. 6.2 Peri-coronary fat as quantified from non-contrast cardiac CT exams. For quantification of peri-coronary fat here, for example, the peri-coronary adipose tissue around the proximal LAD is manually traced as region of interest. (**a**) Within this region of interest, pixels between −195 and −45 Hounsfield units are accounted as fat. (**b**) After three-dimensional reconstruction, peri-coronary fat volume is calculated by summation of all pixels accounted as fat. Peri-coronary adipose tissue attenuation is defined as mean Hounsfield units of all fat pixels of the epicardial adipose tissue volume

proximal to bifurcation, proximal LAD = 5 mm distal from bifurcation, mid LAD = 5 mm distal from origin of the first diagonal branch, proximal LCX = 5 mm distal from bifurcation, mid/distal LCX = 5 mm distal from origin of the first obtuse marginal branch, proximal RCA = 5 mm distal from the ostium, and mid RCA = in the middle of the descending part of the RCA (Fig. 6.2) [38, 69].

Contrary to that, Hell et al. used a different method. Attenuation analysis of peri-coronary fat was performed in perpendicular cross-sectional images using multiplanar reformatted CT angiography images orthogonal to the specified coronary artery longitudinal axis on a dedicated off-line workstation. Furthermore, a predefined image display setting (window 450 Hounsfield units, level 50 Hounsfield units) was applied to manually circle the outer vessel contour. Peri-coronary adipose tissue density was measured in circular regions of interest with a radius of 0.25, 0.5, 0.75, 1.0, and 1.25 cm from the outer vessel border [40].

Marwan et al. evaluated data sets of patients who were referred for invasive coronary angiography and in whom intravascular ultrasound of a coronary vessel was performed for clinical reasons. They identified sixty corresponding coronary artery segments in 29 patients within the coronary artery system in both dual source computed tomography and intravascular ultrasound using bifurcation points as fiducial markers. Coronary segments with lipid-rich plaque, fibrous plaque, and normal coronary segments were identified in CT angiography data sets and intravascular ultrasound according to fiducial markers. CT attenuation of peri-coronary adipose tissue for segments with any coronary atherosclerotic plaque was significantly higher as compared to segments without plaque. When comparing mean density of peri-coronary fat surrounding proximal, mid, and distal segments, significantly highest density was observed in proximal segments, followed by mid and distal segments [65].

In addition, the study detected a significantly lower peri-coronary adipose tissue attenuation for normal versus atherosclerotic coronary segments [65], in contrast to Balcer et al., where no correlation between peri-coronary fat attenuation and culprit lesions was described.

In terms of reference values for peri-coronary fat volume and attenuation, it has to be taken into account that its amount varies between different locations of the coronary artery tree. In a recent analysis on patients presenting with acute coronary syndrome, highest peri-coronary adipose tissue volume was observed in proximal right coronary artery, followed by the middle segment of the right coronary artery. Overall, peri-coronary fat volume was found to be significantly higher in RCA than in the other coronary arteries. In contrast, local fat volume was not significantly different among left main, left anterior descending, and left circumflex coronary artery. For the left anterior descending coronary artery, peri-coronary fat volume was significantly higher in segments with culprit lesions, than peri-coronary fat volume for all left anterior descending coronary segments without culprit lesions [38]. Likewise, Balcer et al. observed a trend toward higher peri-coronary fat volume surrounding culprit lesions in the right coronary artery compared to segments in this vessel without culprit lesions, but not reaching statistical significance. Lowest fat attenuation was detected in mid left anterior descending and highest fat attenuation in left main. Overall, peri-coronary fat attenuation was lower in distal segments compared to proximal segments [38]. When interpreting the present results with respect to local differences in peri-coronary fat volume and attenuation, it has to be taken into account that in this analysis most culprit lesions were in the right coronary artery, while according to larger studies, coronary atherosclerosis most frequently occurs in the proximal left anterior descending [70–72]. A study published by Khawaja et al. investigated global and regional EAT volume by determination of the specific amount of perivascular EAT adjacent to each major coronary artery and especially the direct proximity to the coronary arteries. They suggest that regional alterations in EAT may play an important role in the pathogenesis of myocardial ischemia. They found a regional specific adipose tissue distribution with higher EAT volume around the right and left anterior descending coronary artery compared to the left circumflex artery [73].

Following the hypothesis that local peri-coronary fat attenuation as measure of coronary inflammation is linked with coronary artery disease manifestation, Antonopoulos et al. described a method of peri-coronary fat attenuation assessment [66]. They found that inflamed human vessels release cytokines that prevent lipid accumulation in perivascular fat-derived preadipocytes in vitro, ex vivo, and in vivo and validated a three-dimensional analysis method using CT images of human adipose tissue explants from 453 patients undergoing cardiac surgery, relating the ex vivo images with in vivo CT scan information on the biology of the explants. This measure of local perivascular fat attenuation had high sensitivity and specificity for detecting tissue inflammation as assessed by tissue uptake of 18F-fluorodeoxyglucose in positron emission tomography. In addition, in a validation cohort, the fat attenuation around human coronary arteries identified early subclinical coronary artery disease in vivo, as well as detected dynamic changes of peri-coronary adipose tissue in response to variations of vascular inflammation, and inflamed, vulnerable atherosclerotic plaques during acute coronary syndromes. Consecutively, this group evaluated the association of peri-coronary fat attenuation with incidence of all-cause and coronary mortality in two large prospective studies using coronary CT angiography [37]. In the derivation cohort, they first observed that peri-coronary fat attenuation values around the proximal right coronary artery and left anterior descending artery [but not around the left circumflex artery] were predictive of all-cause and cardiac mortality and correlated strongly with each other. They consecutively used the perivascular fat attenuation measured around the right coronary artery as a representative biomarker of global coronary inflammation and found a strong association with cardiac mortality in Cox regression analysis in the derivation cohort and in the validation cohort. Further, they defined optimum cutoff for the perivascular fat attenuation of −70.1 Hounsfield units [HU] or higher in the derivation cohort. This cutoff value was applied in the validation cohort and provided improved prediction of cardiac and all-cause mortality in addition to traditional cardiovascular risk factors, coronary artery calcification score, overall EAT volume, and high-risk plaque characteristics [37].

Machine learning algorithms are now on the horizon [74], which may further evaluate characteristics that have not been determined so far. This may in addition enhance the prognostic value of fat quantification form cardiac CT via imaging of the residual inflammatory cardiovascular risk.

Periaortic Fat

Besides peri-coronary fat, also the fat depot adjacent to the thoracic and abdominal aorta has been investigated as potential risk marker of aortic atherosclerosis. Both thoracic and abdominal periaortic fat depots can be quantified with high reproducibility using CT imaging and show high correlation with visceral abdominal fat, waist circumference, and body mass index [28]. In the Offspring cohort of the Framingham Heart Study, Lehmann et al. examined associations between adipose tissue depots immediately surrounding the thoracic aorta, metabolic risk factors, and vascular calcification [75]. In this cross-sectional analysis including over 1.000 participants free of cardiovascular disease, they found that periaortic fat volume was associated with traditional risk factors including body mass index, waist circumference, visceral abdominal fat volume, hypertension, low HDL cholesterol, serum triglyceride levels, impaired fasting glucose, and presence of diabetes. These associations remained significant after adjustment for body mass index and waist circumference but were attenuated after adjustment for visceral abdominal fat. When comparing periaortic fat with aortic calcification, they found that thoracic aortic fat was associated with thoracic calcification even after adjustment for visceral adipose tissue but effect sizes were attenuated after adjustment for traditional cardiovascular risk factors. In contrast, thoracic aortic fat was associated with abdominal aortic calcification and coronary artery calcification even in models including risk factors and visceral adiposity [75].

Future Perspective

To date, quantification of EAT volume and attenuation as well as peri-coronary fat assessment is not routinely performed in clinical practice. One of the key reasons is the relatively time-consuming manual delineation of the pericardial sac as region of interest in axial images. However, with recently described machine learning approaches for quantification of both epicardial and peri-coronary fat, this obstacle may not be relevant in the future [45, 66]. Currently, non-contrast cardiac CT is routinely performed for risk stratification in primary prevention to quantify coronary artery calcification score as an imaging-based test of subclinical atherosclerosis [12]. In contrast, coronary CT angiography is suggested for symptomatic patients with a low to intermediate pretest likelihood, allowing exclusion of coronary artery disease due to its high negative predictive value [76]. Assessment of peri-coronary fat attenuation as measure of coronary inflammation represents a novel aspect in the evaluation of coronary CT angiography. It improves prediction, discrimination, and reclassification of all-cause and cardiac mortality. These results are in line with findings of other measures from contrast-enhanced cardiac CT such as severity of coronary artery disease and high-risk plaque characteristics to predict future events [77, 78]. When combining epicardial as well as peri-coronary fat volume and attenuation with information on the extent of plaque burden and plaque composition, coronary CT angiography has the potential to allow for a more accurate risk prediction compared to the Agatston score as assessed by non-contrast CT [79]. Therefore, the routine assessment of thoracic fat depots may lead toward extended indications for coronary CT angiography to prevention cohorts.

Conclusion

EAT is a visceral adipose tissue, directly surrounding the heart. It is located within the pericardial sac, which is the anatomical border from extrapericardial fat. The term pericardial fat is frequently defined as the combination of epicardial and extrapericardial adipose tissue, while some researches use it as synonymic for EAT. With its ability of three-dimensional imaging of the heart and the surrounding structures with isometric voxels, cardiac CT allows for reliable assessment of various thoracic fat depots including EAT. Over the last two decades, there has been growing evidence from patient-centered and population-based cohort studies that CT-derived EAT volume is associated with traditional cardiovascular risk factors and markers of coronary artery plaque burden. In addition, existing literature suggests a robust impact of EAT volume on cardiovascular disease manifestation in cross-sectional and longitudinal analyses. In addition to overall fat volume, its CT-derived attenuation via quantification of mean Hounsfield units of the fat depot has gained interest, as it reflects metabolic and most importantly inflammatory activity. Available data suggests that assessment of EAT attenuation provides complemental information to fat volume with regard to prediction of cardiovascular diseases and therefore may enhance the value of quantification of EAT from cardiac CT imaging. Besides overall EAT volume, local perivascular visceral fat depots such as peri-coronary fat have increasingly been described in the recent literature. Available data suggests that the volume and attenuation of local peri-vascular fat may be a more robust measure of risk, supporting the hypothesis of a paracrine effect of metabolites, secreted by EAT, on the development of atherosclerosis in the adjacent vasculature. With the advent of machine learning-based algorithms that allow for automated assessment of epicardial and peri-coronary fat volume as well as fat attenuation within seconds, these CT-derived measures of thoracic fat may play a more prominent role in clinical routine in the near future.

References

1. Kannel WB, Dawber TR, Kagan A, Revotskie N, Stokes J 3rd. Factors of risk in the development of coronary heart disease--six year follow-up experience. The Framingham Study. Ann Intern Med. 1961;55:33–50.
2. Ford I, Murray H, Packard CJ, Shepherd J, Macfarlane PW, Cobbe SM. Long-term follow-up of the West of Scotland Coronary Prevention Study. N Engl J Med. 2007;357:1477–86.
3. Shah T, Swerdlow D. Detecting, predicting and modifying cardiovascular risk: new and developing strategies. Expert Rev Cardiovasc Ther. 2010;8:1519–21.
4. Pencina MJ, D'Agostino RB Sr, Larson MG, Massaro JM, Vasan RS. Predicting the 30-year risk of cardiovascular disease: the Framingham Heart Study. Circulation. 2009;119:3078–84.
5. Ajani UA, Ford ES. Has the risk for coronary heart disease changed among U.S. adults? J Am Coll Cardiol. 2006;48:1177–82.
6. Akosah KO, Schaper A, Cogbill C, Schoenfeld P. Preventing myocardial infarction in the young adult in the first place: how do the National Cholesterol Education Panel III guidelines perform? J Am Coll Cardiol. 2003;41:1475–9.
7. Brindle P, Emberson J, Lampe F, Walker M, Whincup P, Fahey T, et al. Predictive accuracy of the Framingham coronary risk score in British men: prospective cohort study. BMJ. 2003;327:1267.
8. Möhlenkamp S, Böse D, Mahabadi AA, Heusch G, Erbel R. On the paradox of exercise: coronary atherosclerosis in an apparently healthy marathon runner. Nat Clin Pract Cardiovasc Med. 2007;4:396–401.
9. de Las Heras Gala T, Geisel MH, Peters A, Thorand B, Baumert J, Lehmann N, et al. Recalibration of the ACC/AHA Risk Score in two population-based German cohorts. PLoS One. 2016;11:e0164688.
10. Piepoli MF, Hoes AW, Agewall S, Albus C, Brotons C, Catapano AL, et al. 2016 European guidelines on cardiovascular disease prevention in clinical practice: the Sixth Joint Task Force of the European Society of Cardiology and Other Societies on Cardiovascular Disease Prevention in Clinical Practice (constituted by representatives of 10 societies and by invited experts) Developed with the special contribution of the European Association for Cardiovascular Prevention & Rehabilitation (EACPR). Eur Heart J. 2016;37:2315–81.
11. Grundy SM, Stone NJ, Bailey AL, Beam C, Birtcher KK, Blumenthal RS, et al. AHA/ACC/AACVPR/AAPA/ABC/ACPM/ADA/AGS/APhA/ASPC/NLA/PCNA guideline on the management of blood

cholesterol: a report of the American College of Cardiology/American Heart Association Task Force on Clinical Practice Guidelines. J Am Coll Cardiol. 2018;73:e285–350. Erratum in: J Am Coll Cardiol. 2019;73:3237–3241

12. Detrano R, Guerci AD, Carr JJ, Bild DE, Burke G, Folsom AR, et al. Coronary calcium as a predictor of coronary events in four racial or ethnic groups. N Engl J Med. 2008;358:1336–45.
13. Erbel R, Möhlenkamp S, Moebus S, Schmermund A, Lehmann N, Stang A, et al. Coronary risk stratification, discrimination, and reclassification improvement based on quantification of subclinical coronary atherosclerosis: the Heinz Nixdorf Recall study. J Am Coll Cardiol. 2010;56:1397–406.
14. Greenland P, Bonow RO, Brundage BH, Budoff MJ, Eisenberg MJ, Grundy SM, et al. ACCF/AHA 2007 clinical expert consensus document on coronary artery calcium scoring by computed tomography in global cardiovascular risk assessment and in evaluation of patients with chest pain: a report of the American College of Cardiology Foundation Clinical Expert Consensus Task Force (ACCF/AHA Writing Committee to Update the 2000 Expert Consensus Document on Electron Beam Computed Tomography) developed in collaboration with the Society of Atherosclerosis Imaging and Prevention and the Society of Cardiovascular Computed Tomography. J Am Coll Cardiol. 2007;49:378–402.
15. Mahabadi AA, Nasir K, Rassaf T. Routine CAC-scoring prior to initiation of statin therapy – a European perspective. Eur J Prev Cardiol. 2019;26:1559–61.
16. Agatston AS, Janowitz WR, Hildner FJ, Zusmer NR, Viamonte M Jr, Detrano R. Quantification of coronary artery calcium using ultrafast computed tomography. J Am Coll Cardiol. 1990;15:827–32.
17. Mahabadi AA, Möhlenkamp S, Moebus S, Dragano N, Kalsch H, Bauer M, et al. The Heinz Nixdorf Recall study and its potential impact on the adoption of atherosclerosis imaging in European primary prevention guidelines. Curr Artheroscler Rep. 2011;13: 367–72.
18. Montalescot G, Sechtem U, Achenbach S, Andreotti F, Arden C, Budaj A, et al. 2013 ESC guidelines on the management of stable coronary artery disease: the Task Force on the management of stable coronary artery disease of the European Society of Cardiology. Eur Heart J. 2013;34:2949–3003.
19. Baker AR, Silva NF, Quinn DW, Harte AL, Pagano D, Bonser RS, et al. Human epicardial adipose tissue expresses a pathogenic profile of adipocytokines in patients with cardiovascular disease. Cardiovasc Diabetol. 2006;5:1.
20. Laine P, Kaartinen M, Penttila A, Panula P, Paavonen T, Kovanen PT. Association between myocardial infarction and the mast cells in the adventitia of the infarct-related coronary artery. Circulation. 1999;99:361–9.
21. Mazurek T, Zhang L, Zalewski A, Mannion JD, Diehl JT, Arafat H, et al. Human epicardial adipose tissue is a source of inflammatory mediators. Circulation. 2003;108:2460–6.
22. Ouchi N, Kihara S, Arita Y, Okamoto Y, Maeda K, Kuriyama H, et al. Adiponectin, an adipocyte-derived plasma protein, inhibits endothelial NF-kappaB signaling through a cAMP-dependent pathway. Circulation. 2000;102:1296–301.
23. Ouchi N, Kihara S, Funahashi T, Nakamura T, Nishida M, Kumada M, et al. Reciprocal association of C-reactive protein with adiponectin in blood stream and adipose tissue. Circulation. 2003;107:671–4.
24. Fox CS, Massaro JM, Hoffmann U, Pou KM, Maurovich-Horvat P, Liu CY, et al. Abdominal visceral and subcutaneous adipose tissue compartments: association with metabolic risk factors in the Framingham Heart Study. Circulation. 2007;116:39–48.
25. Pou KM, Massaro JM, Hoffmann U, Vasan RS, Maurovich-Horvat P, Larson MG, et al. Visceral and subcutaneous adipose tissue volumes are cross-sectionally related to markers of inflammation and oxidative stress: the Framingham Heart Study. Circulation. 2007;116:1234–41.
26. Rosito GA, Massaro JM, Hoffmann U, Ruberg FL, Mahabadi AA, Vasan RS, et al. Pericardial fat, visceral abdominal fat, cardiovascular disease risk factors, and vascular calcification in a community-based sample: the Framingham Heart Study. Circulation. 2008;117:605–13.
27. Mahabadi AA, Massaro JM, Rosito GA, Levy D, Murabito JM, Wolf PA, et al. Association of pericardial fat, intrathoracic fat, and visceral abdominal fat with cardiovascular disease burden: the Framingham Heart Study. Eur Heart J. 2009;30:850–6.
28. Schlett CL, Massaro JM, Lehman SJ, Bamberg F, O'Donnell CJ, Fox CS, et al. Novel measurements of periaortic adipose tissue in comparison to anthropometric measures of obesity, and abdominal adipose tissue. Int J Obes. 2009;33:226–32.
29. de Vos AM, Prokop M, Roos CJ, Meijs MF, van der Schouw YT, Rutten A, et al. Peri-coronary epicardial adipose tissue is related to cardiovascular risk factors and coronary artery calcification in post-menopausal women. Eur Heart J. 2008;29:777–83.
30. Al Chekakie MO, Welles CC, Metoyer R, Ibrahim A, Shapira AR, Cytron J, et al. Pericardial fat is independently associated with human atrial fibrillation. J Am Coll Cardiol. 2010;56:784–8.
31. Mahabadi AA, Berg MH, Lehmann N, Kälsch H, Bauer M, Kara K, et al. Association of epicardial fat with cardiovascular risk factors and incident myocardial infarction in the general population: the Heinz Nixdorf Recall Study. J Am Coll Cardiol. 2013;61:1388–95.
32. Mahabadi AA, Lehmann N, Möhlenkamp S, Pundt N, Dykun I, Roggenbuck U, et al. Noncoronary measures enhance the predictive value of cardiac CT above traditional risk factors and CAC score in the general population. J Am Coll Cardiol. 2016;9:1177–85.
33. Mahabadi AA, Lehmann N, Kalsch H, Robens T, Bauer M, Dykun I, et al. Association of epicardial

adipose tissue with progression of coronary artery calcification is more pronounced in the early phase of atherosclerosis: results from the Heinz Nixdorf recall study. J Am Coll Cardiol. 2014;7:909–16.

34. Ding J, Hsu FC, Harris TB, Liu Y, Kritchevsky SB, Szklo M, et al. The association of pericardial fat with incident coronary heart disease: the Multi-Ethnic Study of Atherosclerosis (MESA). Am J Clin Nutr. 2009;90:499–504.
35. Ding J, Kritchevsky SB, Harris TB, Burke GL, Detrano RC, Szklo M, et al. The association of pericardial fat with calcified coronary plaque. Obesity (Silver Spring). 2008;16:1914–9.
36. Fox CS, Gona P, Hoffmann U, Porter SA, Salton CJ, Massaro JM, et al. Pericardial fat, intrathoracic fat, and measures of left ventricular structure and function: the Framingham Heart Study. Circulation. 2009;119:1586–91.
37. Oikonomou EK, Marwan M, Desai MY, Mancio J, Alashi A, Hutt Centeno E, et al. Non-invasive detection of coronary inflammation using computed tomography and prediction of residual cardiovascular risk (the CRISP CT study): a post-hoc analysis of prospective outcome data. Lancet. 2018;392: 929–39.
38. Balcer B, Dykun I, Schlosser T, Forsting M, Rassaf T, Mahabadi AA. Pericoronary fat volume but not attenuation differentiates culprit lesions in patients with myocardial infarction. Atherosclerosis. 2018;276:182–8.
39. Mahabadi AA, Balcer B, Dykun I, Forsting M, Schlosser T, Heusch G, et al. Cardiac computed tomography-derived epicardial fat volume and attenuation independently distinguish patients with and without myocardial infarction. PLoS One. 2017;12:e0183514.
40. Hell MM, Achenbach S, Schuhbaeck A, Klinghammer L, May MS, Marwan M. CT-based analysis of pericoronary adipose tissue density: relation to cardiovascular risk factors and epicardial adipose tissue volume. J Cardiovasc Comput Tomogr. 2016;10:52–60.
41. Nichols JH, Samy B, Nasir K, Fox CS, Schulze PC, Bamberg F, et al. Volumetric measurement of pericardial adipose tissue from contrast-enhanced coronary computed tomography angiography: a reproducibility study. J Cardiovasc Comput Tomogr. 2008;2:288–95.
42. Hell MM, Ding X, Rubeaux M, Slomka P, Gransar H, Terzopoulos D, et al. Epicardial adipose tissue volume but not density is an independent predictor for myocardial ischemia. J Cardiovasc Comput Tomogr. 2016;10:141–9.
43. Schlett CL, Ferencik M, Kriegel MF, Bamberg F, Ghoshhajra BB, Joshi SB, et al. Association of pericardial fat and coronary high-risk lesions as determined by cardiac CT. Atherosclerosis. 2012;222:129–34.
44. Maurovich-Horvat P, Kallianos K, Engel LC, Szymonifka J, Schlett CL, Koenig W, et al. Relationship of thoracic fat depots with coronary atherosclerosis and circulating inflammatory biomarkers. Obesity (Silver Spring). 2015;23:1178–84.
45. Commandeur F, Goeller M, Betancur J, Cadet S, Doris M, Chen X, et al. Deep learning for quantification of epicardial and thoracic adipose tissue from non-contrast CT. IEEE Trans Med Imaging. 2018;37:1835–46.
46. Chevalier M, Moran P, Ten JI, Fernandez Soto JM, Cepeda T, Vano E. Patient dose in digital mammography. Med Phys. 2004;31:2471–9.
47. Vonder M, Vliegenthart R, Kaatee MA, van der Aalst CM, van Ooijen PMA, de Bock GH, et al. High-pitch versus sequential mode for coronary calcium in individuals with a high heart rate: potential for dose reduction. J Cardiovasc Comput Tomogr. 2018;12:298–304.
48. Thanassoulis G, Massaro JM, Hoffmann U, Mahabadi AA, Vasan RS, O'Donnell CJ, et al. Prevalence, distribution, and risk factor correlates of high pericardial and intrathoracic fat depots in the Framingham Heart Study. Circ Cardiovasc Imaging. 2010;3: 559–66.
49. Alexopoulos N, Melek BH, Arepalli CD, Hartlage GR, Chen Z, Kim S, et al. Effect of intensive versus moderate lipid-lowering therapy on epicardial adipose tissue in hyperlipidemic post-menopausal women: a substudy of the BELLES trial (Beyond Endorsed Lipid Lowering with EBT Scanning). J Am Coll Cardiol. 2013;61:1956–61.
50. Greif M, Becker A, von Ziegler F, Lebherz C, Lehrke M, Broedl UC, et al. Pericardial adipose tissue determined by dual source CT is a risk factor for coronary atherosclerosis. Arterioscler Thromb Vasc Biol. 2009;29:781–6.
51. Taguchi R, Takasu J, Itani Y, Yamamoto R, Yokoyama K, Watanabe S, et al. Pericardial fat accumulation in men as a risk factor for coronary artery disease. Atherosclerosis. 2001;157:203–9.
52. Raggi P, Zona S, Scaglioni R, Stentarelli C, Ligabue G, Besutti G, et al. Epicardial adipose tissue and coronary artery calcium predict incident myocardial infarction and death in HIV-infected patients. J Cardiovasc Comput Tomogr. 2015;9:553–8.
53. Kunita E, Yamamoto H, Kitagawa T, Ohashi N, Oka T, Utsunomiya H, et al. Prognostic value of coronary artery calcium and epicardial adipose tissue assessed by non-contrast cardiac computed tomography. Atherosclerosis. 2014;233:447–53.
54. Wong CX, Abed HS, Molaee P, Nelson AJ, Brooks AG, Sharma G, et al. Pericardial fat is associated with atrial fibrillation severity and ablation outcome. J Am Coll Cardiol. 2011;57:1745–51.
55. Thanassoulis G, Massaro JM, O'Donnell CJ, Hoffmann U, Levy D, Ellinor PT, et al. Pericardial fat is associated with prevalent atrial fibrillation: the Framingham Heart Study. Circ Arrhythm Electrophysiol. 2010;3:345–50.
56. Mahabadi AA, Lehmann N, Kalsch H, Bauer M, Dykun I, Kara K, et al. Association of epicardial adipose tissue and left atrial size on non-contrast CT with atrial fibrillation: the Heinz Nixdorf Recall Study. Eur Heart J Cardiovasc Imaging. 2014;15:863–9.

57. Sacks HS, Fain JN. Human epicardial adipose tissue: a review. Am Heart J. 2007;153:907–17.
58. Cavalcante JL, Tamarappoo BK, Hachamovitch R, Kwon DH, Alraies MC, Halliburton S, et al. Association of epicardial fat, hypertension, subclinical coronary artery disease, and metabolic syndrome with left ventricular diastolic dysfunction. Am J Cardiol. 2012;110:1793–8.
59. Iacobellis G, Leonetti F, Singh N, Sharma AM. Relationship of epicardial adipose tissue with atrial dimensions and diastolic function in morbidly obese subjects. Int J Cardiol. 2007;115:272–3.
60. Mahabadi AA, Kahlert HA, Dykun I, Balcer B, Kahlert P, Rassaf T. Epicardial adipose tissue thickness independently predicts severe aortic valve stenosis. J Heart Valve Dis. 2017;26:262–7.
61. Hajer GR, van Haeften TW, Visseren FL. Adipose tissue dysfunction in obesity, diabetes, and vascular diseases. Eur Heart J. 2008;29:2959–71.
62. Torriani M, Oliveira AL, Azevedo DC, Bredella MA, Yu EW. Effects of Roux-en-Y gastric bypass surgery on visceral and subcutaneous fat density by computed tomography. Obes Surg. 2015;25:381–5.
63. Konishi M, Sugiyama S, Sato Y, Oshima S, Sugamura K, Nozaki T, et al. Pericardial fat inflammation correlates with coronary artery disease. Atherosclerosis. 2010;213:649–55.
64. Goeller M, Achenbach S, Marwan M, Doris MK, Cadet S, Commandeur F, et al. Epicardial adipose tissue density and volume are related to subclinical atherosclerosis, inflammation and major adverse cardiac events in asymptomatic subjects. J Cardiovasc Comput Tomogr. 2018;12:67–73.
65. Marwan M, Hell M, Schuhback A, Gauss S, Bittner D, Pflederer T, et al. CT Attenuation of pericoronary adipose tissue in normal versus atherosclerotic coronary segments as defined by intravascular ultrasound. J Comput Assist Tomogr. 2017;41:762–7.
66. Antonopoulos AS, Sanna F, Sabharwal N, Thomas S, Oikonomou EK, Herdman L, et al. Detecting human coronary inflammation by imaging perivascular fat. Sci Transl Med. 2017;9:eaal2658.
67. Mahabadi AA, Reinsch N, Lehmann N, Altenbernd J, Kalsch H, Seibel RM, et al. Association of pericoronary fat volume with atherosclerotic plaque burden in the underlying coronary artery: a segment analysis. Atherosclerosis. 2010;211:195–9.
68. Raggi P, Gadiyaram V, Zhang C, Chen Z, Lopaschuk G, Stillman AE. Statins reduce epicardial adipose tissue attenuation independent of lipid lowering: a potential pleiotropic effect. J Am Heart Assoc. 2019;8:e013104.
69. Raff GL, Abidov A, Achenbach S, Berman DS, Boxt LM, et al. SCCT guidelines for the interpretation and reporting of coronary computed tomographic angiography. J Cardiovasc Comput Tomogr. 2009;3:122–36.
70. Achenbach S, Ropers D, Möhlenkamp S, Schmermund A, Muschiol G, Groth J, et al. Variability of repeated coronary artery calcium measurements by electron beam tomography. Am J Cardiol. 2001;87: 210–3, A8.
71. Fuernau G, Fengler K, Desch S, Eitel I, Neumann FJ, Olbrich HG, et al. Culprit lesion location and outcome in patients with cardiogenic shock complicating myocardial infarction: a substudy of the IABP-SHOCK II-trial. Clin Res Cardiol. 2016;105:1030–41.
72. Moustafa A, Abi-Saleh B, El-Baba M, Hamoui O, AlJaroudi W. Anatomic distribution of culprit lesions in patients with non-ST-segment elevation myocardial infarction and normal ECG. Cardiovasc Diagn Ther. 2016;6:25–33.
73. Khawaja T, Greer C, Thadani SR, Kato TS, Bhatia K, Shimbo D, et al. Increased regional epicardial fat volume associated with reversible myocardial ischemia in patients with suspected coronary artery disease. J Nucl Cardiol. 2015;22:325–33.
74. Antoniades C, Antonopoulos AS, Deanfield J. Imaging residual inflammatory cardiovascular risk. Eur Heart J. 2019; https://doi.org/10.1093/eurheartj/ehz474. [Epub ahead of print].
75. Lehman SJ, Massaro JM, Schlett CL, O'Donnell CJ, Hoffmann U, Fox CS. Peri-aortic fat, cardiovascular disease risk factors, and aortic calcification: the Framingham Heart Study. Atherosclerosis. 2010;210:656–61.
76. Hoffmann U, Truong QA, Schoenfeld DA, Chou ET, Woodard PK, Nagurney JT, et al. Coronary CT angiography versus standard evaluation in acute chest pain. N Engl J Med. 2012;367:299–308.
77. Ferencik M, Mayrhofer T, Bittner DO, Emami H, Puchner SB, Lu MT, et al. Use of high-risk coronary atherosclerotic plaque detection for risk stratification of patients with stable chest pain: a secondary analysis of the PROMISE randomized clinical trial. JAMA Cardiol. 2018;3:144–52.
78. Nielsen LH, Botker HE, Sorensen HT, Schmidt M, Pedersen L, Sand NP, et al. Prognostic assessment of stable coronary artery disease as determined by coronary computed tomography angiography: a Danish multicentre cohort study. Eur Heart J. 2017;38:413–21.
79. Mahabadi AA, Rassaf T. Imaging of coronary inflammation for cardiovascular risk prediction. Lancet. 2018;392:894–6.

Magnetic Resonance Imaging of the Epicardial Adipose Tissue

7

Gianluca Iacobellis

Key Points

- Cardiac magnetic resonance (CMR) imaging provides a precise and noninvasive assessment of both epicardial adipose tissue (EAT) thickness and volume.
- Steady-state free precession (SSFP) CMR can measure EAT filling in different and deeper heart areas.
- Proton magnetic resonance spectroscopy (^{1}H-MRS) is the gold standard technique to measure myocardial triglyceride content that is independently correlated with EAT thickness

Introduction

Epicardial fat (EAT) is a measurable risk factor and marker of visceral adiposity. It can be easily and not invasively measured with echocardiography, as proposed by Iacobellis et al. [1, 2]. However this method has some limitations, such as the operator dependency and the linear measurement. The echocardiographic measurement of EAT has been validated with magnetic resonance imaging (MRI) and actually showed a good agreement. MRI is considered the gold standard technique to measure the adipose tissue [3]. MRI is noninvasive and does not use ionizing radiation, and therefore it is well suitable to measure EAT in both research and clinical setting.

Cardiac MRI of the Epicardial Fat

A dedicated cardiac magnetic resonance (CMR) imaging has been developed to assess EAT volume. Flüchter et al. were the first to develop a protocol to measure EAT using CMR [4]. EAT was measured using a dark blood prepared T1-weighted multislice turbo spin-echo pulse sequence with a water suppression prepulse to obtain a transversal four-chamber view and short-axis images in the same orientations used for the cine short-axis images. Both EAT thickness and volume were measured using CMR by Flüchter and colleagues. Following the anatomical findings and the method previously described by Iacobellis et al. [1, 2], EAT thickness was measured on the right ventricular free wall. Maximum epicardial fat thickness at the right ventricular free wall was measured in different views: in a transversal four-chamber view (Fig. 7.1a) and in consecutive short-axis views (EFT-SAX) covering the whole ventricle (Fig. 7.1b) [4]. Epicardial fat in and near the atrioventricular and interventricular

G. Iacobellis (✉)
Division of Endocrinology, Diabetes and Metabolism, Department of Medicine, University of Miami, Miller School of Medicine, Miami, FL, USA
e-mail: giacobellis@med.miami.edu

G. Iacobellis (ed.), *Epicardial Adipose Tissue*, Contemporary Cardiology,
https://doi.org/10.1007/978-3-030-40570-0_7

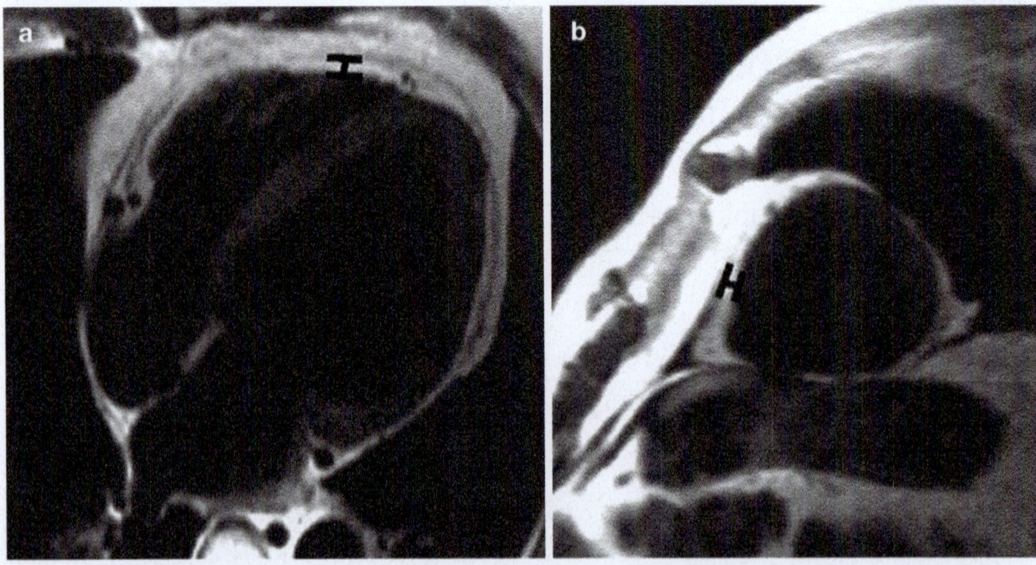

Fig. 7.1 Epicardial fat thickness of the right ventricular free wall measured in the four-chamber view (**a**) and in a representative short-axis view (**b**). (From Flüchter et al. [4], with permission from John Wiley & Sons)

grooves was not considered. While EAT thickness measured with CMR well correlated with autopsy [5], results were different from the EAT thickness values, measured according to the ultrasound methodology proposed by Iacobellis [1, 2]. This discrepancy could be attributed to the measurement of EAT thickness from the four-chamber view with the CMR rather than from the long-axis view as described in the echocardiographic method. The population studies by Flüchter and Iacobellis were also quite different, as some of the patients assessed with CMR presented with congestive heart failure. The left ventricular remodeling could have therefore influenced EAT measurements from the four-chamber view.

In the CMR study, EAT volume was calculated by using the modified Simpson's rule with integration over the image slices: EAT contours were outlined at end-diastole in the short-axis views covering the entire left and right ventricle [4]. The area subtended by the manual tracings was determined in each slice and multiplied by the slice thickness to yield the fat volume. Total EAT volume was obtained after the summation of data of all slices (Fig. 7.2). CMR-measured EAT volume showed excellent agreements with autopsy results [6].

Overall, CMR provides a precise and noninvasive assessment of both EAT thickness and volume. However, the method used by Flüchter may have some limitations. A recent study raised up the concern and need of detecting the diverse EAT anatomy and distribution [7]. EAT is not equally distributed through the heart. EAT is located at the interatrial groove, the atrioventricular septum, and the inferior pyramidal space, the left lateral ridge, the atrioventricular grooves, and the transverse pericardial sinus. Leo et al. recently proposed to use balanced steady-state free precession (SSFP) sequences of CMR to measure the different EAT locations [7]. SSFP sequences have the ability to distinguish the fat from the blood and the muscle, so providing a great quality imaging of EAT distribution. The authors nicely underline that EAT, particularly when abundant, should not be considered as accumulation of layers covering the surface of the heart, but rather fat deeply penetrating into the heart and filling any possible folding. SSFP CMR can catch and detect the folding appearance of human EAT.

Regional fat distribution of EAT plays an important role in the development and potentially

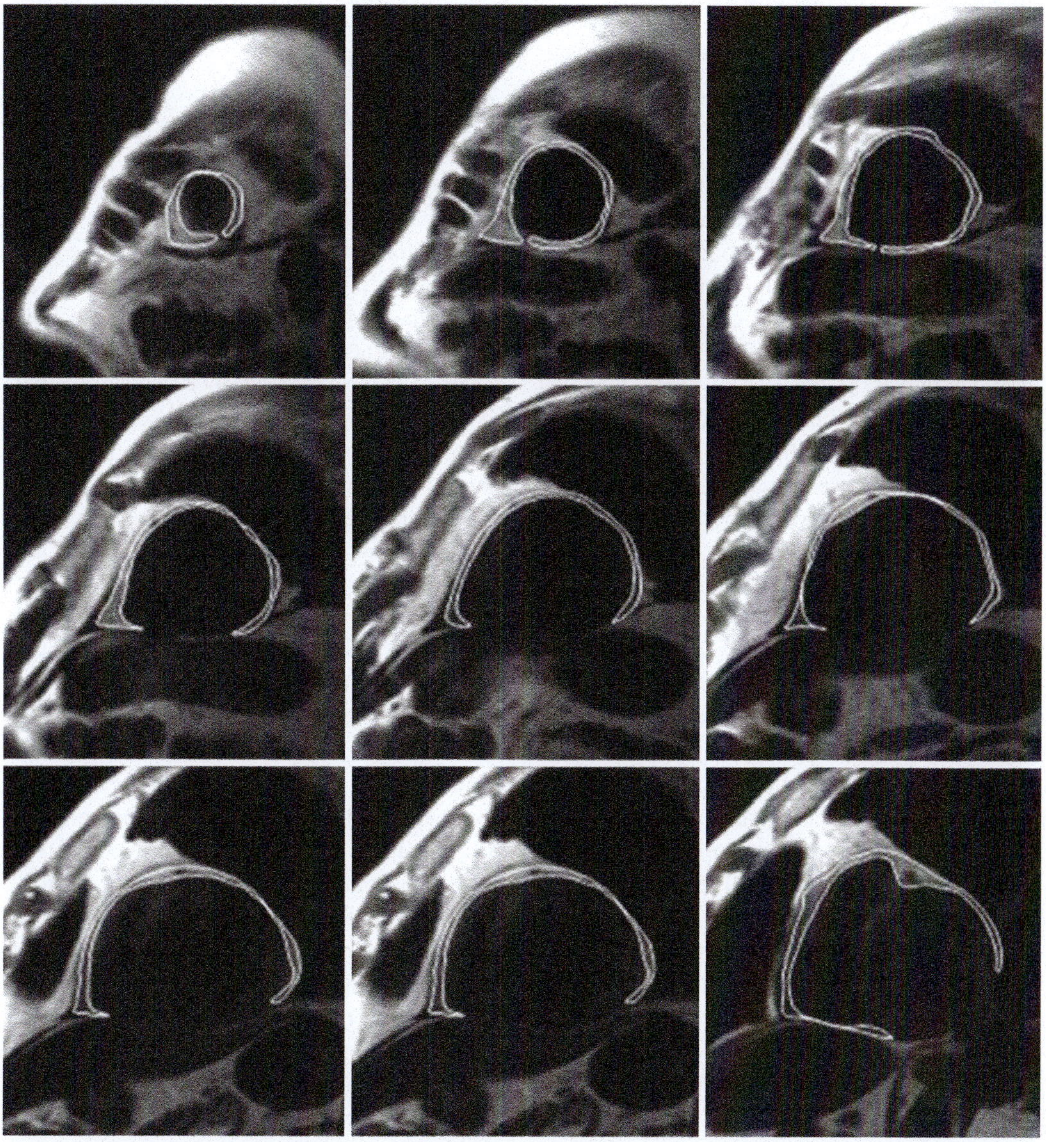

Fig. 7.2 Volumetric measurement of epicardial fat mass. The contours of epicardial adipose tissue were outlined in end-diastolic images of short-axis views covering the whole left and right ventricle. (From Flüchter et al. [4], with permission from John Wiley & Sons)

stratification of different conditions. For example, peri-atrial EAT has shown to be strongly correlated with atrial fibrillation. Hence, clinical assessment of peri-atrial EAT could be instrumental in the prognosis of patients with atrial fibrillation. One study validated the use of a semiautomated three-dimensional atrial PAT model utilizing standard (clinical) CMR sequences for accurate and reproducible assessment of atrial PAT [8].

Nelson et al. also criticized the method proposed by Flüchter [9]. They used an ovine model, to validate a CMR-derived paracardial adipose tissue volume assessment [9]. The measurement was not limited to the adipose thickness over the RV free wall, but included epicardial, paracardial, and pericardial adipose depots. Starting at the mitral annulus, consecutive end-diastolic ventricular images were used to determine the area and volume of epicardial, paracardial, and pericardial adipose tissue included paracardial adipose tissue mass. Unquestionably this method allows the measurement of the entire cardiac adiposity. Nevertheless, this approach is argumentative, as EAT, pericardial, and paracardial adipose tissue are embryologically, anatomically, and functionally very different. The inclusion of the three fat depots as one single entity may not reflect the separate functions and clinical implications of each single adipose tissue.

CMR has been used in several studies to evaluate EAT in patients with different cardiac diseases, such as CAD, HF, and dilated cardiomyopathy [10–12]. CMR imaging can not only measure EAT but also detect myocardial fat infiltration [13–15]. In patients with aortic stenosis, CMR imaging myocardial steatosis correlated with the degree of left ventricular strain impairment [14]. CMR study using variable projection water/fat separation showed a relation between left ventricular function and fat accumulation within the septal myocardium in patients with dilated cardiomyopathy [15]. Additionally, multiparametric CMR provides imaging of cardiac function and myocardial fibrosis by late gadolinium enhancement.

Advantages of CMR Imaging of Epicardial Fat

CMR allows a clear visualization of EAT. CMR imaging using SSFP allows a clear distinction between muscular and adipose tissue. This sequence provides a high signal/noise ratio and an optimal blood/myocardial contrast, which allows a precise definition of the endocardial borders. When using SSFP CMR, the strength of the signal comes from different tissues and depends on T1/T2 ratio. Water (blood) and fat have the same high T1/T2 ratio; then both tissues produce a very high signal. On the contrary, the muscular tissue has a low T1/T2 ratio and produces weak signal. SSFP CMR can distinguish the different EAT locations better than any other noninvasive imaging technique.

Limitations of CMR Imaging of Epicardial Fat

When abundant, EAT not only covers the entire epicardial surface but also invades spaces and folds that usually are almost virtual [7]. Some CMR protocols may be not able and reliable in depicting the exact and deeper EAT distribution. CMR images side by side with corresponding anatomic specimens should be used. CMR is more expensive than echocardiography and requires different skills and labor in measuring EAT. CMR may not be readily available in non-academic hospitals or non-research centers.

Proton Magnetic Resonance Spectroscopy and Epicardial Fat

Myocardial fat accumulation has gained growing attention as independent and direct cause of cardiac diseases. The presence of myocardial fat deposition, otherwise called cardiac steatosis, could represent an additional CMR imaging feature of prognostic importance in high-risk patients. The significance of cardiac steatosis in normal hearts remains to be determined. Proton magnetic resonance spectroscopy (^{1}H-MRS) is the gold standard technique to measure myocardial triglyceride content [16, 17]. ^{1}H-MRS is used as a noninvasive, non-radiation exposure technique for the clinical assessment of myocardial lipid content. The recent use of high-field scanners (3.0 T) has improved the chemical shift resolution and signal-to-noise ratio of cardiac 1H-MRS. This feature allows the discrimination between fatty acid (FA) and unsaturated fatty acid (UFA) deposition in the myocardium. Myocardial TG signals and the water signal are acquired from spectra with water suppression and without water suppression, respectively (Fig. 7.3). The spectroscopic signals are acquired at end-systole and end-expiration with electrocardiographic triggering and respiratory navigator gating.

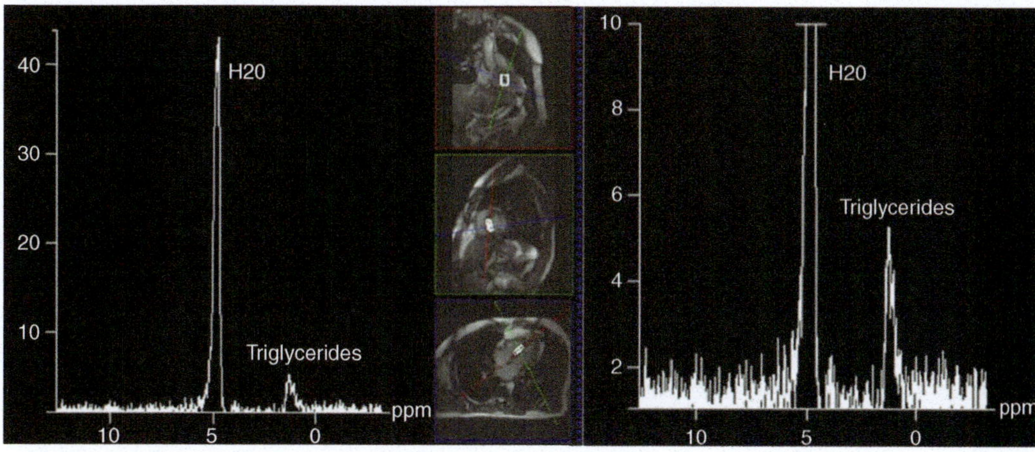

Fig. 7.3 (*Left*) Proton MR spectroscopic image of septal myocardial fat. (*Right*) Example of nonwater-suppressed proton MR spectrum of interventricular septal fat in an obese study patient. Amplitude is expressed in arbitrary units and with two different scales (left of images). (*Center*) Two-chamber plane (*top*), short-axis plane (*middle*), and four-chamber plane (bottom) MR images show voxel positioning in the septum. (From Malazavos et al. [20], with permission from Elsevier)

In clinical studies with ^{1}H-MRS, myocardial triglyceride content is correlated with left ventricular mass and systolic function in patients with heart failure and left ventricular hypertrophy [18, 19]. Ultrasound measured EAT thickness has shown to independently correlate with ^{1}H-MRS myocardial triglyceride content ($R = 0.79$, $p < 0.01$) in subjects with a wide range of obesity and body fat distribution [20]. EAT, as measured by standard cardiac ultrasound, may serve a predictor of triglyceride fat content better than waist circumference and other more traditional biochemical risk factors. This statistical correlation is based on the lack of barrier separating EAT from the underlying myocardium. Hence, EAT excessive free fatty acid influx can reach directly the myocardium via paracrine or vasocrine pathways. It is plausible to speculate that the consensual increase in EAT and myocardial fat might affect the heart morphology and function.

References

1. Iacobellis G, Willens HJ. Echocardiographic epicardial fat: a review of research and clinical applications. J Am Soc Echocardiogr. 2009;22:1311–9.
2. Iacobellis G, Assael F, Ribaudo MC, Zappaterreno A, Alessi G, Di Mario U, et al. Epicardial fat from echocardiography: a new method for visceral adipose tissue prediction. Obes Res. 2003;11:304–10.
3. Gronemeyer SA, Steen RG, Kauffman WM, Reddick WE, Glass JO. Fast adipose tissue (FAT) assessment by MRI. Magn Reson Imaging. 2000;18:815–8.
4. Flüchter S, Haghi D, Dinter D, Heberlein W, Kühl HP, Neff W, et al. Volumetric assessment of epicardial adipose tissue with cardiovascular magnetic resonance imaging. Obesity (Silver Spring). 2007;15: 870–8.
5. Schejbal V. Epicardial fatty tissue of the right ventricle--morphology, morphometry and functional significance. Pneumologie. 1989;43:490–9.
6. Iacobellis G, Corradi D, Sharma AM. Epicardial adipose tissue: anatomic, biomolecular and clinical relationships with the heart. Nat Clin Pract Cardiovasc Med. 2005;2:536–43.
7. Leo LA, Paiocchi VL, Schlossbauer SA, Ho SY, Faletra FF. The intrusive nature of epicardial adipose tissue as revealed by cardiac magnetic resonance. J Cardiovasc Echogr. 2019;29:45.
8. Mahajan R, Kuklik P, Grover S, Brooks AG, Wong CX, Sanders P, et al. Cardiovascular magnetic resonance of total and atrial pericardial adipose tissue: a validation study and development of a 3-dimensional pericardial adipose tissue model. J Cardiovasc Magn Reson. 2013;29(15):73.
9. Nelson AJ, Worthley MI, Psaltis PJ, Carbone A, Dundon BK, Duncan RF, et al. Validation of cardiovascular magnetic resonance assessment of pericardial adipose tissue volume. J Cardiovasc Magn Reson. 2009;11:15.
10. Doesch C, Haghi D, Flüchter S, Suselbeck T, Schoenberg SO, Michaely H, et al. Epicardial adi-

pose tissue in patients with heart failure. J Cardiovasc Magn Reson. 2010;12:40.

11. Doesch C, Haghi D, Suselbeck T, Schoenberg SO, Borggrefe M, Papavassiliu T. Impact of functional, morphological and clinical parameters on epicardial adipose tissue in patients with coronary artery disease. Circ J. 2012;76:2426–34.
12. Doesch C, Streitner F, Bellm S, Suselbeck T, Haghi D, Heggemann F, et al. Epicardial adipose tissue assessed by cardiac magnetic resonance imaging in patients with heart failure due to dilated cardiomyopathy. Obesity (Silver Spring). 2013;21: E253–61.
13. Ng A, Strudwick M, van der Geest RJ, Ng ACC, Gillinder L, Goo SY, et al. Impact of epicardial adipose tissue, left ventricular myocardial fat content and interstitial fibrosis on myocardial contractile function. Circ Cardiovasc Imaging. 2018;11:e007372.
14. Mahmod M, Bull S, Suttie JJ, Pal N, Holloway C, Dass S, et al. Myocardial steatosis and left ventricular contractile dysfunction in patients with severe aortic stenosis. Circ Cardiovasc Imaging. 2013;6: 808–16.
15. Lu M, Zhao S, Jiang S, Yin G, Wang C, Zhang Y, et al. Fat deposition in dilated cardiomyopathy assessed by CMR. JACC Cardiovasc Imaging. 2013;6:889–98.
16. Szczepaniak LS, Babcock EE, Schick F, Dobbins RL, Garg A, Burns DK, JD MG, Stein DT. Measurement of intracellular triglyceride stores by H spectroscopy: validation in vivo. Am J Physiol Endocrinol Metab. 1999;276:E977–89.
17. Reingold JS, McGavock JM, Kaka S, Tillery T, Victor RG, Szczepaniak LS. Determination of triglyceride in the human myocardium by magnetic resonance spectroscopy: reproducibility and sensitivity of the method. Am J Physiol Endocrinol Metab. 2005;289:E935–9.
18. Liao PA, Lin G, Tsai SY, Wang CH, Juan YH, Lin YC, et al. Myocardial triglyceride content at 3 T cardiovascular magnetic resonance and left ventricular systolic function: a cross-sectional study in patients hospitalized with acute heart failure. J Cardiovasc Magn Reson. 2016;18:9.
19. Sai E, Shimada K, Yokoyama T, Hiki M, Sato S, Hamasaki N, et al. Myocardial triglyceride content in patients with left ventricular hypertrophy: comparison between hypertensive heart disease and hypertrophic cardiomyopathy. Heart Vessel. 2017;32:166–74.
20. Malavazos AE, Di Leo G, Secchi F, Lupo EN, Dogliotti G, Coman C, et al. Relation of echocardiographic epicardial fat thickness and myocardial fat. Am J Cardiol. 2010;105:1831–5.

Coronary Artery Disease and Epicardial Adipose Tissue

8

Gianluca Iacobellis

Key Points

- Epicardial adipose tissue (EAT) can locally affect the coronary arteries and play a significant role in the development and progression of coronary artery disease (CAD).
- The incidence of major adverse cardiace event (MACE) increases with higher EAT independently of coronary calcium calcification score and obesity.
- Clinical imaging of EAT provides prognostic information and improves the prediction of first coronary events.

Introduction

Epicardial adipose tissue (EAT) can locally affect the coronary arteries and play a significant role in the development and progression of coronary artery disease (CAD), as emerged only recently. The mechanisms through which EAT can cause atherosclerosis are complex, multifactorial, and not completely understood. However, several players have been already identified such as its anatomical proximity to the heart, lack of muscle fascia and shared microcirculation, the unique transcriptome, and the intense proteasome [1]. EAT lies in direct contiguity with the myocardium without fascial barrier such that some EAT adipocytes even appear to invaginate the epicardial surface. EAT directly surrounds the adventitia and is supplied by branches of the coronary arteries. The absence of anatomical barriers allows a direct interaction and bidirectional cross talk between the epicardial fat and the coronary arteries. In addition to being an anatomically unique adipose depot, EAT demonstrates a transcriptome markedly different from that of subcutaneous fat in the same subjects. EAT secretosome can go directly into the coronary lumen through paracrine or vasocrime mechanisms. The atherogenicity of epicardial fat can be grossly caused and associated to inflammation, innate immunity, oxidative stress, lipotoxicity, and glucotoxicity.

G. Iacobellis (✉)
Division of Endocrinology, Diabetes and Metabolism, Department of Medicine, University of Miami, Miller School of Medicine, Miami, FL, USA
e-mail: giacobellis@med.miami.edu

Epicardial Fat Inflammation

Inflammation is a major player in the development and progression of CAD. EAT should be considered a highly inflammatory organ [2]. Microarray analysis yields the transcriptional identity of EAT in CAD versus no CAD patients (Fig. 8.1) [3]. Epicardial adipocytes are enriched with pro-inflammatory and pro-atherogenic genes [3]. Upregulated EAT genes code for

G. Iacobellis (ed.), *Epicardial Adipose Tissue*, Contemporary Cardiology,
https://doi.org/10.1007/978-3-030-40570-0_8

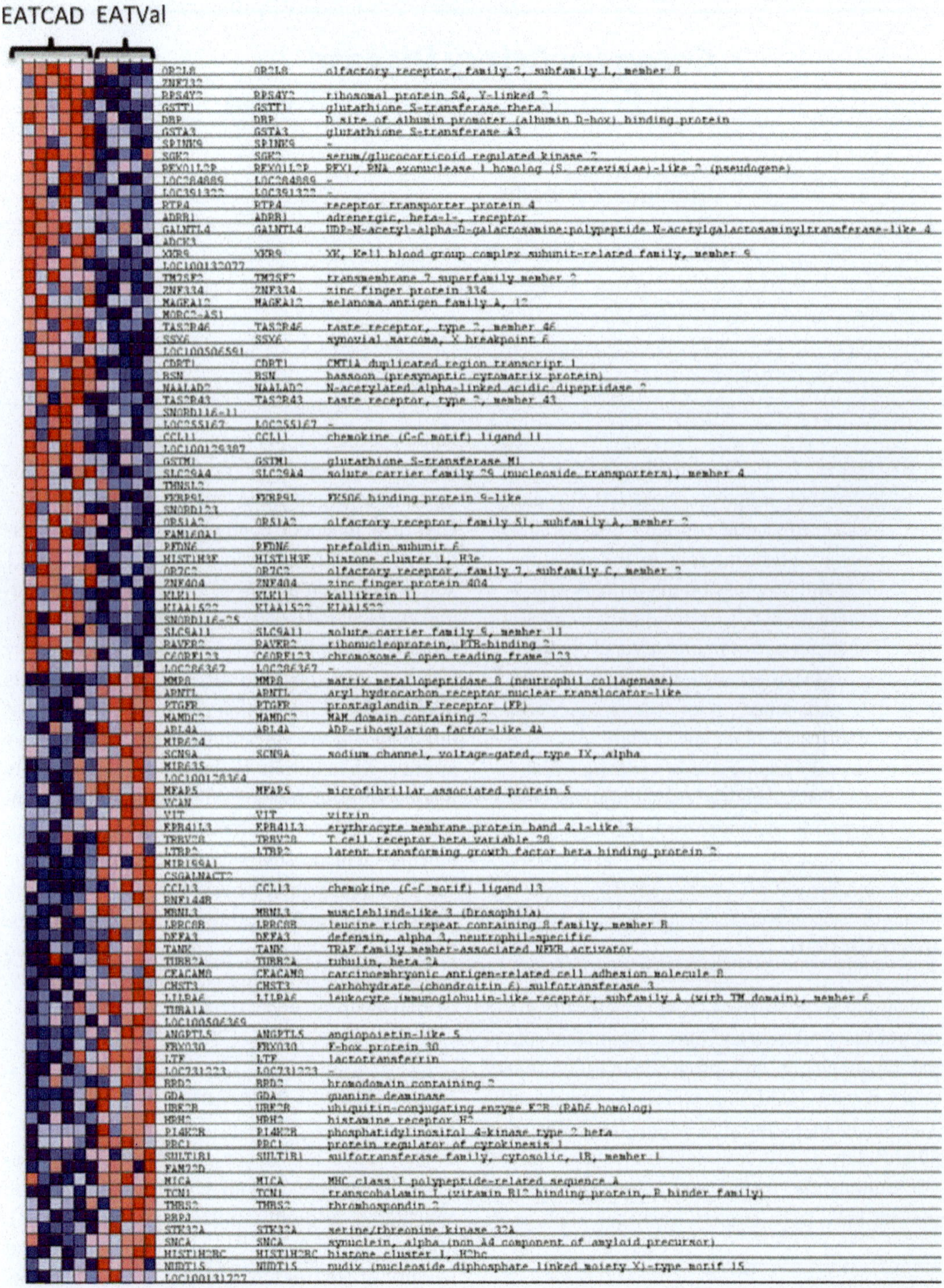

Fig. 8.1 Heat map of the 50 most enriched genes in EATCAD samples compared with EATVal samples. Heat mapping demonstrates the unique features of EAT, where expression values are represented as colors (red: increased expression; blue: decreased expression) with the degree of color saturation indicating the degree of expression. Heat map generated by Broad Institute's Gene Set Enrichment Analysis. EAT epicardial adipose tissue, CAD coronary artery disease, and Val valvulopathy. (From McAninch et al. [3], with permission from John Wiley & Sons)

pro-inflammatory cytokines, such as T cell and macrophage markers and B cell-associated factors, like tumor growth factor (TGF)beta2, multiple chemokine ligands, and chemokine receptors. Multiple chemokine ligands and chemokine receptors are over expressed in EAT of CAD subjects. The high inflammatory infiltrates in the EAT has been described in several studies [2–6]. Most of the analyses found EAT with higher inflammatory activity than any other visceral fat depots. EAT CD45 expression is significantly higher than omental fat depot indicating a unique and significant infiltration of macrophages within epicardial adipocytes [4]. Messenger RNA (mRNA) expression of interleukin 6 (IL-6) and monocyte chemoattractant protein-1 (MCP-1) and tumor necrosis factor alpha (TNF-α) was higher in EAT collected from patients who underwent cardiac surgery for CAD [5].

This intense pro-inflammatory proteasome is directly secreted into the coronary lumen. The secretion of epicardial inflammatory molecules into the coronary bloodstream promotes atherogenesis, more likely through vasocrine rather than paracrine pathways as the plaque built-up tends to increase the arterial wall thickness. Regardless of the pathway, inflammatory cells secreted by the epicardial fat surrounding the adventitia may stimulate the proliferation of vasa vasorum and ultimately cause intramural changes. Coronary atherosclerotic plaque seems to be more prominent where epicardial fat deposit is more abundant [7, 8]. The pro-inflammatory transcriptome is higher and specific in the epicardial fat depot adjacent to severe, but stable coronary plaques [8].

The atherogenic effect of the epicardial fat is exerted not only but its anatomical vicinity to the plaque, but also mostly by its intense activity. Epicardial fat could affect the coronary arteries via multiple pathways including macrophage activation, oxidative stress, innate inflammatory response, and plaque destabilization. A dense inflammatory infiltrate, mainly represented by macrophages, pro-inflammatory M1 macrophages, and mast cells is commonly detected in epicardial fat of subjects with CAD (Fig. 8.2) [9]. Under pathological circumstances, epicardial adipocytes display an intrinsic pro-inflammatory and atherogenic profile. Interestingly, the ratio of epicardial fat pro-inflammatory M1 macrophages and anti-inflammatory M2 macrophages is unbalanced in patients with CAD [9]. The presence of macrophages and mast cells in epicardial adipose tissue could also be reactive to underlying plaque rupture and instability. EAT of CAD patients showed higher infiltration of macrophages and CD8-positive T cells than in EAT samples obtained from non-CAD patients [10]. Epicardial fat expresses adhesion molecules contributing to different phases of the atherosclerotic process, such as MCP-1, growth-related oncogene α, and regulated upon activation T cell and secreted (RANTES) [2–5].

The imbalance between anti- and pro-inflammatory epicardial fat adipokines secretion

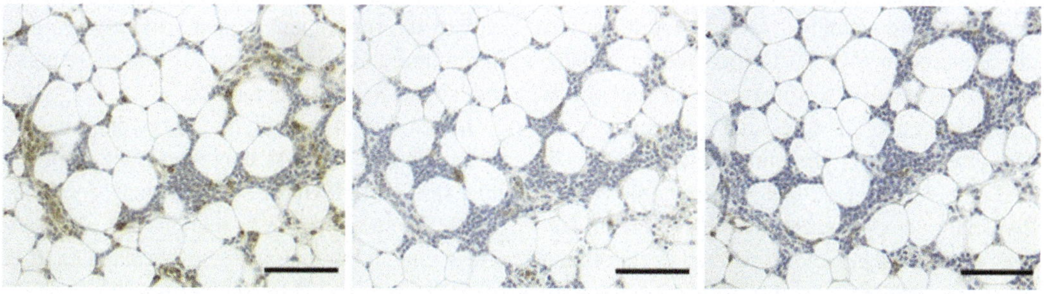

Fig. 8.2 Epicardial adipose tissue (EAT) presents with intense inflammatory infiltrate in coronary artery disease (CAD). Immunohistochemical staining showing accumulation of CD68-, CD11c-, and CD206-positive cells in EAT of patients with CAD. Scale bar = 100 μm. (From Hirata et al. [9], with permission from Elsevier)

is strongly linked to human coronary atherosclerosis [11]. In fact, epicardial fat production of pro-inflammatory adipokines is significantly higher than that of the subcutaneous fat in patients with coronaropathies. IL6, interleukin 8 (IL8), MCP-1, plasminogen activator inhibitor 1, growth-related oncogene-alpha, and macrophage migration inhibitory factor are the most abundant inflammatory cytokines, whereas anti-inflammatory adiponectin was downregulated [11]. Both adiponectin gene and protein expression were significantly lower in patients with coronary artery disease [12]. However, not always the messenger RNAs (mRNAs) of the EAT inflammatory genes was associated with the circulating levels of the proteins [8].

The innate inflammatory response is also an active component of the atherogenicity of the epicardial adipose tissue. Epicardial fat inflammation and innate immunity response are closely interrelated. Nuclear factor-kappaB (NFκB), c-Jun N-terminal kinase (JNK) activity, and toll-like receptors (TLRs) expression are higher in EAT as compared to other visceral fat depots of individuals with CAD [13]. The activated TLRs lead the translocation of NFκB into the nucleus. This cascade causes an upregulation and higher release of inflammatory cytokines such as interleukins (IL) 1 and 6, TNF-α, and resistin [14].

EAT plays a role in the endothelial damage. Higher expression and secretion of EAT resistin was associated with increased in vitro endothelial cell permeability in subjects with CAD [14]. EAT secreted resistin plays a role in the endothelial damage. Interestingly, vasodilator-stimulated phosphoprotein (VASP) is involved in resistin-related endothelial dysfunction and the phenotype conversion of epicardial adipocytes [15]. The modulation of the endothelial function by EAT was investigated and further demonstrated the inflammatory properties of this tissue. In fact, EAT is enriched in factors involved in endothelial function such as, among others, bradykinin receptor B2 which mediates vasodilatation, natriuresis, nitric oxide, prostaglandin release and is involved in cross talk with the renin–angiotensin system [3]. EAT is also implicated in the oxidative stress. KCNN3 involved in endothelial function is also overexpressed in EAT from CAD subjects [3]. The enrichment of these endothelial related genes in the EAT likely reflects a difference in gene expression between peripheral and the cardiac vasculature, as the EAT is supplied by branches of the coronary arteries. Interestingly, EAT-conditioned media caused a migration of monocytic tryptophan hydroxylase 1 (THP-1) cells to human coronary artery endothelial cells in subjects with CAD [10].

EAT is subject of oxidative stress and in a higher extent than subcutaneous fat in patients with cardiovascular disease. Higher reactive oxygen species (ROS) and lower expression of anti-oxidant enzymes, such as catalase, glutathione S-transferase P, and protein disulfide isomerase, are observed in the epicardial fat of individuals with CAD [16]. Lower catalase and higher ROS trigger the local inflammation and secretion of inflammatory factors, such as TNFα, IL8, and neutrophil-binding adhesion molecules. As compared to subcutaneous fat, proteomic analysis showed posttranslational modification of EAT antioxidant markers GSTP1 and PDIA1 that display protective effects against oxidative and endoplasmic reticulum stress [16].

Microarray analysis showed that EAT is also enriched with genes involved in the hemostasis and coagulation. These genes included tissue plasminogen activator, an inhibitor of 6 endogenous fibrinolysis that links fibrinolysis and inflammation in fat and impairs adipose tissue development. Evidence that EAT represents a highly inflammatory fat depot is supported not only by the enrichment of genes directly involved in the immune response, but also by these endothelial and coagulation factors.

In addition to the inflammatory component of this adipose depot, EAT expresses markers of cellular stress. MAP kinase stress response including *MAP2K3* and *MAP3K5*, markers of adipocyte stress and inflammation were enriched in EAT [3]. ER stress markers including *ERN1*, *ATF6*, *EIF2AK3*, *DNAJC1*, and *PDIA3* are also enriched in EAT [3]. Multiple proteases that play roles in lysosomal degradation and apoptosis including cathepsins K, S, G, H, B, and K as well as caspase

8 were also upregulated EAT [3]. Cathepsin B activation in adipocytes contributes to adipocyte cell death and macrophage infiltration in obesity.

The pro-atherogenic activity of EAT is also mediated by recently discovered inflammatory cytokines. One study showed that EAT of CAD patients had significantly higher levels of chemerin than that of controls [17]. Chemerin mRNA expression in EAT was positively correlated with Gensini score. Significantly higher expression of serglycin, a pro-inflammatory adipokine, was reported in in EAT [18]. Serglycin expression was induced during adipocytic differentiation of 3T3L1 cells. TNF-α stimulates serglycin expression and secretion in adipocytes. Omentin-1, a novel adipocytokine mainly expressed in visceral adipose tissue, mRNA, and protein expression were found to be higher in EAT than in paired subcutaneous fat [19]. EAT from CAD subjects have lower omentin-1 mRNA levels than those with no CAD. Omentin-1 expression in patients with CAD is lower in EAT adjacent to coronary stenotic segments than non-stenotic segments.

Epicardial Fat Lipotoxicity

The mechanisms underlying the atherogenicity of epicardial fat involve also the lipid homeostasis. Toll-like receptors (TLRs), located within epicardial fat macrophages and adipocytes response to excessive FFAs, recognized as endogenous antigens, by upregulating the expression of transcription factors, such as NF-κ B and FOS, and then enhancing their translocation of into the nucleus of epicardial adipocytes. The upregulation of these transcription factors causes an overexpression of epicardial fat inflammatory factors such as IL-1, IL-8, IL-6, and TNF-α. Inflammatory mediators then activate macrophages derived from transdifferentiated adipocytes, inducing lipolysis and upregulation of intracellular adhesion molecule-1 (ICAM-1), IL-6, and MCP-1, ultimately leading to the lipid accumulation within the atherosclerotic plaque. Lipase G (LIPG), solute carrier family 7 member 5 (SLC7A5), and solute carrier family 16 member 10 (SLC16A10), all involved in lipid metabolism and nutrient transport, are among the top upregulated genes in diabetic epicardial fat [20]. Epicardial fat could contribute to the lipid accumulation within the atherosclerostic plaque thanks to the higher secretion of the secretory type II phospholipase A2 (sPLA2-II) [21]. A microarray of EAT compared to subcutaneous adipose tissue (SAT) in both CAD and non-CAD subjects found the highest ranked gene encoding for a secreted protein to be secretory type II phospholipase A2 (sPLA2-IIA), the rate-limiting enzyme in the synthesis of a pro-inflammatory lipid mediator. Epicardial fat is highly enriched in sPLA2-IIA in CAD subjects (Fig. 8.3) [21]. The upregulation of sPLA2 is cer-

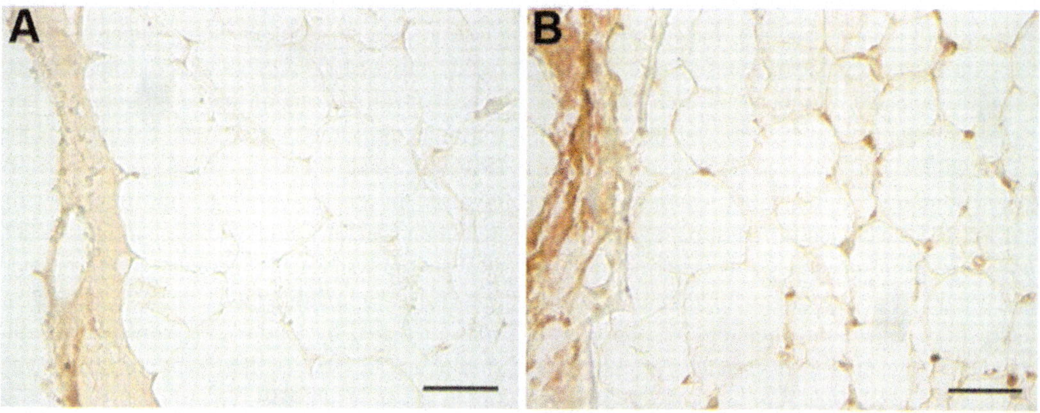

Fig. 8.3 Immunohistochemical staining of $sPLA_2$ in epicardial adipose tissue (EAT) (**b**) and subcutaneous adipose tissue (SAT) (**a**), showing a stronger signal in EAT than SAT. Bar, 50 μm. (From Dutour et al. [21], with permission of Oxford University Press)

tainly an additional factor contributing to the lipid build-up in the coronary arteries. The lipogenic effect of epicardial fat has also been attributed to its highest fat content of conjugated fatty acids [22]. EAT overexpression of low-density lipoprotein receptor-related protein 1 and very low-density lipoprotein receptor has been suggested to play a role diabetic dyslipidemia [23].

Epicardial Fat Glucotoxicity

While insulin resistance and hyperglycemia are traditional and well-established risk factors, EAT recently emerged as novel player in the development and progression of diabetes atherosclerosis. Epicardial fat per se can be considered a relatively insulin resistant fat depot. In fact, the rate of insulin-stimulated lipogenesis in epicardial fat tissue is significantly greater than other visceral fat depots, but insulin had little or no effects on epicardial fat fatty acids incorporation and glucose uptake. Epicardial adipose tissue glucose utilization is about half that of the intra-abdominal fat depots in monkeys [24].

However, the peculiarity of EAT in subjects with diabetes is in its genetic profile. In fact recent RNA-seq analysis from Iacobellis's group showed that diabetic epicardial fat transcriptome is unique and markedly different from that of subcutaneous fat, suggesting a novel atherogenic pathway in diabetes [20]. Omentin (ITLN1) is the most upregulated gene and secreted adipokine in both diabetic and not diabetic epicardial fat. The top upregulated genes (based on fold changes) appeared to have diverse functions. RNA-sequencing analysis showed that diabetic epicardial fat is highly enriched in genes involved in inflammation. Upregulated genes in diabetic epicardial fat included different pathways of the inflammatory response such as cytokine production, leukocyte migration, cytokine–cytokine interaction, innate inflammatory response, and advanced glycation end products/receptor for advanced glycation end products (AGE-RAGE) signaling [20]. Gene enrichment analysis of transcription factors showed that diabetic epicardial fat genes expression is mostly due to the action of upregulated transcription factors, such as those belonging to NF-κB family and FOS family [20]. KEGG pathway analysis further confirmed that the upregulated genes were involved in inflammatory related pathways, such as cytokine–cytokine interaction, TNF, NF-κB, JAK-STAT, and AGE-RAGE signaling. Notably, 20 upregulated genes in diabetic EAT belonged to the AGE-RAGE pathway. Important ligands of this pathway include *S100A8* and *S100A9*, which were increased in diabetic EAT. Enlargement of adipocyte size was related to S100A9 expression levels in stromal cells, but not in epicardial cells [25]. The correlation between RAGE and CAD was observed in another study [26].

EAT could also contribute to create a local coronary insulin resistance. Interestingly, glucose transporter-4 (GLUT4) mRNA levels are lower in epicardial fat, whereas renitol-binding protein 4 (RBP4) are higher than those in subcutaneous fat in patients with coronary artery disease [27]. Interestingly, the expression of p53, another gene involved in adipogenesis, in epicardial stromal cells is related to adipocyte enlargement in obese patients with cardiovascular disease [26].

Diabetic epicardial fat glucose and lipid metabolism are closely interrelated. Epicardial fat endothelial LIPG is upregulated in diabetes, as recently reported [20]. LIPG is a gene involved in the lipid uptake, endothelium regulation and may contribute to the pathogenesis of diabetic cardiomyopathy. LIPG expression was higher in epicardial fat from diabetic compared with non-diabetic patients [27]. Diabetic epicardial fat is highly enriched in GOS2, another protein coding gene, considered one of the target genes of peroxisome proliferator-activated receptor alpha (PPARα) and PPARγ, transcription factors involved in the regulation of lipid metabolism, mitochondrial fatty acid oxidation, inflammation, and immunity. Notably, a recent study pointed out a role of epicardial fat in type 1 diabetes possibly mediated by leptin [28]. Remarkably, epicardial adipocytes size has been correlated with serum leptin levels [29]. The lipotoxic effects of palmitate, highly enriched in diabetic epicardial fat, could increase serum soluble leptin receptor levels and consequently circulating leptin levels.

PTX3, a key component of innate and adaptive immune responses is upregulated in diabetic EAT, as only recently discovered [20]. However, the role of PTX3 in atherosclerosis is controversial, as recent observations suggested PTX3 may actually have cardiovascular protective functions. The upregulation of PTX3 in diabetic EAT may be an adaptive response to CAD.

Long intergenic nonprotein coding RNA 1348 (LINC01348) was upregulated in diabetic EAT, as only recently detected [20]. LINC01348 belongs to long noncoding RNAs (lncRNAs) genes. Although their function is unclear, lncRNAs can regulate gene expression at epigenetic, transcription, and posttranscription levels.

Epicardial fat fatty acid composition is also peculiar in patients with diabetes. Diabetic epicardial fat shows a significant increase in unsaturated fatty acids 12:0 and16:0 and a significant decrease in unsaturated fatty acid 20:4*n*–6 levels [14]. Epicardial fat in diabetic patients displays a significant decrease in palmitic acid (16:0) level and ω3 fatty acids (20:5*n*–3 and 22:6*n*–3) and their precursor, 18:2*n*–6, and increase in trans- and conjugated fatty acids that could contribute to the diabetic cardiomyopathy mediated by the excessive epicardial fat. Diabetic EAT atherogenicity is also linked to its elevated content of sphingolipids and ceramide [30]. The content of EAT sphingolipids (SPA, S1P, C14-Cer, C16-Cer, C18:1-Cer, C18-Cer, and C24:1-Cer) is higher in the obese diabetic comparing to the lean nondiabetic group. Total ceramide content was higher in both obese groups comparing to the lean nondiabetic group and was significant higher in the obese diabetic group as compare to the obese nondiabetic group ($p < 0.01$). All measured DAG species are higher in the EAT of obese diabetic subjects as compared to the lean nondiabetic subjects.

Epicardial Fat Downregulation in Advanced Coronary Artery Disease

Notably, a large number of genes and gene sets involved in housekeeping cellular functions are underrepresented in the EAT of CAD patients, suggesting a global downregulation of the tissue. These genes are related to a broad spectrum of cellular processes including intracellular trafficking, proliferation/transcription regulation, protein catabolism, innate immunity, and lectin pathway [3]. The EAT transcriptome is primarily characterized by markers of inflammation but goes into a relative state of cellular inactivity in subjects with CAD. The most downregulated gene in diabetic EAT was *LINC01105*, an ncRNA [20]. Adaptive, or better maladaptive, mechanisms of CAD progression might result in depletion of the EAT cellular activities. EAT could also encounter fibrotic and apoptotic changes in advanced stages of atherosclerosis and ischemic cardiomyopathies. The chronic hypoxia and unfavorable hemodynamic milieu can eventually affect the regulatory component of EAT proteasome. Future studies of EAT taken from individuals with variable stages of CAD, or in which samples are collected from the same individuals as disease progresses, would further clarify which transcriptional changes occur with disease progression aid in determining causation.

Clinical Role of Epicardial Fat in Coronary Artery Disease

In addition to the above-described complex and multifactorial causative mechanisms, epicardial fat plays a clinical role in the prediction, stratification and progression of coronary artery disease. The association between epicardial fat and CAD was investigated and confirmed in several large population studies. EAT, regardless whether it is measured as volume or thickness, is higher in patients with CAD as compared to individuals without atherosclerosis. Patients with a coronary artery calcium (CAC) score > 10 had significantly higher CT measured EAT volume than patients with calcium scores ≤10 [31]. In that early study by Djaberi et al., a cutoff EAT volume of 75 ml provided the sensitivity and specificity of 72% and 70%, respectively, to detect the presence of atherosclerosis [31]. CT measured pericoronary EAT thickness showed a graded relation with CAD and coronary calcification in healthy postmenopausal women and only in subjects with lower degree of obesity [32–33]. The suggestion that the relation of EAT and CAD is not simply explained by the concurrence of obesity, but rather by independent effects, was confirmed by echocardiographic studies [34]. In fact EAT thickness was significantly higher in CAD patients despite these subjects presented a significantly lower BMI than obese subjects [34]. The lack of a linear correlation between obesity, EAT, and CAD is also due to the fact that obesity is still defined by BMI categories that could not reflect body fat distribution, and discriminate between visceral and subcutaneous fat accumulation. Although, CT is the gold standard technique to measure EAT, echocardiography confirmed that epicardial fat was an independent factor of CAD [35–36].

The presence and amount of calcium within the coronary arteries have a great importance in the development of CAD. Imaging and quantification with coronary calcium score (CAC) is a milestone of the screening of CAD in asymptomatic, but potentially at high cardiovascular risk individuals. The interaction between EAT and CAC has been object of investigations, although results are not univocal. After adjusting for all considered confounders, an independent association with a CAC increase of 3.7% per additional 10 ml of EAT was detected in patients without known CAD [37]. EAT was associated with CAC score irrespective of body size, body fat, and cardiovascular risk factors in men but not in women in the EPICHEART study [38]. Subjects with more severe CAC had higher EAT volume than those with lower CC in the Heinz Nixdorf Recall cohort study [39]. Interestingly, the strongest association of EAT with CAC progression was found in younger individuals (<55 years old) and in those with lower BMI. These findings suggest that EAT is independent of obesity, at least as defined by BMI, and may promote early atherosclerosis development. The role of EAT in causing and predicting early atherosclerosis in high-risk subjects was also confirmed in other studies also including diabetic patients asymptomatic for CAD [40–41].

Of note, the correlation of epicardial fat with risk of CAD can also be independent of coronary calcification. A multivariate analysis showed that EAT volume as a predictor of the presence of an obstructive and a CT-derived vulnerable plaque in symptomatic patients with a zero-calcium score [42]. Higher EAT volume was associated with the presence of noncalcified vulnerable, unstable plaques (Fig. 8.4) [43, 44]. It is, therefore, plausible that EAT plays an earlier, and possibly independent of coronary calcium, role in promoting atherosclerotic plaque and plaques with high-risk

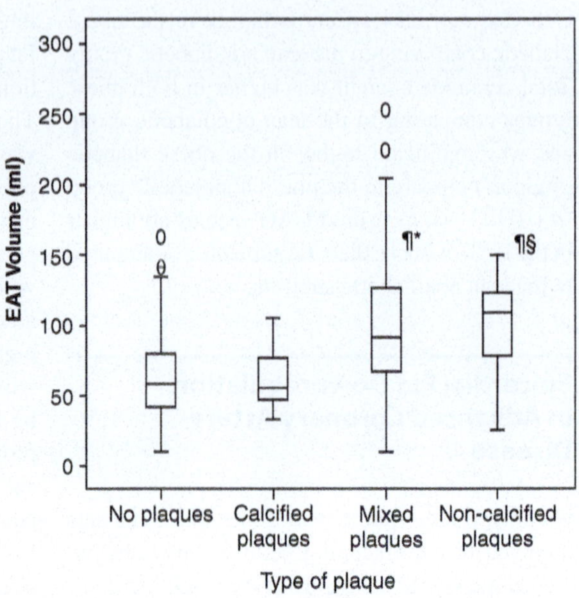

Fig. 8.4 Epicardial adipose tissue (EAT) volume is higher in non-calcified plaques indicating the atherosclerotic effect of EAT can be independent of coronary calcium content. (From Alexopoulos et al. [44], with permission from Elsevier)

features. The prevalence of obstructive plaques and MDCT-derived vulnerable features of coronary plaques were significantly elevated in patients with increased EAT [45]. The correlation of EAT with indices of microvascular dysfunction in the absence of obstructive plaques suggests the earlier atherogenic effect of this fat depot [46]. EAT may be linked to early plaque components or noncalcified plaque burden in the underlying coronary artery.

EAT is not equally distributed through the heart. The importance of regional EAT depots has only recently emerged. Pericoronary EAT has a direct effect on the proximal coronary arteries due to the anatomical proximity (Fig. 8.5). Unlike the echocardiography, computed tomography or MRI allows the detection and measurement of EAT in different locations. Pericoronary fat thickness correlates with stenotic coronary vessels and more severe CAC [33]. Another study showed that EAT thickness in the left atrioventricular groove, but not total EAT volume, was significantly associated with coronary atherosclerosis [47]. Regional epicardial fat rather than total volume was associated with active myocardial ischemia [48]. EAT inflammatory activity also differs with fat distribution. As extensively discussed, inflammation is a key component of both CAD and EAT. The dense EAT inflammatory infiltrate and secretosome leads to higher inflammation atheromatous plaques in underlying coronary vessels. This effect has been confirmed also clinically. 18F-fluoro-2-deoxyglucose positron emission tomography/computed tomography (18F-FDG PET/CT) studies showed that inflammatory activity of pericoronary adipose tissue was higher than any other EAT locations [49]. Pericoronary adipose tissue inflammation correlates also with the plaque burden and necrotic core component of coronary plaque [50].

More importantly, epicardial fat has shown not only to correlate with marker of atherosclerosis, but also to predict major cardiovascular events. CT measured EAT volume was prospectively evaluated in subjects with no history of CAD from the Heinz Nixdorf Recall cohort study [51]. The incidence of fatal or nonfatal coronary event significantly increased by quartile of EAT and

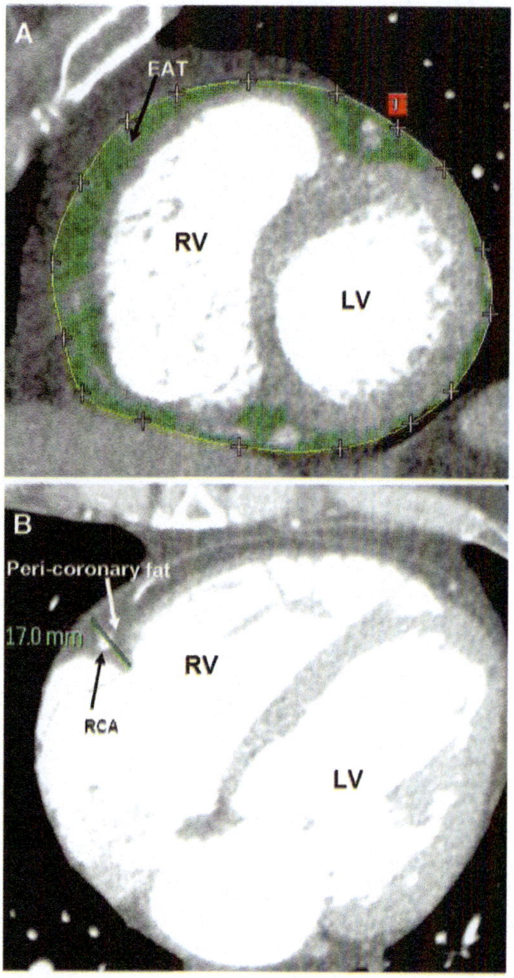

Fig. 8.5 Pericoronary epicardial adipose tissue (EAT) has a direct effect on the proximal coronary arteries due to the anatomical proximity. (**a**) Region of interest (*yellow*) on a cross-sectional image determines EAT area (*green*). (**b**) Pericoronary fat thickness (*green*). LV left ventricle, RCA right coronary artery, RV right ventricle. (From Gorter et al. [33], with permission from Elsevier)

remained significant even after adjustment for coronary calcium calcification (CAC) score [51]. More than 4000 patients were followed for 8.0 ± 1.5 years, and fatal or nonfatal coronary events occurred in 130 subjects. EAT volume was higher in subjects with events (121 ml vs. 95 ml, $p < 0.001$) [51] (Fig. 8.6). In the Heinz Nixdorf Recall cohort study, individuals in the highest quartile of EAT had a fivefold higher risk of new major coronary events compared with subjects in the lowest quartile (Fig. 8.7). The independent

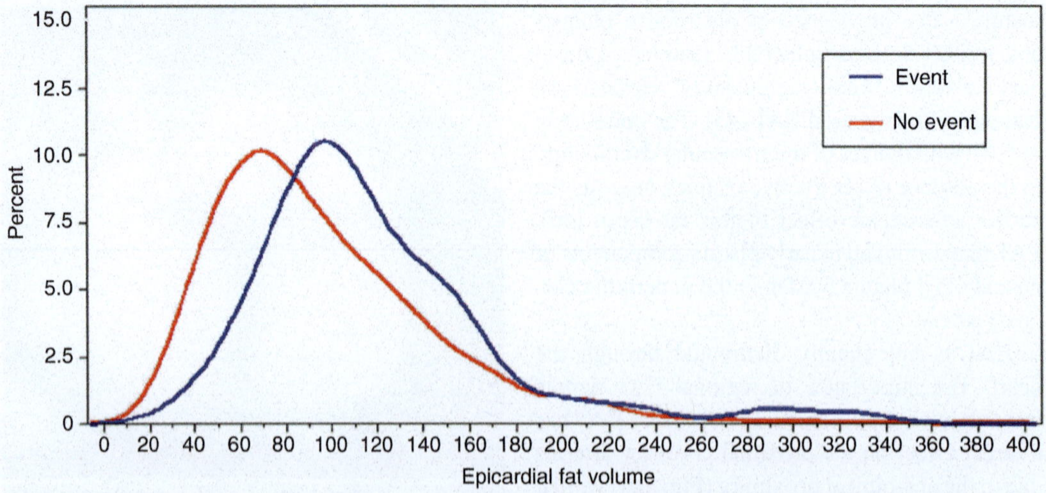

Fig. 8.6 Epicardial fat volume and incident coronary events. Smoothed kernel estimate for distribution of epicardial fat volume, stratified by incident coronary events. Epicardial fat volume was higher in subjects with events (121 ml vs. 95 ml, $p < 0.001$). (From Mahabadi et al. [51], with permission from Elsevier)

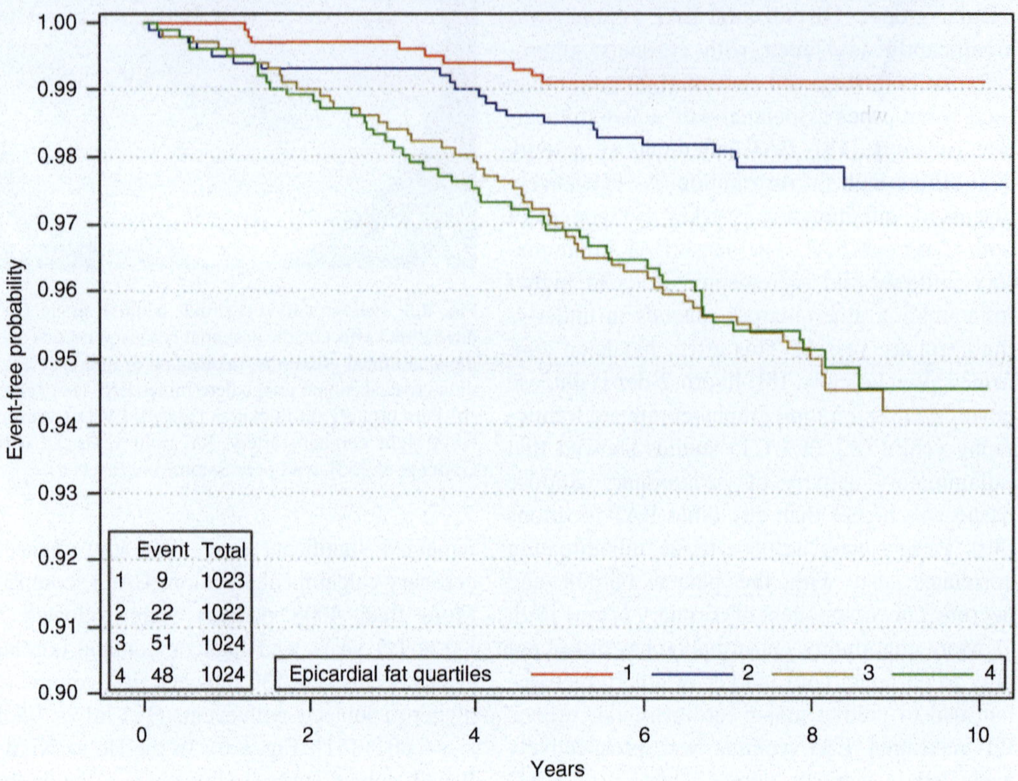

Fig. 8.7 Event-free survival by quartiles of epicardial fat. Kaplan-Meier curves for survival free of coronary events by quartiles of epicardial fat. Incident coronary events increased with the amount of epicardial adipose tissue (EAT), with subjects in the highest quartile of EAT having a fivefold higher risk compared with subjects in the lowest quartile. (From Mahabadi et al. [51], with permission from Elsevier)

correlation of EAT with major adverse cardiac event (MACE), defined as myocardial infarction or cardiovascular death, was confirmed by another study of 48-month follow-up [52]. The Multi-Ethnic Study of Atherosclerosis (MESA) and another large-size population study found that an independent relation of EAT with the incidence of acute coronary events [53–54]. EAT provides prognostic information and improves the prediction of first coronary events. EAT volume was greater in subjects with incident coronary heart disease. Remarkably, in the unadjusted analysis, a 1-SD increment in pericardial fat was associated with a 33% greater risk of developing incident coronary heart disease. MESA participants in the highest quartile of pericardial fat had more than double the risk of CAD than those in the lowest pericardial fat quartile. It is worthy to note that these large studies measured the fat depot within the pericardial sac, so inclusive of both pericardial and epicardial fats. However, MESA investigators measured EAT in a random sample of 159 participants and found a strong correlation between pericardial and epicardial fats [53].

Finally, whether EAT could be related signs and symptoms of CAD was investigated. Notably, epicardial fat was significantly correlated with chest pain, unstable angina and with coronary flow reserve [55–57]. Patients with acute coronary events have significantly higher EAT volume than patients with stable angina pectoris [55]. Of note, EAT volume was associated with lipid-rich plaque in patients with acute coronary syndrome, whereas no correlation between EFV and coronary plaque occurred in patients with stable angina [55].

While many studies clearly showed an association between EAT and CAD, some failed to demonstrate this relation. One study found no significant associations between EAT volume and CAC, severity of ≥50% stenosis by quantitative coronary angiography, or abnormal myocardial perfusion [58].

Impact of Epicardial Adipectomy on CAD

The question whether removing epicardial fat could benefit or even resolve CAD was tempting. One experimental study by McKenney-Drake et al. tried to address this challenging issue. In Ossabaw miniature swine, the selective surgical excision of adipose tissue in direct contiguity with one of the epicardial coronary arteries attenuated the progression of atherosclerosis [59]. This complex experimental study supports the hypothesis that cEAT could contribute to underlying coronary atherogenesis. However, results should be taken with caution, as several limitations can be identified. The findings may be applicable to the early stages of CAD because of the relatively young age of the animals, the short duration of atherogenic diet feeding, and the lack of observed flow-limiting coronary stenosis typical of advanced clinical disease. Also the obese pigs had substantially high LDL cholesterol levels (>500 m/dL). The authors initially suggested the potential mechanisms whereby selective EAT removal could attenuate the progression of CAD. The hypotheses include the (a) removal of pro-inflammatory and atherogenic factors secreted by cEAT that could contribute to atherogenesis by direct diffusion through the adventitia into the coronary intima-media and (b) the disruption of vasa vasorum in the adventitia and in the closely adjacent cEAT and, therefore, affect the vasocrine cross talk between EAT and the coronary arteries. However, the same authors performed another experiment in a different sample of female Ossabaw miniature swine [60]. In this study, they found that cEAT resection was not associated with a decrease in the inflammatory cytokines, whereas increased positive outward remodeling and arrest of atherogenesis could be the most putative mechanism. These hypotheses are intriguing, but they should be proven and confirmed in humans. Given the fact that EAT has also a physiological and cardioprotective role, the indications for its complete surgical removal are questionable. Pharmacological manipulation to restore EAT physiological function may be a more desirable strategy.

Conclusion

From the basic scientist perspective, EAT is clearly and independently associated with the coronary atherosclerosis. In addition to being an anatomically unique adipose depot, EAT demonstrates a transcriptome markedly pro-atherogenic and different from that of subcutaneous fat. The EAT transcriptome is highly enriched with genes encoding for inflammatory factors more actively involved in the early development of lipid-rich and noncalcified coronary plaque, rather than in the advanced and calcified atheroma. These findings provide the basis for new hypothesis generation in the understanding of the physiologic role of EAT and its pathophysiologic involvement in CAD. In the clinical setting, the incidence of MACE increases with higher EAT independently of coronary calcium calcification score and obesity. Clinical imaging of EAT provides important prognostic information and improves the prediction of first coronary events. Routine assessment of EAT could be implemented for a better prediction and stratification of CAD.

References

1. Iacobellis G. Local and systemic effects of the multifaceted epicardial adipose tissue depot. Nat Rev Endocrinol. 2015;11:363–71.
2. Mazurek T, Zhang L, Zalewski A, Mannion JD, Diehl JT, Arafat H, et al. Human epicardial adipose tissue is a source of inflammatory mediators. Circulation. 2003;108:2460–6.
3. McAninch EA, Fonseca TL, Poggioli R, Panos AL, Salerno TA, Deng Y, et al. Epicardial adipose tissue has a unique transcriptome modified in severe coronary artery disease. Obesity. 2015;23:1267–78.
4. Baker AR, Silva NF, Quinn DW, Harte AL, Pagano D, Bonser RS, et al. Human epicardial adipose tissue expresses a pathogenic profile of adipocytokines in patients with cardiovascular disease. Cardiovasc Diabetol. 2006;5:1.
5. Kremen J, Dolinkova M, Krajickova J, Blaha J, Anderlova K, Lacinova Z, et al. Increased subcutaneous and epicardial adipose tissue production of proinflammatory cytokines in cardiac surgery patients: possible role in postoperative insulin resistance. J Clin Endocrinol Metab. 2006;91:4620–7.
6. Cheng KH, Chu CS, Lee KT, Lin TH, Hsieh CC, Chiu CC, et al. Adipocytokines and proinflammatory mediators from abdominal and epicardial adipose tissue in patients with coronary artery disease. Int J Obes. 2008;32:268–74.
7. Mazurek T, Opolski G. Pericoronary adipose tissue: a novel therapeutic target in obesity-related coronary atherosclerosis. J Am Coll Nutr. 2015;34:244–54.
8. Sacks HS, Fain JN, Cheema P, Bahouth SW, Garrett E, Wolf RY, Wolford D, Samaha J. Depot-specific overexpression of proinflammatory, redox, endothelial cell, and angiogenic genes in epicardial fat adjacent to severe stable coronary atherosclerosis. Metab Syndr Relat Disord. 2011;9:433–9.
9. Hirata Y, Tabata M, Kurobe H, Motoki T, Akaike M, Nishio C, et al. Coronary atherosclerosis is associated with macrophage polarization in epicardial adipose tissue. J Am Coll Cardiol. 2011;58:248–55.
10. Hirata Y, Kurobe H, Akaike M, Chikugo F, Hori T, Bando Y, et al. Enhanced inflammation in epicardial fat in patients with coronary artery disease. Int Heart J. 2011;52:139–42.
11. Karastergiou K, Evans I, Ogston N, Miheisi N, Nair D, Kaski JC, et al. Epicardial adipokines in obesity and coronary artery disease induce atherogenic changes in monocytes and endothelial cells. Arterioscler Thromb Vasc Biol. 2010;30:1340–6.
12. Iacobellis G, Pistilli D, Gucciardo M, Leonetti F, Miraldi F, Brancaccio G, Gallo P, di Gioia CR. Adiponectin expression in human epicardial adipose tissue in vivo is lower in patients with CAD. Cytokine. 2005;29:251–5.
13. Baker AR, Harte AL, Howell N, Pritlove DC, Ranasinghe AM, da Silva NF, et al. Epicardial adipose tissue as a source of nuclear factor-kappaB and c-Jun N-terminal kinase mediated inflammation in patients with coronary artery disease. J Clin Endocrinol Metab. 2009;94:261–7.
14. Langheim S, Dreas L, Veschini L, Maisano F, Foglieni C, Ferrarello S, et al. Increased expression and secretion of resistin in epicardial adipose tissue of patients with acute coronary syndrome. Am J Physiol Heart Circ Physiol. 2010;298:H746–53.
15. Wang J, Jia Y, Wang L, Li D, Wang L, Zhu Y, Liu J, Gong J. Vasodilator-stimulated phosphoprotein: regulators of adipokines resistin and phenotype conversion of epicardial adipocytes. Med Sci Monit. 2018;24:6010–20.
16. Salgado-Somoza A, Teijeira-Fernández E, Fernández AL, González-Juanatey JR, Eiras S. Proteomic analysis of epicardial and subcutaneous adipose tissue reveals differences in proteins involved in oxidative stress. Am J Physiol Heart Circ Physiol. 2010;299:H202–9.
17. Gao X, Mi S, Zhang F, Gong F, Lai Y, Gao F, Zhang X, Wang L, Tao H. Association of chemerin mRNA expression in human epicardial adipose tissue with coronary atherosclerosis. Cardiovasc Diabetol. 2011;10:8.
18. Imoto-Tsubakimoto H, Takahashi T, Ueyama T, Ogata T, Adachi A, Nakanishi N, Mizushima K, Naito Y, Matsubara H. Serglycin is a novel adipocytokine highly expressed in epicardial adipose tissue. Biochem Biophys Res Commun. 2013;432:105–10.
19. Du Y, Ji Q, Cai L, Huang F, Lai Y, Liu Y, Yu J, Han B, Zhu E, Zhang J, Zhou Y, Wang Z, Zhao Y. Association between omentin-1 expression in human epicar-

dial adipose tissue and coronary atherosclerosis. Cardiovasc Diabetol. 2016;15:90.
20. Camarena V, Sant D, Mohseni M, Salerno T, Zaleski ML, Wang G, Iacobellis G. Novel atherogenic pathways from the differential transcriptome analysis of diabetic epicardial adipose tissue. Nutr Metab Cardiovasc Dis. 2017;27:739–50.
21. Dutour A, Achard V, Sell H, Naour N, Collart F, Gaborit B, et al. Secretory type II phospholipase A2 is produced and secreted by epicardial adipose tissue and overexpressed in patients with CAD. J Clin Endocrinol Metab. 2010;95:963–7.
22. Pezeshkian M, Mahtabipour MR. Epicardial and subcutaneous adipose tissue fatty acids profiles in diabetic and non-diabetic patients candidate for coronary artery bypass graft. Bioimpacts. 2013;3:83–9.
23. Nasarre L, Juan-Babot O, Gastelurrutia P, Llucia-Valldeperas A, Badimon L, Bayes-Genis A, Llorente-Cortés V. Low density lipoprotein receptor-related protein 1 is upregulated in epicardial fat from type 2 diabetes mellitus patients and correlates with glucose and triglyceride plasma levels. Acta Diabetol. 2014;51:23–30.
24. Marchington JM, Pond CM. Site-specific properties of pericardial and epicardial adipose tissue: the effects of insulin and high-fat feeding on lipogenesis and the incorporation of fatty acids in vitro. Int J Obes. 1990;14:1013–22.
25. Dozio E, Vianello E, Briganti S, Lamont J, Tacchini L, Schmitz G, Corsi Romanelli MM. Expression of the receptor for advanced glycation end products in epicardial fat: link with tissue thickness and local insulin resistance in coronary artery disease. J Diabetes Res. 2016;2016:2327341.
26. Agra RM, Fernández-Trasancos Á, Sierra J, González-Juanatey JR, Eiras S. Differential association of S100A9, an inflammatory marker, and p53, a cell cycle marker, expression with epicardial adipocyte size in patients with cardiovascular disease. Inflammation. 2014;37:1504–12.
27. Salgado-Somoza A, Teijeira-Fernández E, Rubio J, Couso E, González-Juanatey JR, Eiras S. Coronary artery disease is associated with higher epicardial retinol-binding protein 4 (RBP4) and lower glucose transporter (GLUT) 4 levels in epicardial and subcutaneous adipose tissue. Clin Endocrinol. 2012;76:51–8.
28. Iacobellis G, Diaz S, Mendez A, Goldberg R. Increased epicardial fat and plasma leptin in type 1 diabetes independently of obesity. Nutr Metab Cardiovasc Dis. 2014;24:725–9.
29. Kaneda H, Nakajima T, Haruyama A, Shibasaki I, Hasegawa T, Sawaguchi T, et al. Association of serum concentrations of irisin and the adipokines adiponectin and leptin with epicardial fat in cardiovascular surgery patients. PLoS One. 2018;13:e020149.
30. Błachnio-Zabielska AU, Baranowski M, Hirnle T, Zabielski P, Lewczuk A, Dmitruk I, Górski J. Increased bioactive lipids content in human subcutaneous and epicardial fat tissue correlates with insulin resistance. Lipids. 2012;47:1131–41.
31. Djaberi R, Schuijf JD, van Werkhoven JM, Nucifora G, Jukema JW, Bax JJ. Relation of epicardial adipose tissue to coronary atherosclerosis. Am J Cardiol. 2008;102:1602–7.
32. de Vos AM, Prokop M, Roos CJ, Meijs MF, van der Schouw YT, Rutten A. Peri-coronary epicardial adipose tissue is related to cardiovascular risk factors and coronary artery calcification in post-menopausal women. Eur Heart J. 2008;29:777–83.
33. Gorter PM, de Vos AM, van der Graaf Y, Stella PR, Doevendans PA, Meijs MF, et al. Relation of epicardial and pericoronary fat to coronary atherosclerosis and coronary artery calcium in patients undergoing coronary angiography. Am J Cardiol. 2008;102:380–5.
34. Iacobellis G, Lonn E, Lamy A, Singh N, Sharma AM. Epicardial fat thickness and CAD correlate independently of obesity. Int J Cardiol. 2011;146:452–4.
35. Ahn SG, Lim HS, Joe DY, Kang SJ, Choi BJ, Choi SY, Yoon MH, Hwang GS, Tahk SJ, Shin JH. Relationship of epicardial adipose tissue by echocardiography to coronary artery disease. Heart. 2008;94:e7.
36. Eroglu S, et al. Epicardial adipose tissue thickness by echocardiography is a marker for the presence and severity of CAD. Nutr Metab Cardiovasc Dis. 2009;19:211–7.
37. Bettencourt N, Toschke AM, Leite D, Rocha J, Carvalho M, Sampaio F, et al. Epicardial adipose tissue is an independent predictor of coronary atherosclerotic burden. Int J Cardiol. 2012;158:26–32.
38. Mancio J, Pinheiro M, Ferreira W, Carvalho M, Barros A, Ferreira N, et al. Gender differences in the association of epicardial adipose tissue and coronary artery calcification: EPICHEART study: EAT and coronary calcification by gender. Int J Cardiol. 2017;249:419–25.
39. Mahabadi AA, Lehmann N, Kälsch H, Robens T, Bauer M, Dykun I, et al. Association of epicardial adipose tissue with progression of coronary artery calcification is more pronounced in the early phase of atherosclerosis: results from the Heinz Nixdorf recall study. JACC Cardiovasc Imaging. 2014;7:909–16.
40. Yerramasu A, Dey D, Venuraju S, Anand DV, Atwal S, Corder R, et al. Increased volume of epicardial fat is an independent risk factor for accelerated progression of sub-clinical coronary atherosclerosis. Atherosclerosis. 2012;220:223–30.
41. Bachar GN, Dicker D, Kornowski R, Atar E. Epicardial adipose tissue as a predictor of coronary artery disease in asymptomatic subjects. Am J Cardiol. 2012;110:534–8.
42. Ito T, Suzuki Y, Ehara M, Matsuo H, Teramoto T, Terashima M, et al. Impact of epicardial fat volume on coronary artery disease in symptomatic patients with a zero calcium score. Int J Cardiol. 2013;167:2852–8.
43. Oka T, Yamamoto H, Ohashi N, Kitagawa T, Kunita E, Utsunomiya H, et al. Association between epicardial adipose tissue volume and characteristics of non-calcified plaques assessed by coronary computed tomographic angiography. Int J Cardiol. 2012;161:45–9.

44. Alexopoulos N, McLean DS, Janik M, Arepalli CD, Stillman AE, Raggi P. Epicardial adipose tissue and coronary artery plaque characteristics. Atherosclerosis. 2010;210:150–4.
45. Nakanishi K, Fukuda S, Tanaka A, Otsuka K, Jissho S, Taguchi H, et al. Persistent epicardial adipose tissue accumulation is associated with coronary plaque vulnerability and future acute coronary syndrome in non-obese subjects with coronary artery disease. Atherosclerosis. 2014;237:353–60.
46. Alam MS, Green R, de Kemp R, Beanlands RS, Chow BJ. Epicardial adipose tissue thickness as a predictor of impaired microvascular function in patients with non-obstructive coronary artery disease. J Nucl Cardiol. 2013;20:804–12.
47. Wang TD, Lee WJ, Shih FY, Huang CH, Chen WJ, Lee YT, et al. Association of epicardial adipose tissue with coronary atherosclerosis is region-specific and independent of conventional risk factors and intra-abdominal adiposity. Atherosclerosis. 2010;213:279–87.
48. Khawaja T, Greer C, Thadani SR, Kato TS, Bhatia K, Shimbo D, et al. Increased regional epicardial fat volume associated with reversible myocardial ischemia in patients with suspected coronary artery disease. J Nucl Cardiol. 2015;22:325–3.
49. Mazurek T, Kobylecka M, Zielenkiewicz M, Kurek A, Kochman J, Filipiak KJ, et al. PET/CT evaluation of 18F-FDG uptake in pericoronary adipose tissue in patients with stable coronary artery disease: independent predictor of atherosclerotic lesions' formation? J Nucl Cardiol. 2017;24:1075–84.
50. Mazurek T, Kochman J, Kobylecka M, Wilimski R, Filipiak KJ, Królicki L, et al. Inflammatory activity of pericoronary adipose tissue may affect plaque composition in patients with acute coronary syndrome without persistent ST-segment elevation: preliminary results. Kardiol Pol. 2014;72:410–6.
51. Mahabadi AA, Berg MH, Lehmann N, Kälsch H, Bauer M, Kara K, Dragano N, et al. Association of epicardial fat with cardiovascular risk factors and incident myocardial infarction in the general population: the Heinz Nixdorf Recall Study. J Am Coll Cardiol. 2013;61:1388–95.
52. Hajsadeghi F, Nabavi V, Bhandari A, Choi A, Vincent H, Flores F, et al. Increased epicardial adipose tissue is associated with coronary artery disease and major adverse cardiovascular events. Atherosclerosis. 2014;237:486–9.
53. Ding J, Hsu FC, Harris TB, Liu Y, Kritchevsky SB, Szklo M, et al. The association of pericardial fat with incident coronary heart disease: the Multi-Ethnic Study of Atherosclerosis (MESA). Am J Clin Nutr. 2009;90:499–504.
54. Cheng VY, Dey D, Tamarappoo B, Nakazato R, Gransar H, Miranda-Peats R, et al. Pericardial fat burden on ECG-gated noncontrast CT in asymptomatic patients who subsequently experience adverse cardiovascular events. JACC Cardiovasc Imaging. 2010;3:352–60.
55. Harada K, Harada K, Uetani T, Kataoka T, Takeshita M, Kunimura A, et al. The different association of epicardial fat with coronary plaque in patients with acute coronary syndrome and patients with stable angina pectoris: analysis using integrated backscatter intravascular ultrasound. Atherosclerosis. 2014;236:301–6.
56. Picard FA, Gueret P, Laissy JP, Champagne S, Leclercq F, Carrié D, et al. Epicardial adipose tissue thickness correlates with the presence and severity of angiographic coronary artery disease in stable patients with chest pain. PLoS One. 2014;9:e110005.
57. Sade LE, Eroglu S, Bozbaş H, Ozbiçer S, Hayran M, Haberal A, et al. Relation between epicardial fat thickness and coronary flow reserve in women with chest pain and angiographically normal coronary arteries. Atherosclerosis. 2009;204:580–5.
58. Tanami Y, Jinzaki M, Kishi S, Matheson M, Vavere AL, Rochitte CE, et al. Lack of association between epicardial fat volume and extent of coronary artery calcification, severity of coronary artery disease, or presence of myocardial perfusion abnormalities in a diverse, symptomatic patient population: results from the CORE320 multicenter study. Circ Cardiovasc Imaging. 2015;8:e002676.
59. McKenney ML, Schultz KA, Boyd JH, Byrd JP, Alloosh M, Teague SD, et al. Epicardial adipose excision slows the progression of porcine coronary atherosclerosis. J Cardiothorac Surg. 2014;9:2.
60. McKenney-Drake ML, Rodenbeck SD, Bruning RS, Kole A, Yancey KW, Alloosh M, et al. Epicardial adipose tissue removal potentiates outward remodeling and arrests coronary Atherogenesis. Ann Thorac Surg. 2017;103:1622–30.

Perivascular Adipose Tissue and Atherosclerosis

9

Christos P. Kotanidis
and Charalambos Antoniades

Key Points

- Perivascular adipose tissue (PVAT) is a diverse structure surrounding the human vessels, with a highly diverse secretome, including adipokines, cytokines, gaseous messengers, and miRNAs, among others, and is implicated in a bi-directional interplay with the adjacent vascular wall, affecting and being affected by aspects of its biology, mainly vascular inflammation.
- Coronary inflammation, a key component of atherosclerosis, induces molecular, transcriptional and structural changes to PVAT, which alter PVAT's phenotype, creating concentric three-dimensional gradients characterized by small adipocytes with low lipid content, interstitial space expansion, edema, fibrosis and neovascularization, around inflamed vessels.
- PVAT phenotypic changes can be tracked non-invasively utilizing imaging techniques that capture three-dimensional attenuation and texture changes in the visualized adipose tissue and that have important implications in cardiovascular disease diagnosis and prognosis. The Fat Attenuation Index (FAI), an artificial-intelligence enhanced biomarker, captures weighted attenuation gradients in the perivascular space inherent to coronary inflammation, providing an excellent surrogate of both baseline inflammatory burden in the vasculature as well as localized inflammation around the vulnerable plaque. Fat radiomic profiling has also emerged as another promising marker for non-invasively describing permanent structural changes in PVAT that arise from direct inflammation aftereffects, such as fibrosis and neovascularization.

C. P. Kotanidis
Division of Cardiovascular Medicine, Radcliffe Department of Medicine, University of Oxford, Oxford, UK

C. Antoniades (✉)
Division of Cardiovascular Medicine, Radcliffe Department of Medicine, University of Oxford, Oxford, UK

Oxford Academic Cardiovascular CT Core Laboratory, John Radcliffe Hospital, Headley Way, Oxford, UK
e-mail: charalambos.antoniades@cardiov.ox.ac.uk

G. Iacobellis (ed.), *Epicardial Adipose Tissue*, Contemporary Cardiology,
https://doi.org/10.1007/978-3-030-40570-0_9

Introduction

Perivascular adipose tissue is a metabolically active and dynamic structure surrounding most vessels in the human body. It comprises adipocytes, nerves, microvasculatvvure, stem cells, and inflammatory cells. Its close proximity to the vascular wall, being a natural continuation of the vascular adventitia, allows a continuous crosstalk, which has been highlighted recently as an important factor in the pathogenesis and natural course of a range of pathologies [1]. Despite being regarded until recently as simply a structural unit providing mechanical support to the vasculature, its role as modulator of vascular biology is gaining attention, especially in the case of vascular inflammation and coronary artery disease [2].

Coronary artery disease (CAD) continues to claim a spot at the top of the table with leading causes of death in the western world, as demonstrated by the World Health Organization's (WHO) most recent report [3]. Being responsible for 1 in 7 deaths in the USA, killing over 366,800 people a year, it is a major contributor to the ever-increasing medical costs associated with its management, which are projected to amount to $1.1 trillion by 2035 [4]. Despite the fact that mortality rates have seen major declines during recent years compared to past decades, reflecting advances made in primary and secondary prevention [5], the disease remains a significant mortality contributor, and the so-called residual cardiovascular risk persists [6]. Indeed, residual cardiovascular risk has been proposed as a promising target in many large clinical trials utilizing novel, effective but at the same time costly therapies, such as anti-PCSK9 monoclonal antibodies [7] or antibodies targeting chemokines [8]. These therapeutic agents have proven to be rather robust and promising, successfully reducing the global inflammatory burden in patients at high cardiovascular risk; however, their high cost hinders the clinical adaptation by healthcare systems, highlighting the imperative need for early and accurate detection of the target populations [9]. As we move further into the era of personalized medicine, the development and deployment of new "companion diagnostics," will enable the detection of the true "vulnerable patient," meaning the patient that is indeed at the greatest risk and will therefore benefit the most out of these new and expensive therapeutics. These applications will revolutionize the prevention of development of clinical cardiovascular disease, including ischemic heart disease, and at the same time prevent the use of unnecessary invasive therapy in patients with severe but stable CAD, who may mistakenly be considered "vulnerable" under current traditional diagnostics.

This chapter elaborates on the biology of perivascular adipose tissue (PVAT) and its contribution to atherosclerosis, with a special focus on its bidirectional interplay with the vascular wall, and how imaging of perivascular fat can be a window to vascular inflammation and a promising marker of cardiovascular disease with diagnostic and prognostic value.

Atherogenesis and Inflammation

Inflammation is a key player in the natural history of atherogenesis, especially the development of the vulnerable atherosclerotic plaque [10]. The links between inflammatory processes and atherosclerosis are well established, with both innate and adaptive immunity involved in a complex network of molecular and cellular interactions [11, 12]. Components of the innate arm of immunity can be triggered by pathogens in a non-specific manner, leading to the activation of mast cells, neutrophils, macrophages (respiratory burst), and the complement [13]. At the same time, antigen-presenting cells are activated by toll-like receptors (TLRs), leading to pro-inflammatory signaling responses, and cross-linking with adaptive immunity, which is highly organized and more relevant to atherogenesis. T-cell activation, antibody production, and secretion of a range of pro-inflammatory cytokines, such as IFN-γ, IL-1, IL-6, are all responses related to the state of systemic low-grade inflammation inherent to atherosclerosis. This state still accounts for residual risk for cardiovascular events in the population [14].

Low-grade inflammation is induced by the release of pro-inflammatory cytokines that lead to endothelial dysfunction, depletion of nitric oxide bioavailability, and accumulation of cell adhesion molecules to the vascular bed, which attract circulating leukocytes into the arterial intima [15]. Reactive oxygen species produced in the sub-endothelial space, as part of the localized inflammatory cascade, oxidize LDL, which is taken up by macrophages, turning them into foam cells and initiating plaque development [16]. Activated T-lymphocytes are brought into action, while vascular smooth muscle cells (VSMCs) exhibit an increase in proliferation and migration, reaching the intima and differentiating into osteoblasts, contributing to the local deposition of calcium and overall stabilization of the plaque [17]. Nevertheless, perpetuating excess local inflammation and sheer stress induce metalloproteinases and lead to extracellular matrix degradation, remodeling, and ultimately destabilization of the plaque, resulting in fissures, erosion, rupture, occlusive thrombosis, and fatal complications [15, 16].

The inflammatory hypothesis in atherosclerosis development and progression has ignited the search for inflammation markers used as surrogate markers of presence and prognosis of cardiovascular disease. Systemic indices, mainly high sensitivity C-reactive protein (hsCRP) and proinflammatory cytokines in the plasma, have been associated with cardiovascular risk prediction, beyond traditional cardiovascular risk factors, supporting the concept of residual inflammatory risk [18]. This hypothesis became ever more prominent when large trials such as the JUPITER and CANTOS trials were reported. JUPITER [19] showcased a reduction in cardiovascular risk in individuals with elevated hsCRP following treatment with the statin rosuvastatin. However, the full extent of rosuvastatin's pleiotropic anti-inflammatory effects was not fully documented, as LDL levels were also reduced in line with the risk reduction observed, obscuring the true size effect. More recently, the CANTOS trial [8] reported for the first time in humans that targeting IL-1β using the monoclonal antibody canakinumab reduces the risk for cardiovascular events. However, fatal infections and sepsis were observed more frequently in the treatment group, raising safety concerns regarding the targeting of central key players of innate immunity. Importantly, inflammation should not be perceived as a singular therapeutic target, but rather as a spectrum of signaling pathways, each one constituting a singular target with variant therapeutic potential. This remark was underlined by the Cardiovascular Inflammation Reduction Trial (CIRT) [20], in which low-dose methotrexate failed to reduce events versus placebo as well as by a post-hoc analysis of the CANTOS trial data which showed that substantial residual inflammatory risk related to both IL-18 and IL-6 remains after IL-1β inhibition with canakinumab [21]. It is consequently evident that, despite its well-established connection with vascular disease pathogenesis, inflammation needs to be further studied, both as a marker aiding the selection of the vulnerable patient, who would benefit the most from novel expensive therapies, and at the same time as a consistent therapeutic target [22]. Circulating biomarkers, like hsCRP or IL6, have excellent capacity in detecting systemic inflammation but are often driven by other systemic (obesity, diabetes, cancer) or local inflammatory conditions (arthritis, infection) that usually co-exist with coronary inflammation. Therefore, unveiling the role of inflammation in atherogenesis to its full extent, both from a diagnostic as well as a therapeutic point of view, is of key importance. Studying in particular the localized inflammation-induced changes in the human arteries as well as in their perivascular space, may lead to the development of new, local biomarkers of inflammation, driving restratification protocols and revolutionizing the management of CAD. Perivascular adipose tissue – its biology and imaging – has recently emerged as a promising player, projected to provide reliable and promising insight into the detection of vascular inflammation, in a localized and specific manner.

Defining Perivascular Adipose Tissue

Adiposity in the human body is distributed anatomically into two major compartments, subcutaneous fat (SAT) and visceral fat (VAT). In terms of functionality, adipose tissue can be categorized into three depots: white, brown, and "beige" or "brite" [23]. White adipose tissue acts mainly as metabolic energy storage, brown adipose tissue is primarily tasked with non-shivering thermogenesis, whereas the term "beige" refers to brown-like adipocytes inside white adipose tissue that present the ability to produce heat via uncoupling of mitochondrial respiration [24].

The term epicardial adipose tissue (EAT) refers to white adipose tissue located between the myocardium and the visceral layer of the pericardium. It differs embryologically from pericardial (or paracardial) fat, which is the part of intrathoracic visceral adipose tissue attached to the outside of the parietal layer of the pericardium [25]. EAT derives from the splachnopleuric mesoderm, as does the heart, and is supplied with blood by the coronary circulation [26]. On the other hand, intrathoracic VAT originates from the primitive thoracic mesenchyme and is vascularized by non-coronary arteries [25]. In addition, EAT differs greatly from VAT and SAT at a functional level. Low expression levels of adiponectin and high levels of IL-6 and C-C motif chemokine ligand 2 (CCL2) have been associated with higher infiltration of macrophages in coronary artery disease and also linked to other phenotypes such as hypertension [27]. Furthermore, macroscopic measures of EAT, such as thickness and volume, are considered surrogates for metabolically unhealthy obesity and have been used for cardiovascular risk stratification [28].

The need for a separate and clear definition for adipose tissue around the human arteries originated from the observation that the part of EAT in close proximity to the coronary arteries has different morphological and functional characteristics compared to the rest of the depot [29]. In bulk literature, PVAT is vaguely defined as adipose tissue surrounding the blood vessels. However, recently a series of experiments examining the molecular phenotype of pericoronary fat at increasing distances from the coronary artery wall revealed regional variability, resulting from complex, paracrine vessel–PVAT interactions [29]. This led to the proposal of a new robust definition of pericoronary fat – and by extension PVAT in general – as any adipose tissue located within a radial distance from the outer vessel wall equal to the whole vessel diameter of the adjacent coronary artery [29]. This definition highlights the importance of biology, as opposed to crude anatomical borders, in defining distinct fat depots and has the potential to address the contradicting variable definitions of PVAT that have appeared in literature so far (Fig. 9.1).

Perivascular adipose tissue (PVAT) is a highly dynamic and metabolically active tissue surrounding most vascular beds in the human body, except for neural and pulmonary vasculature [30]. In large vessels, PVAT is contiguous with the adventitial layer, whereas in small vessels and microvessels, PVAT adipocytes are an integral part of the vascular wall itself [31]. Typically, healthy PVAT comprises adipocytes, microvasculature, nerves, stem cells, and inflammatory cells, although the exact phenotype depends on anatomical location and will vary significantly with pathogenesis [32]. Also, despite containing predominantly WAT, it has been reported to exert BAT thermogenic capabilities after exposure to cold [31].

PVAT Effects on the Vascular Wall – Outside to Inside Signaling

Adipose tissue produces a wide variety of bioactive molecules, including adipokines (such as adiponectin, leptin, apelin) and inflammatory cytokines, jointly referred to as adipocytokines. A summary of the main roles and clinical relevance of the key adipocytokines secreted by PVAT can be found in Table 9.1. PVAT further secrets micro-RNAs, microvesicles, inorganic molecules such as hydrogen sulfide, reactive oxygen species, fatty acid metabolites, and others (Fig. 9.2). Products from remote depots, such as the subcutaneous adipose tissue, act on distant sites of the cardiovascular system in an endocrine manner, after being released into the bloodstream through the adipose tissue microvessels [23]. Perivascular fat, on the other hand, can utilize other, more direct routes, so as to affect vascular biology. Given its close anatomical affinity with vessels, PVAT has the unique ability to exert

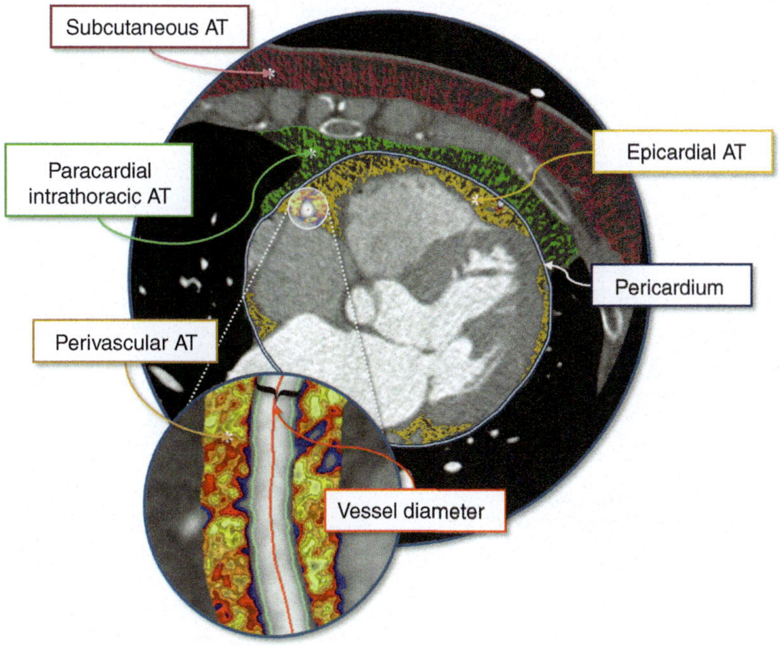

Fig. 9.1 Defining distinct adipose tissue depots. Axial cross-sectional slice of a coronary CTA, depicting the distinct adipose tissue (AT) depots within the thorax. Adiposity in the human body is distributed anatomically into two major compartments, subcutaneous fat (SAT) and visceral fat (VAT). VAT within the thoracic cavity can be further divided into paracardial or pericardial fat, which is the part of intrathoracic visceral adipose tissue located outside of the parietal layer of the pericardium, and epicardial fat which is located between the myocardium and the visceral layer of the pericardium. PVAT is defined as any adipose tissue located within a radial distance from the outer vessel wall equal to the whole vessel diameter of the adjacent coronary artery. (CTA computed tomography angiography, PVAT perivascular adipose tissue)

direct effects on the adjacent vascular wall through the paracrine release of bioactive mediators. Furthermore, PVAT is implicated in a third form of signaling, vasocrine signaling, in which PVAT-derived adipokines can travel through the underlying vascular wall and reach the lumen, thereby being able to circulate in downstream microcirculation and potentially act upon entire vascular beds [33].

Regardless of the route they employ, adipose tissue-derived products influence many aspects of vascular biology, including vascular tone, inflammation, vascular smooth muscle cell migration, endothelial function, and vascular redox state [34, 35]. It has been shown that the secretome of PVAT contains anti-inflammatory and antioxidant components, and it may host defense mechanisms for the vascular wall [36, 37]. Adiponectin induces 5′-AMP-activated protein kinase (AMPK) or RACα serine/threonine-protein kinase (AKT)-mediated endothelial nitric oxide synthase (eNOS) phosphorylation acting as a vasorelaxant [34]. Hydrogen sulfide (H_2S) and palmitic acid methyl ester also influence vascular tone, by activating ATP-regulated and voltage-gated potassium channels, respectively [38, 39]. PVAT also regulates angiotensinogen expression and the ensuing increase in angiotensin II, which acts on smooth muscle cells in the vessel walls to regulate vasoactivity and blood pressure in a circadian fashion, through the production of the aryl hydrocarbon receptor nuclear translocator-like protein 1 (known as BMAL1) in brown adipocytes [40]. The anti-contractile effects of PVAT include also the uptake and metabolism of vasoactive amines, such as norepinephrine [41], whereas the gaseous messenger nitric oxide (NO), which is produced by adipocyte or macrophage NOS, exerts paracrine anti-inflammatory effects [42]. Finally, adipokines adiponectin and

Table 9.1 Summary of key adipokines secreted by perivascular adipose tissue (PVAT)

Adipokine	Producing cells	Vasoconstrictor or vasodilator	Pro- or anti-inflammatory	Other biological roles	Clinical relevance
Adiponectin	Adipocytes	Vasodilator	Anti-	Improves insulin sensitivity Increases glucose uptake Normalizes BP in obese mice	*Normal subjects:* Low plasma levels reflect high CAD risk; gene polymorphisms associated with CAD *Advanced CAD subjects:* High plasma levels predict adverse outcomes
Leptin	Adipocytes	Vasodilator	Pro-	Deficiency/resistance associated with hypertension and IR Energy storage regulation	Polymorphisms in its gene and receptors inked to obesity and CVD
Apelin	Adipocytes	Unclear (vasodilator in small arteries/vasoconstrictor in vein)	Anti-	Apelin-13 increases BP Apelin-12 and apelin-17 reduce BP Increases glucose utilization	Upregulated as a compensatory mechanism in early heart failure
Visfatin	Stromal cells	Vasoconstrictor	Pro-	Insulin mimetic in cultured human osteoblasts	Elevated plasma levels in hypertension Obesity alters production patterns Circulating visfatin is enhanced in many cancers
Omentin	Adipocytes	Vasodilator	Anti-	Antioxidant Reduces BP Enhances insulin-mediated glucose uptake	Plasma levels associated with favorable CVD outcomes
Resistin	Monocytes/ macrophages	Vasoconstrictor	Pro-	Pro-oxidant Pro-atherogenic Impairs insulin-stimulated glucose transport	Elevated in human hypertensive patients
Palmitic acid methyl ester	Adipocytes	Vasodilator	Pro-	Reduces glucose transport	Obesity associated with decreased expression
Angiotensin-(1–7)	Adipocytes produce ACE2	Vasodilator	Anti-	Component of RAAS Enhances insulin signaling pathway	Angiotensin-(1–7) stimulates brown adipose tissue and reduces diet-induced obesity

Chemerin	Adipocytes	Vasoconstrictor	Pro-	Reduces glucose uptake and insulin secretion Chronic treatment of mice with chemerin increases BP	Circulating chemerin is increased in psoriasis, obesity, type 2 diabetes, metabolic syndrome, and CAD. Chemerin is associated with endothelial activation and atherosclerosis in rheumatoid arthritis
TNFa	Monocytes/ macrophages	Unclear	Pro-	Inflammatory cascade Pro-oxidant	Global inflammation marker No specificity for CVD
IL-6	Monocytes/ macrophages	Vasodilator (as part of inflammatory response)	Pro-	Inflammatory cascade Pro-oxidant	Key component of low-grade inflammation inherent to CVD
Endothelin-1	All types	Vasoconstrictor	Pro-	Pro-oxidant	Its implication in the pathogenesis of CVD is established

BP blood pressure, *CAD* coronary artery disease, *CVD* cardiovascular disease, *IR* insulin resistance, *RAAS* renin-angiotensin-aldosterone system, *TNFa* tumor necrosis factor alpha, *IL-6* interleukin 6, *ACE2* angiotensin-converting enzyme 2

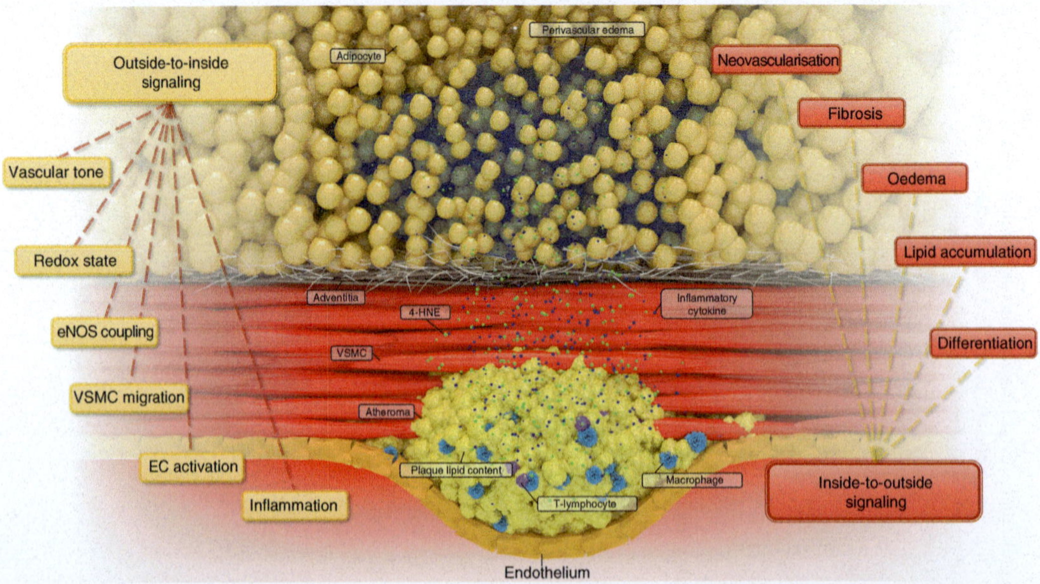

Fig. 9.2 Illustration of the major components of the bidirectional interplay between the vascular wall and fat in the perivascular space. Perivascular adipose tissue (PVAT) is involved in a crosstalk with the vascular wall. Outside to inside signals, including hormones (adiponectin, visfatin, leptin, apelin, etc.), cytokines (IL-6, TNFa, etc.), gaseous messengers (hydrogen sulfide and nitric oxide), fatty acids, reactive oxygen species, microRNAs, and other molecules, are implicated in the regulation of vascular tone, vascular smooth muscle cell (VSMC) migration, regional redox state (NADPH oxidase (NOX) activity and endothelial nitric oxide synthase (eNOS) coupling status), inflammation (M1–M2 macrophage polarization), and local endothelial cell (EC) activation. Inside to outside signals, including components of vascular inflammation (such as pro-inflammatory cytokines), can in turn affect PVAT biology, and more specifically lead to increased edema and decreased adipocyte size, differentiation and lipid accumulation, fibrosis, and neovascularization. Conversely, vascular oxidative stress products, such as 4-hydroxynonenal (4-HNE), upregulate adiponectin's ADIPOQ gene in PVAT via a peroxisome proliferator-activated receptor-γ (PPARγ)-dependent mechanism allowing it to exert its beneficiary antioxidant and vasoprotective effects

omentin act as antioxidants by inhibiting the activity of the NOX1 and NOX2 isoforms of NADPH oxidase in the vascular wall, by preventing the activation and membrane translocation of RAC1 and by downregulating the p22phox (also known as CYBA) regulatory protein, consequently reducing superoxide production [43].

On the other hand, PVAT may also contribute to inflammatory processes. Pro-oxidant adipokines such as leptin and resistin promote activation of NADPH oxidase isoforms and lead to increased vascular oxidative stress, which is a key contributor of vascular inflammation and has been linked with senescence and adverse clinical outcomes [37]. eNOS coupling status may also be modulated by adipose tissue, leading either to the beneficiary production of NO or to the damaging production of superoxide; chemerin in particular reduces the bioavailability of the enzyme's cofactor tetrahydrobiopterin (BH4) promoting the enzyme's uncoupling and decreasing nitric oxide (NO) production in favor of superoxide [36, 44]. Vascular inflammation can be promoted further by expression of endothelial cell adhesion molecules, which is induced by adipokines such as visfatin and adipose tissue-derived pro-inflammatory cytokines such as IL-1β and tumor necrosis factor (TNF) [23]. The nuclear factor-κB pathway is yet again implicated as a central signaling pathway exerting a critical role in orchestrating the wide range of pro-atherogenic effects from the PVAT to the vascular wall [45]. Moreover, the migration of inflammatory cells into the adventitia promotes the deposit of collagen and leads to localized upregulation of inflammatory chemokines, TGF-β-dependent differentiation of fibroblasts to migratory myofibroblasts, and increased vasa vasorum neovascularization [46]. Also, we have recently shown that WNT5A, a wingless-related integration site (WNT) signaling pathway molecule, secreted by PVAT is implicated in vascular redox signaling in obesity. Circulating WNT5A is increased in obese individuals, who also present with increased release of WNT5A from PVAT and upregulation of WNT5A receptors in the arterial wall. These receptors increase arterial sensitivity to the non-canonical WNT signaling pathway and enhance arterial NADPH oxidase activity, increasing superoxide generation and inducing endothelial dysfunction and eNOS uncoupling (Fig. 9.3) [47].

In addition, microRNAs, which comprise a vast spectrum of small RNA molecules involved in post-transcriptional regulation, are also produced by PVAT. MicroRNAs have been implicated in several processes, ranging from the recruitment of inflammatory cells to adipose tissue browning, myocardial fibrosis, atherosclerosis, and vascular smooth muscle cell activation, and their profile changes in response to obesity, insulin resistance, and coronary artery disease [48]. Furthermore, PVAT-derived exosomes have been shown to promote M1 pro-inflammatory polarization of macrophages and to accelerate atherosclerosis in

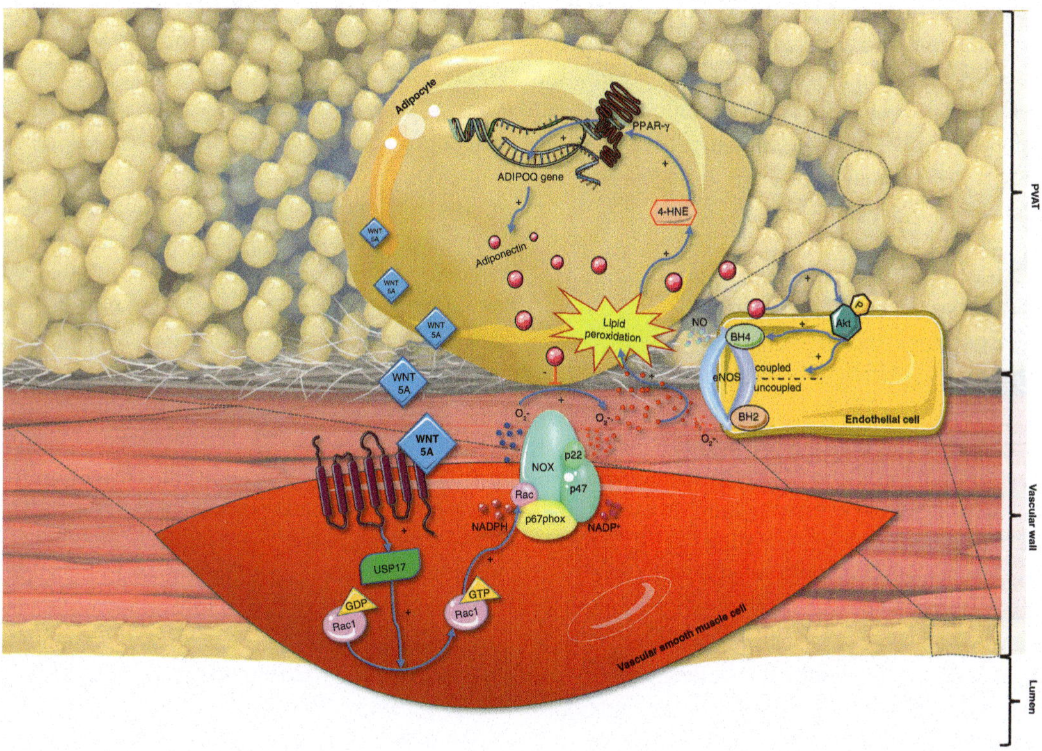

Fig. 9.3 The adiponectin and WNT5A paradigms of PVAT and vascular wall interactions. WNT5A is released from PVAT and binds to Frizzled receptors on the arterial wall, activating the non-canonical WNT signaling pathway. This leads to a USP17/RAC1-mediated increase in NADPH oxidase activity and superoxide generation and induces endothelial dysfunction via eNOS uncoupling. Enhanced production of superoxide leads to increased local production of lipid peroxidation products such as 4-HNE, which are able to diffuse to PVAT and upregulate adiponectin's ADIPOQ gene expression via a PPARγ-mediated mechanism, that leads to adiponectin secretion. Adiponectin, in turn, secreted by PVAT, exerts antioxidant and vasoprotective roles in the adjacent vasculature by inhibiting the activity of NADPH-oxidases as well as through Akt-mediated stimulation of eNOS activity and coupling, resulting in increased production of NO. (PVAT perivascular adipose tissue, NADPH nicotinamide adenine dinucleotide phosphate, eNOS endothelial nitric oxide synthase, BH4 tetrahydrobiopterin, BH2 dihydrobiopterin, NO nitric oxide, O_2^- superoxide, 4HNE 4-hydroxynonenal, PPARγ peroxisome proliferator-activated receptor gamma, ADIPOQ adiponectin)

ApoE−/− mice [49]. The differential regulation of adipose tissue-derived exosomes and microRNAs in obesity and diabetes mellitus, as well as the proven effects of weight loss and exercise on the levels of specific micro-RNAs in the adipose tissue, has highlighted microRNAs as potential therapeutic targets in obesity-related CVD.

Finally, the immunologic state of adipose tissue, mainly macrophage infiltration and polarization, is described as a crucial regulator of its function, as PVAT inflammation, through the release of a range of cytokines and chemokines, is associated with vascular dysfunction [50]. It is becoming evident that adipose tissue, with its highly diverse secretome, can be critical to both health and disease. PVAT exerts anti-contractile, anti-inflammatory, and antioxidant effects to the adjacent vasculature, while at the same time retaining the ability to undergo remodeling, and adapt an inflamed, pro-oxidant profile, shifting its phenotype from protective to detrimental for the vessels [24].

Adipose Tissue Remodeling in Response to Signals Form the Circulation

Shifts in adipose tissue phenotype and biology are observed in the presence of cardiometabolic disease, including obesity, insulin resistance, diabetes mellitus, and inflammation [51]. The nature of these changes dictates whether adiposity will exert protective or adverse effects in the course of cardiovascular disease pathogenesis. Obesity is characterized by excessive calorie uptake, in response to which the adipose tissue undergoes an increase in adipocytes number (hyperplasia) and/or size (hypertrophy) [52]. Pre-adipocytes are mobilized and differentiated into mature adipocytes as part of a traditionally considered healthy mechanism of adipose tissue expansion, whereas at the same time hypertrophy causes adipocytes to acquire a more dysfunctional, lipid-laden phenotype in the setting of adipose tissue inflammation [53]. The latter happens in many chronic diseases such as obesity, diabetes mellitus, and atherosclerosis, where the adipose tissue is infiltrated by increasing populations of inflammatory cells, such as lymphocytes (including T helper 1 (TH1) cells and B cells), neutrophils, macrophages, and mast cells, whereas the population of eosinophils, TH2 cells, and regulatory T cells remains unchanged or reduces [53]. This balance between the different types of inflammatory cells and immune responses affects also macrophage polarization, with TH2 cytokines promoting the M2 anti-inflammatory macrophage phenotype, while the dominant production of TH1 cytokines (mainly IFNγ) shifts the macrophage phenotype toward the M1 pro-inflammatory type [54]. The M1 phenotype is also involved in localized neoangiogenesis through secretion of platelet-derived growth factor-β, which activates pericytes [55].

Dysfunction of the expanded adipose tissue in obesity is further characterized by endothelial cell activation with increased expression of adhesion molecules (*P*-selectin and *E*-selectin) that promote inflammatory cell infiltration, and vasomotor dysfunction of the vasculature, resulting in capillary rarefaction. The reduced delivery of nutrients and oxygen to the adipose tissue creates a hypoxic microenvironment that triggers adipose tissue fibrosis, through increased expression of the hypoxia-inducible factor 1α, and eventually promotes further its dysfunction and insulin resistance [56, 57]. In addition, the escape of chyle from lymphatic vessels into the dysfunctional adipose tissue has been implicated in its phenotypic shifts. Lipids are known to be adipogenic and the leakage of lipid-rich lymph in visceral adipose tissue has been shown to stimulate adipose tissue hypertrophy and ectopic adipose tissue expansion [58].

Metabolic disease may also alter adipose tissue qualitative composition between the relatively protective BAT and beige adipose tissue phenotypes and the deleterious WAT phenotype. BAT is characterized by increased metabolic activity, thermogenic capacity, and the release of BAT-specific adipokines, which exert beneficial autocrine, paracrine, and endocrine effects on peripheral tissues, including the cardiovascular system [59]. Obesity is associated with lower BAT volumes [60]. Beiging of WAT – characterized by increased expression of mitochondrial brown fat uncoupling protein 1 (UCP1) in adipocytes – is associated with weight loss and improved insulin resistance, whereas its downregulation in human epicardial adipose tissue leads to increased adipose tissue oxidative stress and dysfunction [61].

Finally, the secretome of adipose tissue is another factor undergoing changes in response to signals from the periphery. Obesity, insulin resistance, and diabetes mellitus are linked to a secretory and biochemical profile, consistent with a shift toward a more pro-inflammatory phenotype [62]. Higher circulating levels of visfatin, chemerin, vaspin, and resistin and lower levels of omentin and adiponectin are between the changes occurring. It should be noted though that circulating adipokine levels are not always correlated with the expression levels in the adipose tissue itself, underlying the existence of complex paracrine mechanisms governing crosstalks in the adipo–vascular axis [34].

Overall, it becomes evident that adipose tissue has the ability to sense and respond to signals originating from other tissue's pathologies. Diseases with chronicity, such as cancer, congestive heart failure, infectious and inflammatory disease (i.e., tuberculosis, rheumatoid arthritis, Crohn's disease, etc.), as well as advanced age, are characterized by cachexia [63]. Cachexia refers to a state of chronic low-grade inflammation, characterized by a hypercatabolic state leading to unintentional weight loss through lipolysis of adipose tissue [64]. Systemic low-grade inflammation suppresses adipose-tissue produced adiponectin levels and abolishes its insulin-sensitizing and anti-atherogenic properties in humans with or without significant cardiovascular disease [65]. Therefore, it is apparent that adipose tissue undergoes changes, ranging from expansion in the presence of high calorie intake in obesity, to atrophy seen in many conditions presenting with cachexia, to transcriptome changes driven by circulating inflammatory molecules. This perception of fat is being highlighted by the so-called obesity paradox. A large-scale meta-analysis including over 30 million individuals showed that the association between BMI and all-cause mortality in the general population can be described as *U*-shaped or *J*-shaped [66]. The obesity paradox can easily be explained if we take into consideration that despite the fact that excess adipose tissue is associated with reduced survival, significantly reduced adipose tissue in chronic disease (such as cancer, heart failure, renal failure, chronic inflammatory diseases, and other conditions) will also lead to poor survival rates. The concept that there is only a positive association between BMI and short-term (5–10 years) survival in the general population is therefore misleading, as it ignores the negative effects of the reduced and dysfunctional adipose tissue in the presence of chronic disease [67, 68].

PVAT as a Sensor of Early Vascular Disease Signals – Inside to Outside Signaling

The concept that cardiovascular biology can affect adipose tissue biology in a localized manner through a bidirectional crosstalk loop has been introduced lately with important implications in our understanding of CVD pathogenesis and diagnosis (see Fig. 9.2). Early studies underlined that overxpression of p22phox – a subunit of the NOX1, NOX2, and NOX4 isoforms of NADPH oxidase – in vascular smooth muscle cells (VSMC) exaggerates obesity and insulin resistance in mice with high-fat feeding [69]. Intravascular injury, balloon-induced or wire-induced, in mice has been described to produce rapid phenotypic modifications of the perivascular adipose tissue through the upregulation of proinflammatory adipocytokines, primarily TNFa [70]. Following these initial observations, we found that increased vascular oxidative stress induces the release of products of lipid peroxidation, such as 4-hydroxynonenal (4-HNE), that diffuse into the perivascular space; adipocytes within PVAT receive these signals, through a process termed "adipose tissue sensing," and upregulate adiponectin's ADIPOQ gene via a peroxisome proliferator-activated receptor-γ (PPARγ)-dependent mechanism. Subsequently, adiponectin is released back to the vessel wall, exerting its beneficiary antioxidant and vasoprotective effects, in a protective loop, that concludes a defense mechanism within the proposed bidirectional crosstalk between PVAT and vasculature [34]. Similar links have also been suggested to govern interactions between the myocardium and epicardial adipose tissue. As in vessels, oxidation products from the myocardium lead to PPARγ-mediated upregulation of adiponectin expression and release in the adjacent epicardial fat, which then exerts antioxidant effects on the cardiomyocytes (see Fig. 9.3) [71].

In addition, we have more recently reported that inflammation in the human vascular wall triggers the release of inflammatory cytokines, such as TNFα, IL-6, and IFNγ, which also diffuse into the perivascular space. PVAT responds by adopting a "cachexia-type" sequence of biologic events within adipocytes; differentiation becomes suppressed and intracellular lipid formation decreases. Adipocytes get smaller in size as their intracellular lipid content depletes due to an increase in lipolysis and simultaneous decrease in adipogenesis, both resulting from the adverse microenvironment inside the perivascular space caused by vascular inflammation [29]. Further to lipolysis and reduced adipogenesis, perivascular edema may also appear around the inflamed artery as a result of increased inflammation-induced permeability in the microcirculation and expansion of the interstitial space in the perivascular space. Finally, vascular inflammation has the potential to induce more permanent changes in the surrounding fat, such as fibrosis and neoangiogenesis, which are known to occur in the setting of chronic inflammation [72]. Indeed, inflammatory changes of coronary PVAT, as assessed in vivo by ^{18}F-fluorodeoxyglucose positron emission tomography (^{18}F-FDG PET), were significantly enhanced at sites of coronary injury caused by everolimus-eluting stents as compared to untouched control sites in an in vivo porcine model [73].

All these biological modifications result in the development of a gradient of adipocyte size around the inflamed human coronary artery, with smaller adipocytes closer to the vessel wall that gradually increase to match the baseline size of the rest of epicardial fat adipocytes moving further away from the vessel. At a macroscopic level, these changes can be identified as a gradual shift in the balance between the lipid and aqueous phase in the adipose tissue directly adjacent to the inflamed artery [29]. As adipocytes get smaller in size through suppression of differentiation and decrease in intracellular lipid content, the lipid phase of the tissue starts to become depleted and gradually the aqueous phase reflecting localized edema and increased interstitial space becomes more apparent. It should be noted though that, although these changes are dynamic and subject to the degree of coronary inflammation, their kinetics are not entirely understood.

However, these observations about macroscopic changes in the PVAT in response to the presence of coronary inflammation and therefore atherosclerosis, have had a substantial impact in highlighting this otherwise neglected adipose tissue depot as a very promising and applicable marker of disease presence in the clinical setting. Taking into account all the above, it becomes evident that vascular inflammation is being communicated to the PVAT close to it, which in turn adjusts its biology by entering a state of hypercatabolism and suppressed adipogenesis, leading ultimately to macroscopic phenotypic alterations. The possibility to detect these molecular changes around the inflamed human artery using noninvasive imaging brings up new potential in using PVAT as a "thermometer," to detect and quantify coronary inflammation.

Imaging Perivascular Adipose Tissue

Taking into account the fact that it was only until recently that PVAT acquired a clear anatomic definition and more knowledge about its biology became available, this adipose tissue depot has been mainly studied in literature so far as part of epicardial adipose tissue. However, during the last few years, interest in this area by the imaging community has sparked and novel techniques and methodologies are being proposed. Adipose tissue imaging has been used for patient risk stratification in clinics and can be visualized by exploiting a wide and diverse range of imaging modalities, which provide quantitative and qualitative information on adipose tissue anatomy.

Dual Energy X-Ray Absorptiometry Dual energy X-ray absorptiometry (DXA) is a method for measuring bone mineral density and soft tissue composition and is commonly used to calculate body fat mass. It utilizes the absorption of two X-ray beams at different energy levels. Although it is a fairly easy, widely available and cheap modality, used as the method of choice for measuring body composition in athletes, DXA cannot provide detailed information about adipose tissue distribution [74].

Ultrasonography Echocardiography is an easy, low-cost method for evaluating the thickness of adipose tissue depots accessible to the ultrasound beam. It can provide an easy assessment of epicardial adipose tissue thickness; it is readily accessible in routine clinical practice but is heavily operator dependent and limited to the two-dimensional plane [75].

Computed Tomography Imaging Computed tomography is considered to be the gold standard for three-dimensional phenotyping of adiposity, with excellent computer-processed algorithms for segmentation and adipose tissue characterization. It can be combined with CT angiography for PVAT phenotyping and also with PET imaging for quantification of radiotracer uptake and provision of functional information on inflammatory and metabolic tissue activity. It is widely used and commonly available in clinical practice, and has received a Class I indication by the European Society of Cardiology (ESC) guidelines as a first-line investigation of suspected CAD [76], but it involves radiation exposure [77].

Magnetic Resonance Imaging MRI includes a range of sequences that provide excellent 3D quantification, while combination with proton spectroscopy can give further characterization of adipose tissue. It avoids radiation exposure but involves long scanning times, complex protocols, and expensive equipment that may not always be available [78]. Importantly its spatial resolution is not enough to allow accurate quantification of epicardial adipose tissue, while it can't visualize pericoronary adipose tissue in humans [79].

Quantitate Imaging Features

EAT thickness has been consistently associated with the metabolic syndrome and relative clinical features such as high blood pressure, high levels of low-density lipoprotein cholesterol, and insulin resistance [80]. However, the most studied quantitative index is EAT volume, with several large-scale cohorts exploring its significance in atherosclerosis. In low-risk asymptomatic populations, EAT volume, measured on non-contrast CT scans, was associated with the presence of ischemic heart disease, coronary calcification, and progression [81, 82]. In cohorts consisting of individuals with intermediate cardiovascular risk, higher EAT volume was described to be associated with coronary stenosis, ischemia, and high-risk plaque features [83–85]. Nonetheless, when analyzing data from subjects in high cardiovascular risk, Tanami et al. found no correlation between EAT volume and obstructive coronary artery disease or coronary calcification [86], highlighting the fact that the significance of EAT volume in characterizing atherosclerosis is highly dependent on the subject's baseline risk profile and the stage of disease progression. Of note, the SMART (Secondary Manifestations of ARTerial disease) study reported that low EAT attenuation, independently of EAT volume, on CT was associated with coronary artery calcification, indicating that quality features of the adipose tissue are also of importance, bearing the potential to add complementary information to that provided by quantitative measures [87].

Qualitative Imaging Features

Evaluation of PVAT inflammation assessed by FDG uptake using positron emission tomography (PET) showed greater standardized uptake values

(SUV) in pericoronary fat compared with other fat depots, while in overweight patients with CAD, a positive correlation between PVAT SUV and respective coronary artery stenosis was described [88]. However, low spatial resolution, high background noise, high exposure to radiation, and low clinical availability are limiting factors for PET imaging and may restrict its extensive use in low-risk populations. Conventional cardiac CT angiography is able to provide information on adipose tissue quality, by analyzing attenuation shifts. In the SMART study, Franssens et al. found a negative association between EAT attenuation and age, BMI, waist circumference, visceral abdominal AT, fasting glucose, and insulin resistance [87]. Similarly, in 609 asymptomatic low to intermediate risk patients, Abazid et al. observed a negative correlation between EAT density and coronary calcification independently of EAT volume [89]. On the contrary, in a cross-sectional analysis of patients with acute myocardial infarction (MI) and stable CAD controls, Mahabadi et al. observed a positive association between EAT attenuation and type I acute MI [90], while Hell et al. did not report a link between EAT attenuation and myocardial ischemia on SPECT [91]. These contradictory findings can be attributed to a number of factors such as small sample size, selection, bias and methodological limitations, but the most significant point to be noted here would be that all aforementioned studies derive attenuation data by analyzing EAT as a whole, without taking into account the regional biological – and therefore imaging – variability of adipose tissue in close proximity to the coronaries, stressing the critical need for a standardized CT-based approach for qualitative analysis of PVAT. Toward that end, phenotypic mapping of PVAT has been recently introduced utilizing algorithms constantly evolving though artificial intelligence processes to capture non-invasively PVAT phenotypic alterations, such as reduction in adipocyte size, edema, fibrosis, and neovascularization, which have been shown to chaperon coronary inflammation [29].

Measuring PVAT Attenuation: Introducing the Fat Attenuation Index (FAI)

In PVAT around the coronaries, the attenuation is affected by inflammatory signals coming from the vascular wall that induce structural changes at a microscopic level, resulting in a gradient of adipocyte size in the first few millimeters around the inflamed coronary arterial wall, as discussed extensively above. This gradient is reflected on PVAT, as its attenuation swings between a more aqueous/less lipophilic phase close to the inflamed artery to a less aqueous/more lipophilic phase in the non-PVAT within the epicardial fat [92]. Indeed, large, fully differentiated, adipocytes with high lipid content drive attenuation values toward the more negative values within the widely accepted Hounsfield Unit (HU) range (−190HU to −30HU) for adipose tissue characterization in computed tomography. The presence of small, less differentiated adipocytes, with low lipid content, causes attenuation to shift to the less negative values (toward the −30HU end), reflecting the shift in tissue composition that can be attributed to several factors: (a) reduced intracellular lipid content, (b) increased intracellular aqueous phase, which replaces intracellular lipids after lipolysis, (c) increased extracellular fluid from the shrinking adipocytes, and (d) edema in the inflamed environment [62]. This important observation led to the creation of the perivascular Fat Attenuation Index (FAI), an imaging tool that measures weighted three-dimensional attenuation gradients of adipose tissue in the perivascular space (Fig. 9.4) [93].

Calculating FAI

Perivascular FAI was developed using a radiotranscriptomic approach to describe molecular changes in the transcriptomic, metabolic, and phenotypic profile of PVAT in response to signals originating from the adjacent vascular wall driven by coronary inflammation [29]. The calculation of FAI is performed using artificial

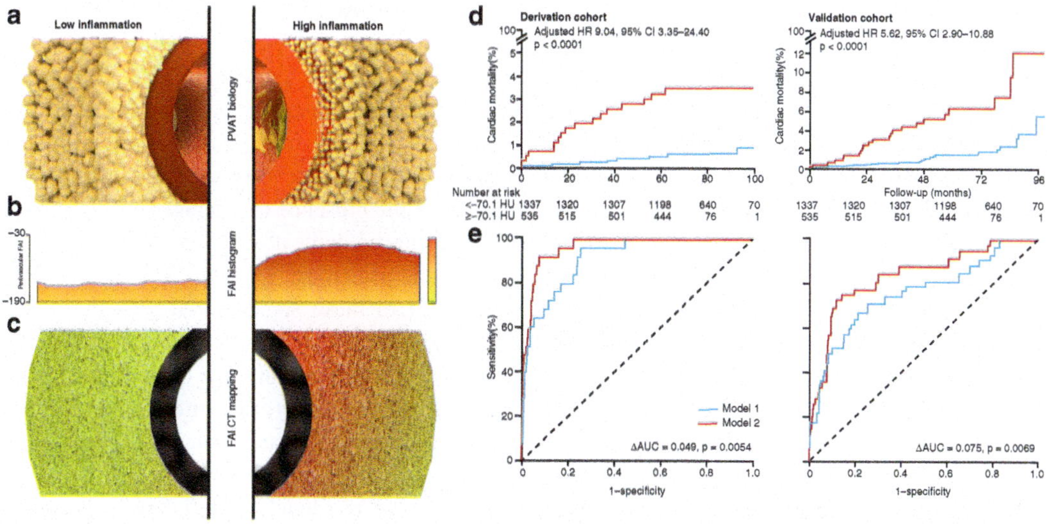

Fig. 9.4 Schematic representation of the biology underlying FAI and its prognostic value. Morphological appearance of perivascular adipose tissue surrounding healthy and inflamed coronary arteries, depicting the gradient of adipocyte size induced by exogenous vascular inflammation (**a**). Illustrative visualization of the perivascular FAI gradient and radial distance from vascular wall in the presence of low versus high inflammation (**b**, **c**). Kaplan–Meier curves of cardiac mortality with high versus low perivascular FAI for the derivation and validation cohorts. HRs are adjusted for risk factors, technical factors, the extent of coronary artery disease, and number of high-risk plaque features (**d**). Comparison of time-dependent ROC curves (at 6 years) and respective AUC of two nested models for discrimination of cardiac mortality in the derivation (top) and validation (bottom) cohorts. Model 1 represents the current state of the art in risk assessment and consists of age, sex, risk factors (hypertension, hypercholesterolemia, diabetes mellitus, smoker status, epicardial adipose tissue volume), modified Duke coronary artery disease index, and number of high-risk plaque features on coronary CTA. Model 2 incorporates perivascular FAI values into model 1 (**e**). AUC area under the curve, FAI Fat Attenuation Index, PVAT perivascular adipose tissue, HR hazard ratio, HU Hounsfield unit, HRP high-risk plaque. (From Oikonomou et al. [93], with permission from Lancet and Elsevier)

intelligence-enhanced algorithms (CaRi-HEART, Caristo Diagnostics, Oxford, UK) that provide accurate and reproducible weighted measures of 3D attenuation gradients within perivascular tissue around the human arterial wall [92]. Quantifying perivascular FAI is a particularly complex process, involving multiple analysis steps. The heart is initially segmented, and the vessel wall of interest is defined in a fully automated way by the CaRi-HEART application, followed by analysis algorithms dependent on the type of analysis requested (standardized proximal segment analysis or plaque-specific). The longitudinal length of PVAT is determined by the vessel segment of interest, and the analysis takes place in multiple layers of PVAT in the perpendicular dimension. This is essential to capture the gradient of PVAT density around the human artery. These analyses are performed within the standard adipose tissue HU range window of −190 to −30HU by algorithms that involve multiple adjustments and are constantly evolving through artificial intelligence processes [92]. Indeed, it should be stressed that FAI differs to the crude "mean CT attenuation (or radiodensity)," since it is appropriately corrected and weighted for parameters related to the coronary segment of interest itself, the patient, such as obesity status and other anatomical factors, and technical scanning parameters, such as scanner type and settings, reconstruction algorithms, tube voltage, etc. All this information is incorporated and extracted by the FAI algorithm from the coronary computed tomography angiography (CCTA) file data. Crude measurement of perivascular attenuation on the other hand, without taking into account attenuation gradients around inflamed arteries, may misinterpret coronary inflammation. Obese individuals have overall larger adipocytes in their epicardial fat driving the attenuation closer to −190HU and leading to underestimations of vascular inflammation. Similarly, in lean individuals, smaller adipocytes, with lower lipid content, lead to less negative crude attenuation values that overestimate the inflammatory burden, even in the absence of local inflammation in the adjacent artery. Furthermore, measurement of absolute attenuation may be affected by the hardware used, CT scan settings, reconstruction algorithms, and many other technical parameters, all of which are corrected for in the CaRi-HEART algorithm. Importantly, FAI is not affected by arterial calcification or lumen attenuation, thus having an advantage over coronary wall biomarkers, although the information provided is complementary to high-risk plaque features [29].

FAI as an Internal "Thermometer" of the Entire Coronary Tree

As suggested by recent translational studies exploring the regional biological variability of EAT, coronary PVAT around the coronary arteries is defined as the adipose tissue located within a radial distance from the outer vessel wall equal to the diameter of the adjacent coronary vessel [29]. Outside this region, the cellular composition and biological signature of epicardial adipose tissue reaches a "steady state" and can no longer be affected by vascular biology. In initial analyses, the measurement of FAI was limited to the proximal 40 mm segments of the three major coronary arteries: right coronary artery (RCA), left anterior descending artery (LAD), and left circumflex artery (LCX) [29]. These areas were chosen due to lack of molecular validation of FAI measurements in other coronary segments, given that the amount of PVAT and its biological characteristics vary from segment to segment in the coronary tree, and that absolute values of perivascular attenuation are highly dependent on the segment under examination. However, it became clear that following this standardized measurement of perivascular FAI in the proximal 40 mm segments of the big coronaries yields comparable results with measurements in the anatomical coronary segments proposed by the Society of Cardiovascular CT guidelines [94]. This standardized measurement provides an excellent surrogate of the background vascular inflammatory burden of the entire coronary tree – independently of the presence of plaque – which may be abnormal even in the absence of any visible coronary atherosclerotic plaque. Perivascular FAI measured in these standardized proximal coronary segments is significantly higher in patients with coronary artery disease compared to individuals with non-atherosclerotic vessels, while it is not related with local coronary calcification or overall coronary calcium score (CCS), after adjusting for age, gender, and other cardiovascular risk factors [29]. Thus, FAI is a robust biomarker of low-grade inflammation that precedes atherosclerotic plaque formation, acting as an internal "thermometer" of the entire coronary arterial tree.

FAI as a Local Biomarker of Coronary Plaque Inflammation and Vulnerability

Apart from standardized segments, FAI analysis can also be performed around atherosclerotic plaques, in an effort to quantify local variability of coronary inflammation that comes along with the vulnerable plaque. Implementing a different type of analysis, FAI measurements around lesions are an excellent surrogate of the localized inflammatory burden on top of any background coronary inflammation [29]. Indeed, FAI is significantly increased around the culprit lesions in patients with acute coronary syndrome as compared with non-culprit lesions of the same patient or around stable lesions in stable patients [29]. Notably, perivascular FAI around the culprit lesion decreases to baseline levels 5 weeks after the acute event, highlighting its ability to tracks changes in coronary inflammation that are inherent to the events leading up to acute myocardial infarction [29]. To correct for any background effects of overall inflammation present in the coronary tree and enable accurate identification of the localized increases in the inflammatory burden around the vulnerable "inflamed" plaque, the change of perivascular FAI, referenced to a segment proximal to the lesion, was found to be superior to crude perivascular attenuation measurement [29], although the magnitude of the changes in PVAT attenuation around culprit lesions during ACS is so high that measurement of the crude PVAT attenuation can also contribute to the detection of vulnerable plaques [95]. Importantly, a shift of perivascular attenuation was observed around coronary segments with atherosclerotic plaques compared with segments without disease [96]. To further confirm the ability of perivascular attenuation shifts to detect coronary inflammation, increased PVAT crude attenuation has been associated with an increase in ^{18}F-NaF PET uptake in stable patients with high-risk plaques on CTA [97]. Also, coronary dissection, a pathology that stems from coronary inflammation, has also been linked with high attenuation values closer to the vascular wall, confirming the proof of principle that acute local inflammation in the vascular wall drives shifts of perivascular attenuation [98].

FAI as a Predictor of Long-Term Outcomes

Perivascular FAI is a biomarker that can detect both baseline background low-grade inflammation in the entire coronary tree (measured in standardized proximal coronary segments) and coronary plaque vulnerability (measured around plaques). We recently reported its predictive value in the CRISP-CT (Cardiovascular RISk Prediction using Computed Tomography) study, which explored the ability of perivascular FAI around the proximal segments of the three main epicardial arteries, to predict clinical outcomes in almost 4000 individuals undergoing CCTA as part of their clinical care in Erlangen, Germany and Cleveland, USA (as derivation and validation cohorts respectively, with ~2000 individuals each) [93]. A *J*-shaped association between perivascular FAI and the risk for cardiac death was observed and perivascular FAI around the proximal segment of the LAD or RCA was strongly predictive of all-cause and cardiac mortality but not non-cardiac mortality [93]. Among individuals with perivascular FAI above −70.1HU, the risk for all-cause mortality was HR (95%CI) 2.55 (1.65–3.92) in the derivation and 3.69 (2.26–6.02) in the validation cohort. When looking into cardiac mortality specifically, patients with "abnormally high" perivascular FAI had ninefold higher risk in the derivation cohort and 5.6 times higher risk in the validation cohort. This predictive value was incremental to the current state of the art in risk assessment using CCTA, as assessed by comparison with a model that includes clinical risk factors, calcium score, the extend of coronary atherosclerosis, and the presence of high-risk plaque features (deltaAUC = 0.049, p = 0.0054 in the derivation and deltaAUC = 0.075, p = 0.0069 in the validation cohorts) (see Fig. 9.4). In addition, abnormal perivascular FAI was also predictive of non-fatal heart attacks but was only weakly correlated with calcium score or plasma hsCRP (marker of systemic inflammation). This permits reclassification of an individual's risk, independently of their background calcium score, the presence of CAD, or any high risk plaque (HRP) features [93]. Importantly, individuals with high FAI but absence of HRP features exerted a higher cardiac risk as opposed to patients with HRP features but low FAI values, highlighting yet again that FAI captures biology not detectable by other indices [92]. With respect to the predictive value of FAI in secondary prevention, it has to be noted that the vast majority of the participants in the CRISP-CT study were low-intermediate risk individuals, which are commonly the ones referred for CCTA. Regarding higher risk populations, although the numbers of patients with CAD in the CRISP-CT study were rather low (467 in the derivation and 286 in the validation cohort), the HR for fatal heart attacks remained significant (8.54 [2.41–30.21] and 3.85 [1.21–12.27] in the derivation and validation cohorts, respectively). The predictive value also remained significant in those with or without high-risk plaque features. Interestingly, perivascular FAI lost its predictive value among those individuals who started treatment with statin and aspirin immediately after CCTA, while among those who didn't change their medication, the hazard ratio for cardiac mortality was more than doubled. This suggests that the risk identified by perivascular FAI is modifiable and could potentially be tracked by repeat CCTA after treatments initiation. This finding was later validated in a cohort of psoriasis patients, in which biologic therapy with anti-TNFα, anti-IL12/23, or anti-IL17 antibodies was associated with a reduction in FAI values used to assess coronary inflammation [99].

Entering the Big Data Era: PVAT Radiomic Phenotyping

Recent advances in computational and imaging processing methodologies have enabled the extraction of large amounts of quantitative data from images. Specialized data-characterization algorithms can identify patterns of data behavior within an image, which are not perceived by the human reader and can have significant clinical relevance [100]. Imaging studies in oncology were the first to identify this new field of potential – termed "radiomics" – linking specific shape- and texture-related patterns within the volume of the tumor to the underlying tumor biology and overall clinical prognosis [101]. These patterns are the product of complex mathematical data transformations that collectively describe the structure imaged in a far more comprehensive way than what is perceived by the human eye.

In a recent large study, we performed a radiotrancriptomic experiment using adipose tissue biopsies in an effort to identify radiomic signatures that best describe non-invasively three major aspects of adipose tissue biology: inflammation – using the expression of TNFa as marker; fibrosis – evidenced by collagen (COL1A1 gene) expression; vascularity – reflected by the expression of endothelial marker CD31 (PECAM1 gene). Features related mostly to tissue attenuation (captured by the FAI) were highly correlated with TNFA expression, confirming yet again the concept that attenuation metrics are descriptive of inflammation. Of note, features associated with the texture of adipose tissue were found to detect more permanent changes in its phenotype, such as fibrosis (COL1A1 expression) and microvascular remodeling (CD31 expression), which are also affecting the histological heterogeneity of adipose tissue. Interestingly, authors report that different radiomic signatures were differentially associated with tissue inflammation, fibrosis, and vascularity, proposing that radiomic phenotypic can provide a comprehensive phenotyping of the biological variation within adipose tissue [102].

Following these initial observations, a machine-learning approach was applied to construct a radiomic-based PVAT signature that would enable increased cardiac risk detection (Fig. 9.5). Indeed, internal validation of this signature – namely the Fat Radiomic Profile (FRP) – showed that it can accurately identify cardiac risk (AUC: 0.77 [0.62–0.93]) [102]. Applying FRP phenotyping to a population of 1575 individuals (CCTA arm of the SCOT-HEART trial) showed a striking 11-fold higher risk for major adverse cardiovascular events for patients classified in the high HRP group, independently of traditional risk factors, presence of coronary artery disease (≥50% stenosis), presence of HRP features, Agatston coronary calcium scoring, and scanner type [102]. Importantly, FRP offered incremental prognostic information beyond current CCTA-based tools (including Agatston CCS, HRP features, and luminal stenosis), suggesting a residual level of cardiac risk that is not detected by traditional risk stratification algorithms (delta-AUC = 0.13, $p < 0.001$). Further analyses revealed that after performing serial CCTA scans in patients with AMI, FRP remained unchanged with FAI significantly decreasing as discussed above, suggesting that FRP captures permanent PVAT structural changes and can be useful for initial screenings, whereas FAI captures the dynamic inflammatory burden of the coronary vasculature [102].

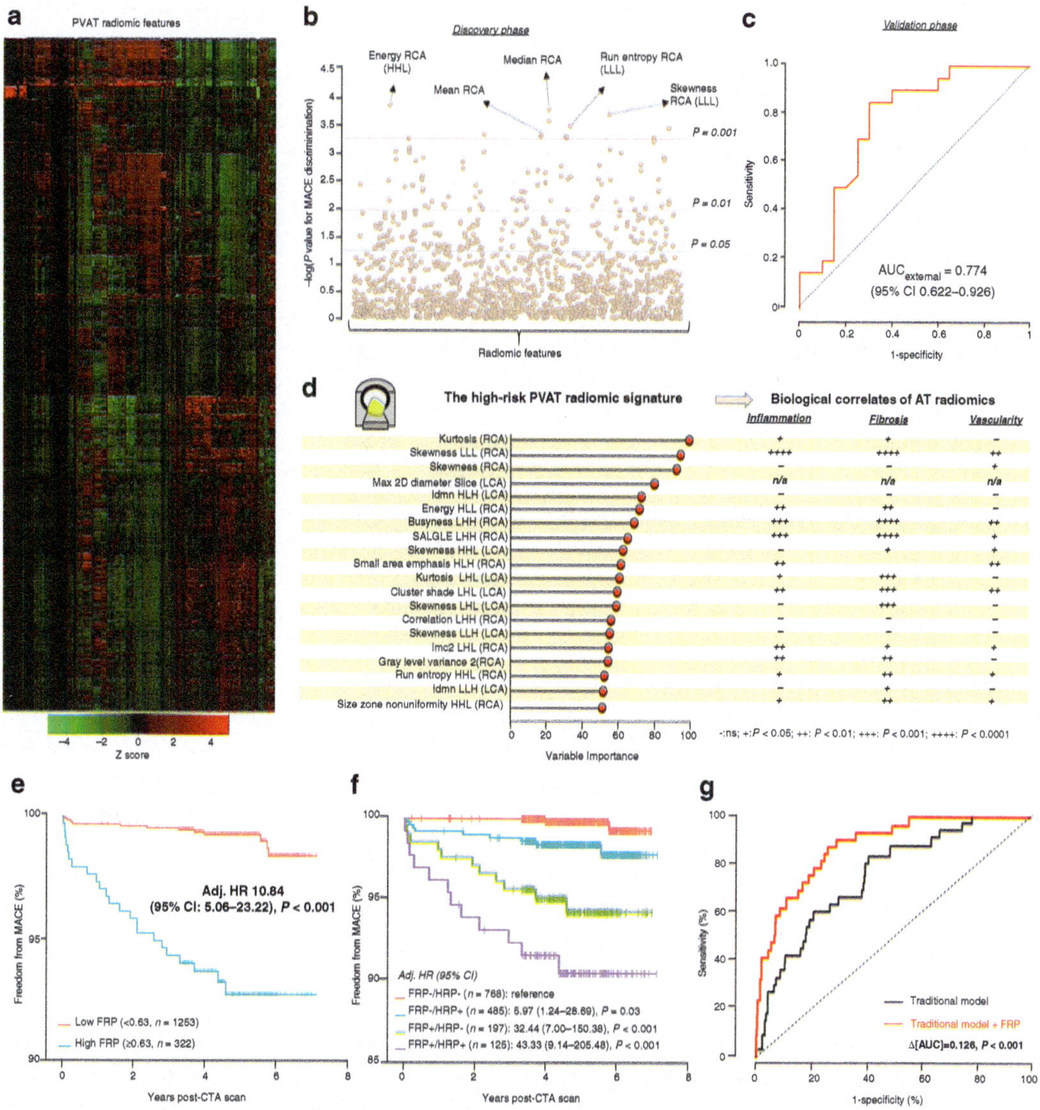

Fig. 9.5 The pericoronary Fat Radiomic Profile. (**a**) Heatmap of scaled radiomic features in the SCOT-HEART population revealing between-patient variance across the cohort. (**b**) A forest plot of the discriminatory value of each radiomic feature in univariable analysis. (**c**) Validation of the final model in the validation set (20% of the initial sample). (**d**) Variable importance of the top 20 radiomic features of the final random forest model and corresponding strength of association with adipose tissue inflammation, fibrosis, and vascularity (**e, f**) Kaplan–Meier curves and adjusted hazard ratios for major adverse cardiac events across strata of FRP and HRP features. (**g**) Time-dependent receiver operating characteristic curves (t = 5 years) for two nested prediction models consisting of age, sex, systolic blood pressure, diabetes mellitus, body mass index, smoking status, presence of coronary artery disease (≥50% stenosis), total cholesterol, high-density lipoprotein levels, scanner type, presence of high-risk plaque, as well as Agatston coronary calcium scoring [log(CCS + 1)] with (AUC: 0.880) or without (AUC: 0.754) FRP. AUC area under the curve, CI confidence interval, CCTA coronary computed tomography angiography, FRP Fat Radiomic Profile, H high filter, Imc2 informational measure of correlation 2, Idmn inverse difference moment normalized, L low filter, LCA left coronary artery, MACE major adverse cardiac events, MI myocardial infarction, RCA right coronary artery, CCS coronary calcium score, HR hazard ratio, HRP high-risk plaque feature. (++++P < 0.0001; +++P < 0.001. ++P < 0.01, +P < 0.05, and –P ≥ 0.05). (From Oikonomou et al. [102], with permission from Oxford University Press)

An increasing number of studies are being reported in cardiovascular medicine utilizing these novel imaging processing methodologies [103]. It was recently shown that radiomic features within the arterial wall can reliably discriminate the napkin-ring HRP sign between metabolically active from inactive lesions [104]. Radiomics is a promising new area of research bridging the fields of imaging and biology, offering tremendous potential for early, effective, and accurate clinical diagnosis.

Summary

Perivascular adipose tissue is a distinct, dynamic fat depot involved in a wide range of interactions with the cardiovascular system. PVAT produces a highly diverse secretome that regulates vascular biology. Hormones, cytokines, gaseous messengers, lipid esters, micro-RNAs, and vesicles, among others, are secreted by PVAT and disseminate into the adjacent vascular wall to regulate vascular tone, inflammatory infiltration, redox state, endothelial activation, and other biological processes that are implicated in the pathogenesis of atherosclerosis. Conversely, PVAT biology is being affected by exogenous signals arising from the inflamed arterial wall. Adipocytes in the perivascular space respond by adopting a cachexia-type phenotype, characterized by reduced adipogenesis and suppressed differentiation, that results in decreased cell size. Furthermore, edema appears, the interstitial space is expanded, and as inflammatory signals persist, the extracellular matrix becomes degraded and fibrosis and neovascularization are induced. All these lead to structural changes in the macroscopic appearance of PVAT with the creation of a gradient of adipocyte size and edema around the coronary artery presenting very early pathological signs of atherosclerosis.

Interestingly, alterations in the PVAT phenotype can be captured non-invasively using computed tomography imaging. The aforementioned changes in the transcriptional and metabolic phenotype of PVAT disturb the balance between the lipid and aqueous phases in the attenuation maps. Consequently, the biological gradient is reflected by a three-dimensional gradient of weighted attenuation values around the vascular wall of the inflamed vessel. This information is captured by the recently developed perivascular Fat Attenuation Index (FAI), which is a biomarker both of baseline background inflammation in the coronary tree and of the increased inflammatory burden around the vulnerable plaque that is likely to rupture and create atherothrombotic events. The relation of FAI with future outcomes has been well described and established, allowing for a unique risk classification system with strong implications for guiding medical management in patients undergoing CCTA. Incorporating perivascular FAI in standard CCTA reporting could guide the use of primary and secondary prevention measures, whereas by assessing vascular inflammation with FAI, abnormal perivascular FAI may provide guidance for expensive, novel risk-reducing therapeutics (e.g., anti-PCSK9 inhibitors or monoclonal antibodies). Nevertheless, FAI analysis can be challenging given the complexity of calculations involved, and its implementation demands dedicated, computationally powerful workstations.

In addition, recent advances in image processing algorithms perusing big data and artificial intelligence applications have enabled the development of radiomic signatures of PVAT biology. For instance, the recently reported Fat Radiomic Profile (FRP) index is a high-risk radiomic signature of coronary PVAT, derived from CCTA scans, which detects adverse structural changes associated with PVAT fibrosis and microvascular remodeling. FRP was shown to have excellent prognostic value for major adverse cardiovascular events, improving risk prediction beyond the current state-of-the-art and discriminates patients with AMI from those with stable disease. It is therefore clear that incorporating PVAT imaging markers, such as FAI and FRP, facilitates the development of a more comprehensive individualized cardiac risk profile for each patient. In conclusion, radiomic characterization of PVAT constitutes a novel, promising approach to capturing coronary inflammation and its associated residual cardiac risk. CCTA recently received a

Class I indication by the European Society of Cardiology (ESC) guidelines as a first-line imaging modality in suspected CAD [76]. Hence, PVAT and its imaging could be used as a "companion diagnostic" streamlined in CCTA, contributing to improved diagnosis and stratification of CAD and guiding the deployment of personalized therapeutic solutions in primary and secondary prevention.

Acknowledgments CPK acknowledges support from the EPSRC, the Scatcherd Fund at the University of Oxford, and the A.G. Leventis Foundation.

CA is supported in part by the British Heart Foundation (FS/16/15/32047, TG/16/3/32687), the Oxford BHF Centre of Research Excellence, the Novo Nordisk Foundation (NNF15CC0018486), and Innovate UK.

Author Contributions CPK performed the literature review, wrote the book chapter, and prepared the figures and table. CA provided scientific direction and wrote and reviewed the book chapter.

Conflict of Interest The CaRi-HEART technology is subject to patent applications PCT/GB2015/052359, GB20161620494.3, GB20181818049.7, GR20180100490, and GR201801005100. CA is a founder and shareholder of Caristo Diagnostics, a CT-image analysis company.

References

1. Saxton SN, Clark BJ, Withers SB, Eringa EC, Heagerty AM. Mechanistic links between obesity, diabetes, and blood pressure: role of perivascular adipose tissue. Physiol Rev. 2019;99:1701–63.
2. Cheng CK, Bakar HA, Gollasch M, Huang Y. Perivascular adipose tissue: the sixth man of the cardiovascular system. Cardiovasc Drugs Ther. 2018;32:481–502.
3. World Health Organization. Disease burden and mortality estimates. Geneva: WHO; 2018.
4. Dunbar SB, Khavjou OA, Bakas T, Hunt G, Kirch RA, Leib AR, et al. Projected costs of informal caregiving for cardiovascular disease: 2015 to 2035: a policy statement from the American Heart Association. Circulation. 2018;137:e558–e77.
5. Kalbacher D, Waldeyer C, Blankenberg S, Westermann D. Beyond conventional secondary prevention in coronary artery disease—what to choose in the era of CANTOS, COMPASS, FOURIER, ODYSSEY and PEGASUS-TIMI 54? A review on contemporary literature. Ann Transl Med. 2018;6:323.
6. Ferrari R, Catapano AL. Residual cardiovascular risk. Eur Heart J Suppl. 2016;18:C1–C.
7. Schmidt AF, Pearce LS, Wilkins JT, Overington JP, Hingorani AD, Casas JP. PCSK9 monoclonal antibodies for the primary and secondary prevention of cardiovascular disease. Cochrane Database Syst Rev. 2017;4:CD011748.
8. Ridker PM, Everett BM, Thuren T, MacFadyen JG, Chang WH, Ballantyne C, et al. Antiinflammatory therapy with canakinumab for atherosclerotic disease. N Engl J Med. 2017;377:1119–31.
9. Sehested TS, Bjerre J, Ku S, Chang A, Jahansouz A, Owens DK, et al. Cost-effectiveness of Canakinumab for prevention of recurrent cardiovascular events. JAMA Cardiol. 2019;4:128–35.
10. Antonopoulos AS, Margaritis M, Lee R, Channon K, Antoniades C. Statins as anti-inflammatory agents in atherogenesis: molecular mechanisms and lessons from the recent clinical trials. Curr Pharm Des. 2012;18:1519–30.
11. Libby P, Ridker PM, Hansson GK. Atherothrombosis LTNo. Inflammation in atherosclerosis: from pathophysiology to practice. J Am Coll Cardiol. 2009;54:2129–38.
12. Tousoulis D, Psarros C, Demosthenous M, Patel R, Antoniades C, Stefanadis C. Innate and adaptive inflammation as a therapeutic target in vascular disease. J Am Coll Cardiol. 2014;63:2491–502.
13. Tousoulis D, Psarros C, Demosthenous M, Patel R, Antoniades C, Stefanadis C. Innate and adaptive inflammation as a therapeutic target in vascular disease: the emerging role of statins. J Am Coll Cardiol. 2014;63:2491–502.
14. Harrington RA. Targeting inflammation in coronary artery disease. N Engl J Med. 2017;377:1197–8.
15. Souilhol C, Serbanovic-Canic J, Fragiadaki M, Chico TJ, Ridger V, Roddie H, et al. Endothelial responses to shear stress in atherosclerosis: a novel role for developmental genes. Nat Rev Cardiol. 2020;17(1):52–63. https://doi.org/10.1038/s41569-019-0239-5. [Epub ahead of print].
16. Antoniades C, Bakogiannis C, Tousoulis D, Antonopoulos AS, Stefanadis C. The CD40/CD40 ligand system: linking inflammation with atherothrombosis. J Am Coll Cardiol. 2009;54:669–77.
17. Durham AL, Speer MY, Scatena M, Giachelli CM, Shanahan CM. Role of smooth muscle cells in vascular calcification: implications in atherosclerosis and arterial stiffness. Cardiovasc Res. 2018;114:590–600.
18. Ridker PM. C-reactive protein and the prediction of cardiovascular events among those at intermediate risk. J Am Coll Cardiol. 2007;49:2129–38.
19. Ridker PM, Danielson E, Fonseca FAH, Genest J, Gotto AM, Kastelein JJP, et al. Rosuvastatin to prevent vascular events in men and women with elevated c-reactive protein. N Engl J Med. 2008;359:2195–207.
20. Ridker PM, Everett BM, Pradhan A, MacFadyen JG, Solomon DH, Zaharris E, et al. Low-dose methotrexate for the prevention of atherosclerotic events. N Engl J Med. 2019;380(8):752–62:NEJMoa1809798.

21. Ridker PM, MacFadyen JG, Thuren T, Libby P. Residual inflammatory risk associated with interleukin-18 and interleukin-6 after successful interleukin-1β inhibition with canakinumab: further rationale for the development of targeted anti-cytokine therapies for the treatment of atherothrombosis. Eur Heart J. 2019; https://doi.org/10.1093/eurheartj/ehz542. [Epub ahead of print].
22. Passacquale G, Di Giosia P, Ferro A. The role of inflammatory biomarkers in developing targeted cardiovascular therapies: lessons from the cardiovascular inflammation reduction trials. Cardiovasc Res. 2016;109:9–23.
23. Oikonomou EK, Antoniades C. The role of adipose tissue in cardiovascular health and disease. Nat Rev Cardiol. 2019;16(2):83–99.
24. Mancio J, Oikonomou EK, Antoniades C. Perivascular adipose tissue and coronary atherosclerosis. Heart. 2018;104:1654–62.
25. Iacobellis G. Local and systemic effects of the multifaceted epicardial adipose tissue depot. Nat Rev Endocrinol. 2015;11:363–71.
26. Antonopoulos AS, Antoniades C. The role of epicardial adipose tissue in cardiac biology: classic concepts and emerging roles. J Physiol. 2017;595:3907–17.
27. Baker AR, Da Silva NF, Quinn DW, Harte AL, Pagano D, Bonser RS, et al. Human epicardial adipose tissue expresses a pathogenic profile of adipocytokines in patients with cardiovascular disease. Cardiovasc Diabetol. 2006;5:1.
28. Sarin S, Wenger C, Marwaha A, Qureshi A, Go BDM, Woomert CA, et al. Clinical significance of epicardial fat measured using cardiac multislice computed tomography. Am J Cardiol. 2008;102:767–71.
29. Antonopoulos AS, Sanna F, Sabharwal N, Thomas S, Oikonomou EK, Herdman L, et al. Detecting human coronary inflammation by imaging perivascular fat. Sci Transl Med. 2017;9:eaal2658.
30. Aghamohammadzadeh R, Withers S, Lynch F, Greenstein A, Malik R, Heagerty A. Perivascular adipose tissue from human systemic and coronary vessels: the emergence of a new pharmacotherapeutic target. Br J Pharmacol. 2012;165:670–82.
31. Akoumianakis I, Antoniades C. The interplay between adipose tissue and the cardiovascular system: is fat always bad? Cardiovasc Res. 2017;113:999–1008.
32. Szasz T, Webb RC. Perivascular adipose tissue: more than just structural support. Clin Sci. 2012;122:1–12.
33. Yudkin JS, Eringa E, Stehouwer CD. "Vasocrine" signalling from perivascular fat: a mechanism linking insulin resistance to vascular disease. Lancet. 2005;365:1817–20.
34. Margaritis M, Antonopoulos AS, Digby J, Lee R, Reilly S, Coutinho P, et al. Interactions between vascular wall and perivascular adipose tissue reveal novel roles for adiponectin in the regulation of endothelial nitric oxide synthase function in human vessels. Circulation. 2013;127:2209–21.
35. Oikonomou EK, Antoniades C. Immunometabolic regulation of vascular redox state: the role of adipose tissue. Antioxid Redox Signal. 2018;29:313–36.
36. Antoniades C, Shirodaria C, Warrick N, Cai S, de Bono J, Lee J, et al. 5-Methyltetrahydrofolate rapidly improves endothelial function and decreases superoxide production in human vessels. Circulation. 2006;114:1193–201.
37. Margaritis M, Sanna F, Lazaros G, Akoumianakis I, Patel S, Antonopoulos AS, et al. Predictive value of telomere length on outcome following acute myocardial infarction: evidence for contrasting effects of vascular vs. blood oxidative stress. Eur Heart J. 2017;38:3094–104.
38. Lee Y-C, Chang H-H, Chiang C-L, Liu C-H, Yeh J-I, Chen M-F, et al. Role of perivascular adipose tissue–derived methyl palmitate in vascular tone regulation and pathogenesis of hypertension. Circulation. 2011;124:1160–71.
39. King AL, Polhemus DJ, Bhushan S, Otsuka H, Kondo K, Nicholson CK, et al. Hydrogen sulfide cytoprotective signaling is endothelial nitric oxide synthase-nitric oxide dependent. Proc Natl Acad Sci U S A. 2014;111:3182–7.
40. Chang L, Xiong W, Zhao X, Fan Y, Guo Y, Garcia-Barrio M, et al. Bmal1 in perivascular adipose tissue regulates resting-phase blood pressure through transcriptional regulation of angiotensinogen. Circulation. 2018;138:67–79.
41. Ayala-Lopez N, Thompson JM, Watts SW. Perivascular adipose tissue's impact on norepinephrine-induced contraction of mesenteric resistance arteries. Front Physiol. 2017;8:37.
42. Graham DB, Jasso GJ, Mok A, Goel G, Ng AC, Kolde R, et al. Nitric oxide engages an anti-inflammatory feedback loop mediated by peroxiredoxin 5 in phagocytes. Cell Rep. 2018;24:838–50.
43. Antonopoulos AS, Margaritis M, Coutinho P, Shirodaria C, Psarros C, Herdman L, et al. Adiponectin as a link between type 2 diabetes and vascular NADPH oxidase activity in the human arterial wall: the regulatory role of perivascular adipose tissue. Diabetes. 2015;64:2207–19.
44. Neves KB, Lobato NS, Lopes RAM, Filgueira FP, Zanotto CZ, Oliveira AM, et al. Chemerin reduces vascular nitric oxide/cGMP signalling in rat aorta: a link to vascular dysfunction in obesity? Clin Sci. 2014;127:111–22.
45. Taube A, Schlich R, Sell H, Eckardt K, Eckel J. Inflammation and metabolic dysfunction: links to cardiovascular diseases. Am J Physiol Heart Circ Physiol. 2012;302:H2148–H65.
46. Maiellaro K, Taylor WR. The role of the adventitia in vascular inflammation. Cardiovasc Res. 2007;75:640–8.
47. Akoumianakis I, Sanna F, Margaritis M, Badi I, Akawi N, Herdman L, et al. Adipose tissue–derived WNT5A regulates vascular redox signaling in

obesity via USP17/RAC1-mediated activation of NADPH oxidases. Sci Transl Med. 2019;11:510.
48. Fischer C, Seki T, Lim S, Nakamura M, Andersson P, Yang Y, et al. A miR-327–FGF10–FGFR2-mediated autocrine signaling mechanism controls white fat browning. Nat Commun. 2017;8:2079.
49. Xie Z, Wang X, Liu X, Du H, Sun C, Shao X, et al. Adipose-derived exosomes exert proatherogenic effects by regulating macrophage foam cell formation and polarization. JAMA. 2018;7:e007442.
50. Lumeng CN, Bodzin JL, Saltiel AR. Obesity induces a phenotypic switch in adipose tissue macrophage polarization. J Clin Invest. 2007;117:175–84.
51. Fuster JJ, Ouchi N, Gokce N, Walsh K. Obesity-induced changes in adipose tissue microenvironment and their impact on cardiovascular disease. Circ Res. 2016;118:1786–807.
52. Krotkiewski M, Björntorp P, Sjöström L, Smith U. Impact of obesity on metabolism in men and women. Importance of regional adipose tissue distribution. J Clin Invest. 1983;72:1150–62.
53. Rutkowski JM, Stern JH, Scherer PE. The cell biology of fat expansion. J Cell Biol. 2015;208:501–12.
54. Fujisaka S, Usui I, Bukhari A, Ikutani M, Oya T, Kanatani Y, et al. Regulatory mechanisms for adipose tissue M1 and M2 macrophages in diet-induced obese mice. Diabetes. 2009;58:2574–82.
55. Onogi Y, Wada T, Kamiya C, Inata K, Matsuzawa T, Inaba Y, et al. PDGFRβ regulates adipose tissue expansion and glucose metabolism via vascular remodeling in diet-induced obesity. Diabetes. 2017;66:1008–21.
56. Chadderdon SM, Belcik JT, Bader L, Kirigiti MA, Peters DM, Kievit P, et al. Proinflammatory endothelial activation detected by molecular imaging in obese nonhuman primates coincides with onset of insulin resistance and progressively increases with duration of insulin resistance. Circulation. 2014;129:471–8.
57. Pasarica M, Sereda OR, Redman LM, Albarado DC, Hymel DT, Roan LE, et al. Reduced adipose tissue oxygenation in human obesity: evidence for rarefaction, macrophage chemotaxis, and inflammation without an angiogenic response. Diabetes. 2009;58:718–25.
58. Escobedo N, Proulx ST, Karaman S, Dillard ME, Johnson N, Detmar M, et al. Restoration of lymphatic function rescues obesity in Prox1-haploinsufficient mice. JCI Insight. 2016;1:e85096.
59. Villarroya F, Cereijo R, Villarroya J, Giralt M. Brown adipose tissue as a secretory organ. Nat Rev Endocrinol. 2017;13:26.
60. Franssens BT, Hoogduin H, Leiner T, van der Graaf Y, Visseren FL. Relation between brown adipose tissue and measures of obesity and metabolic dysfunction in patients with cardiovascular disease. J Magn Reson Imaging. 2017;46:497–504.
61. Chechi K, Voisine P, Mathieu P, Laplante M, Bonnet S, Picard F, et al. Functional characterization of the Ucp1-associated oxidative phenotype of human epicardial adipose tissue. Sci Rep. 2017;7:15566.
62. Antoniades C, Kotanidis CP, Berman DS. State-of-the-art review article. Atherosclerosis affecting fat: what can we learn by imaging perivascular adipose tissue? J Cardiovasc Comput Tomogr. 2019;13(5):288–96. https://doi.org/10.1016/j.jcct.2019.03.006. [Epub ahead of print].
63. Tisdale MJ. Cachexia in cancer patients. Nat Rev Cancer. 2002;2:862–71.
64. Han J, Meng Q, Shen L, Wu G. Interleukin-6 induces fat loss in cancer cachexia by promoting white adipose tissue lipolysis and browning. Lipids Health Dis. 2018;17:14.
65. Antonopoulos AS, Margaritis M, Coutinho P, Digby J, Patel R, Psarros C, et al. Reciprocal effects of systemic inflammation and brain natriuretic peptide on adiponectin biosynthesis in adipose tissue of patients with ischemic heart disease. Arterioscler Thromb Vasc Biol. 2014;34:2151–9.
66. Flegal KM, Kit BK, Orpana H, Graubard BI. Association of all-cause mortality with overweight and obesity using standard body mass index categories. JAMA. 2013;309:71.
67. Antonopoulos AS, Tousoulis D. The molecular mechanisms of obesity paradox. Cardiovasc Res. 2017;113:1074–86.
68. Aune D, Sen A, Prasad M, Norat T, Janszky I, Tonstad S, et al. BMI and all cause mortality: systematic review and non-linear dose-response meta-analysis of 230 cohort studies with 3.74 million deaths among 30.3 million participants. BMJ. 2016;353:i2156.
69. Youn J-Y, Siu KL, Lob HE, Itani H, Harrison DG, Cai H. Role of vascular oxidative stress in obesity and metabolic syndrome. Diabetes. 2014;63:2344–55.
70. Takaoka M, Suzuki H, Shioda S, Sekikawa K, Saito Y, Nagai R, et al. Endovascular injury induces rapid phenotypic changes in perivascular adipose tissue. Arterioscler Thromb Vasc Biol. 2010;30:1576–82.
71. Antonopoulos AS, Margaritis M, Verheule S, Recalde A, Sanna F, Herdman L, et al. Mutual regulation of epicardial adipose tissue and myocardial redox state by PPAR-γ/adiponectin signalling. Circ Res. 2016;118:842–55.
72. Crewe C, An YA, Scherer PE. The ominous triad of adipose tissue dysfunction: inflammation, fibrosis, and impaired angiogenesis. J Clin Invest. 2017;127:74–82.
73. Ohyama K, Matsumoto Y, Amamizu H, Uzuka H, Nishimiya K, Morosawa S, et al. Association of coronary perivascular adipose tissue inflammation and drug-eluting stent–induced coronary hyperconstricting responses in pigs. Arterioscler Thromb Vasc Biol. 2017;37:1757–64.
74. Kaul S, Rothney MP, Peters DM, Wacker WK, Davis CE, Shapiro MD, et al. Dual-energy X-ray absorptiometry for quantification of visceral fat. Obesity. 2012;20:1313–8.

75. Iacobellis G, Ribaudo MC, Assael F, Vecci E, Tiberti C, Zappaterreno A, et al. Echocardiographic epicardial adipose tissue is related to anthropometric and clinical parameters of metabolic syndrome: a new indicator of cardiovascular risk. J Clin Endocrinol Metab. 2003;88:5163–8.
76. Knuuti J, Wijns W, Saraste A, Capodanno D, Barbato E, Funck-Brentano C, ESC Scientific Document Group, et al. 2019 ESC Guidelines for the diagnosis and management of chronic coronary syndromes. Eur Heart J. 2020;41(3):407–77. https://doi.org/10.1093/eurheartj/ehz425. [Epub ahead of print].
77. Davidovich D, Gastaldelli A, Sicari R. Imaging cardiac fat. Eur Heart J Cardiovasc Imaging. 2013;14:625–30.
78. Krumm P, Mangold S, Gatidis S, Nikolaou K, Nensa F, Bamberg F, et al. Clinical use of cardiac PET/MRI: current state-of-the-art and potential future applications. Jpn J Radiol. 2018;36:313–23.
79. Nelson AJ, Worthley MI, Psaltis PJ, Carbone A, Dundon BK, Duncan RF, et al. Validation of cardiovascular magnetic resonance assessment of pericardial adipose tissue volume. J Magn Reson Imaging. 2009;11:15.
80. Pierdomenico SD, Pierdomenico AM, Cuccurullo F, Iacobellis G. Meta-analysis of the relation of echocardiographic epicardial adipose tissue thickness and the metabolic syndrome. Am J Cardiol. 2013;111:73–8.
81. Mahabadi AA, Massaro JM, Rosito GA, Levy D, Murabito JM, Wolf PA, et al. Association of pericardial fat, intrathoracic fat, and visceral abdominal fat with cardiovascular disease burden: the Framingham heart study. Eur Heart J. 2008;30:850–6.
82. Mahabadi AA, Lehmann N, Kälsch H, Robens T, Bauer M, Dykun I, et al. Association of epicardial adipose tissue with progression of coronary artery calcification is more pronounced in the early phase of atherosclerosis. JACC Cardiovasc Imaging. 2014;7:909–16.
83. Versteylen MO, Takx RAP, Joosen IAPG, Nelemans PJ, Das M, Crijns HJGM, et al. Epicardial adipose tissue volume as a predictor for coronary artery disease in diabetic, impaired fasting glucose, and non-diabetic patients presenting with chest pain. Eur Heart J Cardiovasc Imaging. 2012;13:517–23.
84. Ito T, Suzuki Y, Ehara M, Matsuo H, Teramoto T, Terashima M, et al. Impact of epicardial fat volume on coronary artery disease in symptomatic patients with a zero calcium score. Int J Cardiol. 2013;167:2852–8.
85. Bos D, Shahzad R, van Walsum T, van Vliet LJ, Franco OH, Hofman A, et al. Epicardial fat volume is related to atherosclerotic calcification in multiple vessel beds. Eur Heart J Cardiovasc Imaging. 2015;16:1264–9.
86. Tanami Y, Jinzaki M, Kishi S, Matheson M, Vavere AL, Rochitte CE, et al. Lack of association between epicardial fat volume and extent of coronary artery calcification, severity of coronary artery disease, or presence of myocardial perfusion abnormalities in a diverse, symptomatic patient population: results from the CORE320 multicenter study. Circ Cardiovasc Imaging. 2015;8:e002676.
87. Franssens BT, Nathoe HM, Leiner T, van der Graaf Y, Visseren FL, group Ss. Relation between cardiovascular disease risk factors and epicardial adipose tissue density on cardiac computed tomography in patients at high risk of cardiovascular events. Eur Heart J Cardiovasc Imaging. 2017;24:660–70.
88. Mazurek T, Kobylecka M, Zielenkiewicz M, Kurek A, Kochman J, Filipiak KJ, et al. PET/CT evaluation of 18F-FDG uptake in pericoronary adipose tissue in patients with stable coronary artery disease: independent predictor of atherosclerotic lesions' formation? J Nucl Cardiol. 2017;24:1075–84.
89. Abazid RM, Smettei OA, Kattea MO, Sayed S, Saqqah H, Widyan AM, et al. Relation between epicardial fat and subclinical atherosclerosis in asymptomatic individuals. J Thorac Imaging. 2017;32:378–82.
90. Mahabadi AA, Balcer B, Dykun I, Forsting M, Schlosser T, Heusch G, et al. Cardiac computed tomography-derived epicardial fat volume and attenuation independently distinguish patients with and without myocardial infarction. PLoS One. 2017;12:e0183514.
91. Hell MM, Ding X, Rubeaux M, Slomka P, Gransar H, Terzopoulos D, et al. Epicardial adipose tissue volume but not density is an independent predictor for myocardial ischemia. J Cardiovasc Comput Tomogr. 2016;10:141–9.
92. Antoniades C, Antonopoulos AS, Deanfield J. Imaging residual inflammatory cardiovascular risk. Eur Heart J. 2019; https://doi.org/10.1093/eurheartj/ehz474. [Epub ahead of print].
93. Oikonomou EK, Marwan M, Desai MY, Mancio J, Alashi A, Hutt Centeno E, et al. Non-invasive detection of coronary inflammation using computed tomography and prediction of residual cardiovascular risk (the CRISP CT study): a post-hoc analysis of prospective outcome data. Lancet. 2018;392:929–39.
94. Leipsic J, Abbara S, Achenbach S, Cury R, Earls JP, Mancini GJ, et al. SCCT guidelines for the interpretation and reporting of coronary CT angiography: a report of the society of cardiovascular computed tomography guidelines committee. J Cardiovasc Comput Tomogr. 2014;8:342–58.
95. Goeller M, Achenbach S, Cadet S, Kwan AC, Commandeur F, Slomka PJ, et al. Pericoronary adipose tissue computed tomography attenuation and high-risk plaque characteristics in acute coronary syndrome compared with stable coronary artery disease. JAMA Cardiol. 2018;3:858–63.
96. Marwan M, Hell M, Schuhbäck A, Gauss S, Bittner D, Pflederer T, et al. CT attenuation of pericoronary adipose tissue in normal versus

atherosclerotic coronary segments as defined by intravascular ultrasound. J Comput Assist Tomogr. 2017;41:762–7.
97. Kwiecinski J, Dey D, Cadet S, Lee SE, Otaki Y, Huynh PT, et al. Pericoronary adipose tissue density is associated with 18F-sodium fluoride coronary uptake in patients with high-risk plaques. J Am Coll Cardiol Imaging. 2019;12:2000–10.
98. Hedgire S, Baliyan V, Zucker EJ, Bittner DO, Staziaki PV, Takx RAP, et al. Perivascular epicardial fat stranding at coronary ct angiography: a marker of acute plaque rupture and spontaneous coronary artery dissection. Radiology. 2018;287:808–15.
99. Elnabawi YA, Oikonomou EK, Dey AK, Mancio J, Rodante JA, Aksentijevich M, et al. Association of biologic therapy with coronary inflammation in patients with psoriasis as assessed by perivascular fat attenuation index. JAMA Cardiol. 2019; https://doi.org/10.1001/jamacardio.2019.2589. [Epub ahead of print].
100. Gillies RJ, Kinahan PE, Hricak H. Radiomics: images are more than pictures, they are data. Radiology. 2015;278:563–77.
101. Aerts HJ, Velazquez ER, Leijenaar RT, Parmar C, Grossmann P, Carvalho S, et al. Decoding tumour phenotype by noninvasive imaging using a quantitative radiomics approach. Nat Commun. 2014;5:4006.
102. Oikonomou EK, Williams MC, Kotanidis CP, Desai MY, Marwan M, Antonopoulos AS, et al. A novel machine learning-derived radiotranscriptomic signature of perivascular fat improves cardiac risk prediction using coronary CT angiography. Eur Heart J. 2019;40:3529–43.
103. Dey D, Commandeur F. Radiomics to identify high-risk atherosclerotic plaque from computed tomography: the power of quantification. Circ Cardiovasc Imaging. 2017;10:e007254.
104. Kolossváry M, Karády J, Szilveszter B, Kitslaar P, Hoffmann U, Merkely B, et al. Radiomic features are superior to conventional quantitative computed tomographic metrics to identify coronary plaques with napkin-ring sign. Circ Cardiovasc Imaging. 2017;10:e006843.

Atrial Fibrillation and Epicardial Adipose Tissue

10

Ghaith Zaatari and Jeffrey J. Goldberger

Key Points

- Obesity has been associated with atrial fibrillation, while weight loss decreases atrial fibrillation (AF) burden and recurrence post-ablation.
- Epicardial adipose tissue is a risk factor for development of AF and predictor of recurrence after catheter ablation.
- The mechanism by which epicardial adipose tissue contributes to the pathogenesis of atrial fibrillation remains unclear. Various mechanisms have been proposed including fatty infiltration, fibrosis, inflammation, oxidative stress, atrial remodelling, and genetic factors.
- Peri-atrial epicardial adipose tissue (EAT) may play a more prominent role in the pathogenesis of AF due to its proximity to the atrial myocardium and local paracrine effect.

Introduction

Atrial fibrillation (AF) is linked with increased cardiovascular morbidity and mortality [1, 2]. AF is the most common sustained heart rhythm disorder affecting humans [3]. AF affects 5.2 million Americans as of 2010 with projections that it will affect 12.1 million people in the United States by 2030 [4]. Incremental cost related to AF has been estimated at $6–26 billion per year in the United States alone [5]. This rise in AF prevalence is partially connected to a growing elderly population with AF prevalence doubling with each advancing decade of age >50 years [6, 7]. Besides age, various risk factors predispose to the development of AF, such as coronary artery disease [8, 9], obesity [10, 11], hypertension [6, 12–14], diabetes mellitus [15–17], heart failure, [6, 18], and sleep apnea [19–21].

As these risk factors do not directly affect the atrium, their association with AF is likely mediated by intermediate pathways causing disease in the atrial myocardium. Moreover, as in coronary artery disease, the clinical manifestation of AF is likely preceded by years of subclinical progressive atrial disease (atrial myopathy), which may involve inflammation, oxidative stress, fibrosis, and electrical, structural, and autonomic remodelling [22–26]. Multiple studies show that obesity is associated with the development of AF substrate via various mechanisms [27–30]. Obesity may contribute to the

G. Zaatari · J. J. Goldberger (✉)
University of Miami Miller School of Medicine, Department of Medicine, Cardiovascular Division, Miami, FL, USA
e-mail: j-goldberger@miami.edu

G. Iacobellis (ed.), *Epicardial Adipose Tissue*, Contemporary Cardiology,
https://doi.org/10.1007/978-3-030-40570-0_10

development of AF indirectly via its effects on comorbidities such as hypertension (activation of renin-angiotensin-aldosterone system) and obstructive sleep apnea (hypoxia and hypercapnia, systemic information). Obesity may also be directly implicated in the development of AF via local pro-inflammatory effects [27–30].

Obesity is associated with epicardial adipose tissue (EAT) [10, 31–46]. Due to its contiguity to the underlying atrial myocardium, it is possible that epicardial adipose tissue (EAT) is associated with the development of AF. In this chapter, we will explore the nature of the relation between EAT and AF, pathophysiological mechanisms, clinical correlation, and some proposed future therapeutic options targeting EAT.

Obesity and Atrial Fibrillation

The role of adipose tissue in multiple disease states has now been clearly established. Adipose tissue is a heterogeneous tissue that includes mature adipocytes, inflammatory cells of various phenotypic characteristics, fibroblasts, and stem cells as well as vascular cells coming from microvascular structures embedded in the tissue [47]. All cell types contribute to the adipose tissue secretome, which may contain pro-inflammatory and pro-atherogenic adipocytokines (e.g., resistin, leptin, visfatin, and monocyte chemoattractant protein-1) in metabolically unhealthy obesity [48]. The adipocytokines secreted by the adipose tissue can exert paracrine effects on the neighboring vascular wall (i.e., perivascular adipose tissue) [49] or myocardium (i.e., epicardial adipose tissue) [50], as well as endocrine effects (i.e., from "remote" depots like subcutaneous adipose tissue) on the cardiovascular system through the circulation [51].

The most widely used assessment of adiposity is weight/body mass index [52]. The population disease burden due to the obesity epidemic is widely recognized. Obesity rates worldwide have nearly tripled in the last 40 years, with more than a third of the world's population being obese or overweight [53]. As for the United States, 38% of adults are obese, with a body mass index (BMI) over 30 kg/m^2, and an additional 33% are overweight with BMI between 25 and 30 kg/m^2 [54]. In recent years, obesity has been shown to be an independent risk factor for development of AF (Table 10.1) [10, 31–46]. Importantly, the Framingham Heart Study revealed a 4% increased risk in incident AF per unit increase in body mass index in both men and women [31]. A meta-analysis of 51 studies involving more than 600,000 individuals evaluated the impact of obesity on AF [36]. It was found that every 5-unit rise in BMI confers an additional 19–29% risk of incident AF, a 10% risk of postoperative AF, and a 13% risk of post-ablation AF [36]. The association of obesity with other coexisting risk factors for AF (such as diabetes and hypertension) raises uncertainty in the independent association between obesity and AF. To account for this, Lee et al. recently conducted a retrospective study with a cohort of nearly 400,000 obese patients free of comorbidities [37]. The association between AF and obesity remained significant with a hazard ratio of 1.3 (95% confidence intervals 1.14–1.48) when compared to healthy non-obese patients [37]. Additionally, one study that followed 3248 patients for 5.1 years found that BMI independently predicted progression of AF from paroxysmal to permanent – hazard ratio of 1.04 (95% CI, 1.03–1.06; $P < 0.0001$) [38]. BMI was also shown to be an independent predictor of AF relapse post-ablation therapy in a recent multicenter observational study hazard ratio of 1.01 per kg/m^2 (95% CI, 1.01–1.02, $P = 0.002$) [39].

The impact of weight loss on AF is also well established and evident in multiple recent studies [55–60]. Abed et al. conducted a randomized, interventional clinical trial in Australia for overweight or obese patients (body mass index >27 kg/m^2) with symptomatic AF. Patients were randomized into a structured weight management group (intervention) or general lifestyle advice (control) [55]. The interventional group showed a dramatic reduction in weight, AF symptom burden scores, symptom severity scores, and number of AF episodes when compared to control [55]. The Aggressive Risk Factor Reduction Study for Atrial Fibrillation (ARREST-AF) study [59] included a cohort of patients who underwent a structured risk

Table 10.1 Epidemiological studies showing association between obesity and atrial fibrillation

Study	Country	Study design	Population	Follow-up	Key findings for atrial fibrillation
Wang et al. [31]	USA	Community-based prospective observational study	*N* = 5282 Age 57 ± 13 years 55% female	13.7 years	AF adjusted HR 1.04 (95% CI, 1.01–1.04; *P* = 0.02) for men and 1.04 (95% CI, 1.01–1.07; *P* = 0.009) for women per unit increase in BMI
Frost et al. [10]	Denmark	Population-based prospective cohort	*N* = 47,589 Age 56 years (50–64) 53% female	5.7 years	Adjusted HR of 1.08 (95% CI, 1.05–1.11) for men and 1.06 (95% CI, 1.03–1.09) for women for AF/flutter per unit increase in BMI
Tedrow et al. [33]	USA	Prospective women's health study	*N* = 34,309 Age 54.6 ± 7.0 years 100% female	12.9 years	BMI was linearly associated with AF risk, with adjusted HR 1.04 (95% CI, 1.03–1.06)
Huxley et al. [40]	USA	Prospective The Atherosclerosis Risk in Communities study (ARIC)	*N* = 14,598 54.2 ± 5.8 55% female	17.1 years	17.9% AF incident attributed to overweight and obesity
Long et al. [41]	China	Community-based nested case control study Giangzhou Biobank cohort study	*N* = 19,964 Age 62 years 71% female	2.9 years	Adjusted HR 1.06 (95% CI, 1.01–1.11 per unit increase in BMI)
Karasoy et al. [42]	Denmark	Prospective observational study	*N* = 271,203 Age 30.6 ± 4.7 years 100% female	4.6 years	Adjusted HR = 1.07 (95% CI, 1.04–1.11; *P* < 0.0001) per unit increase in BMI
Knuiman et al. [34]	Australia	Prospective observational study	*N* = 4267 56% female	15 years	Adjusted HR 1.34 (95% CI, 1.21–1.49; *P* < 0.0001) per 1 SD increase in BMI
Berkovitch et al. [43]	Israel	Prospective observational study	*N* = 18,290 Age 39 ± 11 years 73% male	6.4 years	Adjusted HR compared to normal weight 1.49 (95% CI, 1.11–2.00; *P* = 0.008) for overweight and 2.34 (95% CI, 1.64–3.34; *P* = 0.001) for obese
Lee et al. [37]	South Korea	Retrospective observational study	*N* = 389,321 Age 45.6 ± 11 years 27% female	7.5 years	Compared to non-obese HR for obesity 1.19 (95% CI, 1.12–1.27)
Foy et al. [44]	USA	Prospective observational cohort study	*N* = 67,278 76.9% female	8 years	Adjusted OR 1.40 (95% CI, 1.26–1.56) for obesity
Lim et al. [45]	South Korea	Korean National Health Insurance Service–Health Screening cohort	*N* = 171,324 39% female	47.4 months	Adjusted HR 1.01 (95% CI, 0.9–1.12; *P* = 0.85) for risk of new onset AF for BMI >25

AF atrial fibrillation, *BMI* body mass index, *CI* confidence interval, *EAT* epicardial adipose tissue, *HR* hazard ratio, *OR* odds ratio, *PAF* paroxysmal atrial fibrillation, *PeAF* persistent atrial fibrillation, *PVI* pulmonary vein isolation

factor management program following catheter ablation for treatment of AF in one arm, and a control group who did not participate in the risk factor management program in the second arm. Patients in the risk factor management program experienced a 13% decrease in body mass index (versus 1% for the control group) after a median follow-up of 42.8 months with significant decline in blood pressure and LA volume index [59]. Additionally, patients in this program after 2 years of follow-up achieved arrhythmia free survival at final follow-up of 32.9% (*P* < 0.001) after a single procedure and

87% ($P < 0.001$) after multiple procedures versus 9.7% ($P < 0.001$) for a single procedure and 17.8% ($P < 0.001$) for patients requiring multiple procedures in the control group [59]. The LEGACY study noted that weight loss ≥10% resulted in six times greater probability of AF-free survival (95% confidence interval: 3.4–10.3; $P < 0.001$) compared to the groups with 3–9% and <3% weight loss [60]. Moreover, the REVERSE-AF study assessed the progression and reversal of AF in the same cohort of the LEGACY study. In patients with ≥10% weight loss, 88% experienced reversal from persistent to paroxysmal or no AF ($P < 0.001$) at final follow-up after individualized arrhythmia management, a striking difference when compared to 49% and 26% reversal in patients who lost 3–9% and <3% of their body weight, respectively ($P < 0.001$) [58]. Despite the uncertainty of the exact mechanisms by which weight loss impacts AF, the evidence seems clear and strong. Hence, and for the first time, the 2019 focused update to the AF guidelines [61] introduced a class I recommendation: "For overweight and obese patients with AF, weight loss, combined with risk factor modification, is recommended" based on emerging data [36, 55, 59].

The mechanisms by which obesity impacts AF require investigation. In theory, obesity may directly (in addition to indirect effects through hypertension and diabetes) contribute to AF via systemic effects of visceral adiposity or from direct effects of the cardiac adipose tissue on the adjacent myocardium. The cardiac adipose tissue has been studied as the epicardial adipose tissue (EAT) or pericardial adipose tissue (PAT) and is associated with the development of AF (see Clinical Evidence of Association between EAT and AF) [62–66]. EAT is associated with increased body mass index (BMI) and is a well-documented risk factor for AF initiation and perpetuation [66–68]. EAT is a unique visceral adipose depot with anatomic and functional proximity to the myocardium and coronary arteries [69–72]. Advanced cardiac imaging has paved the way for better characterization of EAT and studying its effect on cardiovascular health [65, 73]. Under physiologic conditions, EAT has cardioprotective metabolic, thermogenic, and mechanical characteristics [70]. The pathophysiological mechanisms that link EAT to AF, however, remain elusive and are not entirely understood. Atrial electrical and structural remodeling, inflammation, oxidative stress, neural mechanisms, and genetic factors may be pathways mediating EAT effects on AF occurrence [22–26]. This will be discussed in the next section.

EAT and Atrial Fibrillation: Anatomy, Physiology, and Pathophysiological Mechanisms

Anatomy

EAT is a peculiar visceral fat depot with anatomical and functional contiguity to the myocardium and coronary arteries [69–72]. EAT is situated between the myocardium and visceral layer of the pericardium and is present in the atrioventricular and interventricular grooves without a structure or fascia separating it from the myocardium and the epicardial vessels [72, 74–76]. This means EAT and the myocardium share common microcirculation, suggesting a close and strong interaction between the two structures [77]. A paracrine process is one possible biological interaction between EAT and its adjacent myocardium. A vasocrine pathway is also likely via the vasa vasorum [72]. In contrast, pericardial adipose tissue is another cardiac fat deposit situated outside the visceral pericardium and on the outer surface of the parietal pericardium [77]. Although PAT and EAT are close in proximity, they are distinct [77]. Unlike EAT, PAT is separated from the myocardium by visceral pericardium [78]. PAT and EAT are also embryologically different [72]. EAT originates from the splanchnopleuric mesoderm, which also gives rise to mesenteric and omental fat [79], while PAT is derived from the primitive thoracic mesenchyme [79]. EAT is perfused by the coronary arteries, while PAT is supplied by a branch of the internal mammary artery, the pericardiophrenic artery [79]. However, it is noteworthy that the effects of PAT rather than EAT on the heart are often reported [63–65, 80–84]. This likely relates to the methods of quantitation. A more detailed look at anatomy and terminology is described in Chap. 1.

Moreover, recent findings indicate that regional EAT distribution is important. Left atrial EAT (LAEAT) is significantly increased in patients with AF and may be related to the recurrence of AF after catheter ablation [65, 83, 85–89]. LAEAT displays a unique genetic pattern when compared to peri-coronary and peri-ventricular EAT [90]. LAEAT is enriched in genes involved in oxidative phosphorylation, muscular contraction, and calcium signaling when compared to other EAT areas [90].

Physiology

The functional complexity of human EAT is not yet fully understood. However, under physiological conditions, EAT's role in the heart is generally distinguished by mechanical, metabolic, thermogenic, and endocrine/paracrine functions [70]. EAT mechanically serves as a cushion protecting the coronary arteries from extreme distortion caused by arterial pulsation and myocardial contraction via its compressibility and elasticity [91]. Metabolically, EAT differs from other visceral fat in its ability to synthesize and break down free fatty acids (FFA) at a higher rate and a lower rate of glucose utilization [75, 92]. EAT contains abundant saturated fatty acids, and this enrichment and increased metabolism of free fatty acids (FFAs) maintain myocardial energy supplies, particularly during periods of high demand [71, 93]. FFA oxidation is responsible for about 50–70% of the energy production of the heart, and it is proposed that EAT functions as a buffer to protect the heart against excessively high levels of FFAs [72].

Moreover, EAT has higher expression of uncoupling protein-1 (UCP1) genes when compared to fat depots in other parts of the body [94]. This may provide EAT the thermogenic ability to produce heat (like brown adipose tissue) to protect the coronary arteries from hypothermia damage similar to what we see in hibernating animals [75]. EAT also acts as a source for paracrine modulators of myocardial inflammation and oxidative stress by producing multiple bioactive cytokines [95]. Under normal physiological conditions, cytokines such as adiponectin and adrenomedullin have antidiabetic, antiatherogenic, antioxidative, and anti-inflammatory roles exerting cardioprotective functions [96–99]. This is discussed in detail in Chap. 2. However, despite its cardioprotective mechanisms, EAT in the pathological state can be harmful, producing inflammatory factors exacerbating cardiovascular diseases and may participate in the pathogenesis of AF via various mechanisms that will be discussed next.

Pathophysiological Mechanisms

Multiple studies have established an association between EAT and AF (see Clinical Evidence of Association between EAT and AF). However, the exact mechanisms by which EAT contribute to AF development are unresolved and remain an intriguing topic in translational research. Multiple mechanisms have been identified. These mechanisms could include a direct effect of EAT on the atrium (e.g., by the infiltration of adipose tissue into the myocardium leading to altered atrial electrophysiological properties) or indirect mechanisms (e.g., by acting as a source for paracrine modulators of myocardial inflammation and oxidative stress). Altered gene expression may play a role in the contribution of EAT to AF. Alternatively, EAT may influence local atrial and pulmonary vein electrophysiologic properties, such as the refractory period, which interact with a remodeled atrial substrate to sustain AF [100]. These mechanisms are discussed in detail below.

Fatty Infiltration

Given its location and the lack of fascia separating EAT from the underlying myocardium, direct fatty infiltration into the atrium is possible. Multiple previous studies have noted that the abundance of epicardial fat is associated with direct adipocyte infiltration into the underlying atrial myocardium [78, 101]. This may contribute to myocardial functional disorganization and the formation of local arrhythmogenic substrate [102]. Mahajan et al., for example, found an accumulation of epicardial fat with pronounced myocardial infiltration by adipocytes, particularly over the posterior left atrial wall in diet-induced obese sheep [101]. In contrast, non-obese control sheep had less epicardial fat accumulation and minimal adipocyte infiltration into the myocardium. Such direct fatty infiltration can mechanically separate myocytes and could directly result in conduction slowing or could promote side-to-side cell connection loss similar to that seen with microfibrosis [103, 104]. Simultaneous endo-epicardial mapping of atrial electrical activity has shown that breakthrough and micro reentry circuits increase with increasing AF substrate complexity. Losing epicardial layer continuity due to atrial fibrosis appears to be one of the major determinants of the complexity of fibrillatory conduction pathways [105]. In addition to the direct anatomical effect of fatty infiltration, Haemers et al. [106] reported that patients with a history of AF had a higher histological degree of fibrosis of the adipose tissue present in sub-epicardium, with abundance of active inflammatory cells [106]. These observations suggest that this adipose tissue component of the atrial myocardium may not be an innocent bystander.

Inflammation

Inflammation is a potential contributor to the pathogenesis of AF. It may play a role in AF initiation and perpetuation [107]. Notable markers of inflammation, like C-reactive protein (CRP), interleukin-6 (IL-6), interleukin-8 (IL-8), interleukin-1b (IL-1b), and tumor necrosis factor-α (TNF-α), have been associated with the incidence, severity, and recurrence of AF [108–112]. These markers are produced by EAT and may have local pro-inflammatory effects on the adjacent atrial myocardium that facilitate arrhythmogenesis. Aviles et al. first demonstrated that elevated CRP predicted increased risk of developing AF in a large population-based prospective cohort including 5806 patients [111]. In another study, it was found that high levels of CRP were a predictor of arrhythmia recurrence after cardioversion [110]. Li et al. demonstrated that serum TNF-α blood levels were higher in patients with AF compared with those in sinus rhythm and in persistent and permanent AF compared with paroxysmal AF [113].

The immunohistochemistry of the left atrial appendage obtained from 16 patients during cardiac surgery showed immunologically active monocytes, and macrophages with abundance of inflammatory proteins like monocyte chemoattractive protein-1, intracellular adhesion molecule-1, and vascular cell adhesion molecule-1 that were more expressed in the endocardium of patients with AF compared to those in sinus rhythm [114]. This supports the hypothesis of a local immunologic inflammatory response in the atrium of patients with AF [114]. Moreover, the neutrophil-to-lymphocyte ratio was also shown to be an independent predictor for non-valvular AF [115]. Interestingly, it was demonstrated that elevated levels of monocyte chemoattractant protein-1 were found to be associated with increased epicardial fat thickness [116]. A significant correlation was found between EAT thickness and neutrophil-to-lymphocyte ratio [117].

In addition, the inflammatory activity of EAT reflected by maximal standardized uptake value (SUV) of 18-fluorodeoxyglucose(FDG)-positron emission tomography (PET) which reflects glucose metabolism was found to be higher in patients with AF compared to controls, and inflammatory activity of EAT adjacent to the LA, atrioventricular groove, and left main artery was greater than in subcutaneous or visceral thoracic tissue [118]. Kusayama et al. [119] reported that inflammation of EAT around the LA, but not subcutaneous adipose tissue is related to the presence of paroxysmal AF.

In addition to pro-inflammatory cytokines, adipose tissue also secretes adiponectin, an adipocytokine with anti-inflammatory effects [120]. Kourliouros et al. conducted a study to investigate the role of adiponectin in the pathogenesis of postoperative AF. Ninety patients undergoing coronary artery bypass graft (CABG) surgery had adiponectin level measured in serum and EAT. Increased levels of adiponectin were associated with sinus rhythm (SR) following surgery, thus reinforcing the inflammatory hypothesis in the pathogenesis of postoperative AF [121]. Moreover, an inverse relationship between adiponectin and LA size, independent of age, sex, insulin resistance, and left ventricular mass, has been reported, suggesting that adiponectin could influence atrial remodeling [122]. Taken together, if inflammatory pathways in peri-atrial adipose tissue are implicated in the pathogenesis of AF, this could be a potential future target for the prevention of AF. For example, intraoperative dexamethasone administration demonstrated significant protection against AF after cardiac surgery in one large clinical study [123]. A recent meta-analysis demonstrated that steroid therapy reduces the incidence of postoperative AF and the length of stay in the intensive care unit or in the hospital [124]. It is possible that the greatest benefit of anti-inflammatory interventions is limited to settings of inflammatory reaction due to tissue damage such as in cardiac surgery and catheter ablation. More studies are needed to elucidate the role of inflammation and the benefit of anti-inflammatory interventions in patients with AF.

Atrial Remodelling

Electrical Remodelling

Left atrial EAT can directly modulate electrical properties and ion currents of LA myocytes. When LA myocytes were incubated with epicardial adipocytes, they had longer action potential durations, a more-positive resting membrane potential, larger late sodium currents, L-type calcium currents, and transient outward potassium currents (I_{to}), but smaller delayed rectifier potassium and inward rectifier potassium (K_{ir}) currents than control LA myocytes [125]. In the clinical setting, epicardial fat was independently associated with atrial conduction time in a large population study as indicated by P-wave indices [126]. Moreover, left atrial EAT was associated with lower bipolar voltage and electrogram fractionation in 30 patients assessed in sinus rhythm before AF ablation. Multivariate analysis for the potential nonlinear association between EAT and low voltage zones was significant with OR = 1.60 ($P < 0.001$) [127]. Another small study using a 3D merge process and dominant frequency left atrial map identified EAT locations to correspond to high dominant frequency during AF [128, 129]. These data suggest a possible role of EAT on AF electrophysiological substrate that requires further research.

Structural Remodeling

Another potential mechanism is the role of EAT in atrial structural remodeling. Atrial fibrosis is the hallmark of structural remodeling. Interstitial fibrosis leads to heterogeneity of conduction, which provides a substrate for AF [130]. Atrial fibrosis is the primary pathologic abnormality seen in AF-related structural remodeling, and the degree of fibrosis has clinical implications [116, 131]. EAT may contribute to atrial fibrosis by exerting a paracrine effect on the atrium secreting profibrotic cytokines [132] such as activin A and matrix metalloproteinases (MMP) [72, 78, 121, 133, 134].

Activin A is a member of the TGF-ß superfamily. First recognized as an inducer of follicle-stimulating hormone release, activin A is a multifunctional cytokine expressed in various tissue types. A profibrotic effect of activin A has already been described for liver fibrosis [135–137]. In rats, the supplementation of culture media with recombinant human activin A-induced marked rat atrial myocardial fibrosis, while anti-activin A antibody neutralized these profibrotic effects [138]. Both EAT-conditioned medium and activin A induced the expression of TGF-ß1 and -β2 in the atria, which could indirectly mediate the profibrotic effect of activin A [138]. Activin A-induced cardiac effects other than fibrosis have also been described. For instance, this cytokine has anti-hypertrophic and anti-apoptotic properties on the myocardium when it is exposed to ischemia, reperfusion, and pressure overload injuries [139, 140]. Activin A causes a negative inotropic effect on isolated guinea pig cardiac myocytes, suggesting a direct effect of this cytokine on the excitation-contraction coupling process [141].

MMPs are important regulators of extracellular matrix homeostasis, including the various collagen fibers and basement membrane components. During AF, it has been demonstrated that upregulated activity of several MMPs, notably MMP2 and 7, contribute to the accumulation of interstitial fibrosis [142]. Levels of serum MMP2, which has been implicated in atrial remodeling, were higher in patients with greater EAT volume [143]. MMP8, which is abundantly expressed in EAT, is known to be involved in the formation of atherosclerotic plaques [144, 145], whereas little is known of its role in myocardial fibrosis [146]. Venteclef et al. found that the level of both activin A and MMP8 are enhanced in patients with heart failure. Moreover, Greulich et al. [139] report that activin A is more abundantly expressed in the EAT of obese patients with type 2 diabetes.

In a recent study, Wang et al. [147] showed that connective tissue growth factor (cTGF) expression is significantly higher in EAT than in subcutaneous or pericardial adipose tissue from patients with AF and in EAT from patients with sinus rhythm. They concluded that cTGF is associated with atrial fibrosis and can be an essential risk factor for AF [147].

EAT may also affect the atrial cellular components by altering the proliferation of myofibroblasts and the number of dedifferentiated and dystrophic myocytes [148, 149]. In fact, adipose tissue contains abundant stem cells located in the stroma fraction [150, 151] that are capable of differentiating not only into adipocytes but also into cardiomyocytes [152] or myofibroblasts [153]. Therefore, cardiac fatty tissue may constitute a source of precursor cells that can differentiate into myofibroblasts, contributing to atrial structural remodeling.

EAT may contribute to structural remodeling by promoting ventricular diastolic dysfunction. Patients with left ventricular diastolic dysfunction have a significant increase in EAT volume [154]. Suffee et al. [155] demonstrated that adult atrial epicardial progenitor cells can transition to adipocytes and provided evidence that this process is driven by atrial natriuretic peptide (ANP) secreted by the myocardium. EAT accumulation in adult atria is a slow process that could occur in response to chronic alterations of atrial myocardium workload and metabolic conditions. Hence, these data indicate a possible crosstalk between EAT expansion and mechanical function of the atrial myocardium [155].

Oxidative Stress

EAT is known to be a source of reactive oxygen species that could contribute to the pathogenesis of AF [156]. Recently, Antonopoulos et al. [50] demonstrated that products of oxidation, such as 4-hydroxynonenal which is generated in the human cardiac tissue under conditions of increased oxidative stress, can act as signaling molecules and result in adiponectin upregulation in neighboring EAT. Adiponectin has a cardioprotective paracrine effect, and its upregulation is evidence of local defensive response of EAT against oxidative stress. Previous data have shown that the production of reactive oxygen species is higher in human EAT than it is in subcutaneous adipose tissue [156]. Ascorbat, an antioxidant and peroxynitrite decomposition catalyst, inhibited reactive oxygen species in dogs and appeared to attenuate atrial remodeling induced by rapid pacing [157].

Neural Mechanism

The autonomic nervous system plays an important role in the initiation and maintenance of AF. EAT is the anatomic site of the intrinsic cardiac autonomic nervous system, namely, ganglionated plexi (GP) and interconnecting nerves, especially in the posterior wall around pulmonary vein ostia [70]. These ganglia are a critical element responsible for the initiation and maintenance of AF [158, 159]. Sympathovagal imbalance detected by both impaired heart rate variability and heart rate turbulence parameters has been demonstrated to be related to EAT thickness [160]. Activation of the ganglionated plexi (GP) located within the epicardial fat tissue can cause both parasympathetic and sympathetic stimulation, resulting in shortening of action potential duration and increases in calcium transient, respectively, in the atrial myocardium [161]. Recent evidence also suggests that it is the ganglionated plexi activity to the PVs that is important in the pathogenesis of AF [162]. One study demonstrated that stimuli applied to PVs do not induce AF, unless there is simultaneous stimulation of the adjacent GP that does not excite the atrial myocardium [163]. In isolated canine PV preparations, simultaneous administration of acetylcholine plus norepinephrine [164] or local autonomic (both parasympathetic and sympathetic) nerve electrical stimulation [165] has been shown to induce early after depolarizations (EADs) and short surges of triggered firing from the PVs, similar to the pattern recorded from the PVs in patients with paroxysmal AF [164].

Multiple clinical studies have investigated the role that neuromodulation may have in controlling AF, particularly by ablation of ganglionated plexi of the intrinsic cardiac nervous system [166]. It is possible that the encasing epicardial fat influences the ganglionated plexi and thus contributes to arrhythmogenesis. It is interesting to note that botulinum toxin injection into epicardial fat pads during surgery may reduce cardiac autonomic nervous activity and have long-term effects on AF, potentially by suppressing ganglionated plexi [167].

Genetic Factors

Gene expression represents a new perspective in understanding the precise role of EAT in AF pathogenesis. In an experimental study that utilized human and pig atrial samples, both AF and rapid pacing were associated with significant changes in atrial gene expression consistent with the induction of an adipocyte-related expression profile [168]. These genes favor the development of important risk factors for AF like obesity and diabetes mellitus and may facilitate AF substrate formation by increasing atrial ectopic fat and fat infiltration [168].

The peri-atrial EAT transcriptome profile is notable for the expression of genes implicated in oxidative phosphorylation, muscular contraction, and Ca^{2+} signaling [90]. The SERCA1 gene codes for a Ca^{2+}/ATP-dependent intracellular pump that translocates the cytosolic Ca^{2+} into the lumen of the sarcoplasmic reticulum and promotes excitation-contraction coupling [169]. Moreover, EAT secretome was described as a possible substrate for postoperative AF [170]. It encompasses various proteins differentially expressed in patients who later develop postoperative AF. Among those, gelsolin reduction, a protein involved in inflammation and ion channel regulation, was associated with postoperative AF [170].

Clinical Evidence of Association Between EAT and Atrial Fibrillation

Several studies have described the association between cardiac adipose tissue and AF (Table 10.2) [64, 65, 80–82, 85, 86, 102, 171–174] and AF recurrence post-catheter ablation (Table 10.3) [65, 83, 85, 87–89, 175–179]. One of the largest studies that examined the relationship between pericardial fat and AF is from the Framingham Heart study. In this study involving 3217 participants, the investigators characterized pericardial fat (defined as adipose tissue within the pericardial sac) with computed tomography (CT) and observed that pericardial fat volume predicted AF risk independent of other measures of adiposity OR = 1.28 (95% CI, 1.05–1.6; $P = 0.03$) for every standard deviation increase in PAT volume [64]. This relation remained significant despite adjustment for common AF risk factors, including age, sex, myocardial infarction, heart failure, BMI, and other regional fat deposits [64]. Importantly, the study did not show similar association of AF with other fat deposits such as intrathoracic or abdominal visceral fat. This suggests that contiguity of adipose tissue rather than generalized increases in fat depots may be essential in the pathogenesis of AF [64].

Table 10.2 Studies showing association between epicardial and pericardial adipose tissue with atrial fibrillation

Study	Study design and location	Fat depot	Imaging	Population	Findings
Thanassoulis et al. [64]	Retrospective study Framingham Heart Study USA	PAT	CT	$N = 3217$ 54 AF	PAT associated with prevalent AF in multivariable-adjusted models OR 1.28 per SD of PAT volume (95% CI, 1.03–1.58; $P = 0.03$)
Batal et al. [171]	Retrospective study USA	LAEAT	CT	73 no AF 60 PAF 36 PeAF	LAEAT was a multivariate predictor of AF burden (OR 5.30; 95% CI, 1.39–20.24; $P = 0.015$)
Al Chekakie et al. [80]	Retrospective study USA	PAT	CT	76 no AF 126 PAF 71 PeAF	PAT multivariate predictor of PAF (OR = 1.11; 95% CI, 1.01–1.23, $P = 0.04$) and PeAF (OR 1.18, 95% CI, 1.05–1.33; $P = 0.004$)
Tsao et al. [85]	Retrospective study Taiwan	EAT	CT	34 no AF 68 AF	EAT increased in AF (29.9 ± 12.3 vs 20.2 ± 6.5 cm^3; $P < 0.001$)
Nagashima et al. [86]	Retrospective study Japan	EAT	CT	37 no AF 24 PAF 16 PeAF	Increased EAT and LAEAT in PAF vs no AF and PeAF vs PAF and no AF
Shin et al. [172]	Retrospective study South Korea	EAT	CT	80 no AF 40 PAF 40 PeAF	Increased EAT in PAF vs no AF and PeAF vs PAF and no AF
Wong et al. [65]	Retrospective study Australia	PAT	MRI	20 no AF 38 PAF 34 PeAF 30 permanent AF	PAT (OR 11.25; 95% CI, 2.07–61.24; $P = 0.005$) and peri-atrial fat (OR 5.35; 95% CI, 1.25–22.66; $P = 0.02$) are predictors of AF
Nakanishi et al. [173]	Retrospective study USA	EAT volume	CT	262 no AF 16 AF	Peri-atrial EAT a multivariate predictor of AF ($P < 0.001$)
Greif et al. [81]	Retrospective study Germany	PAT	CT	934 no AF 223 PAF 131 PeAF	PAT multivariate predictor of AF (OR 1.52; 95% CI, 1.14–2.00; $P = 0.03$) and of PeAF (OR 2.58; 95% CI, 1.69–3.99; $P < 0.001$)
Drossos et al. [82]	Prospective study Greece	PAT	CT	55 no AF 28 AF	PAT multivariate predictor of AF post-CABG (OR 1.018; 95%, CI, 1.009–1.027; $P = 0.0001$)
Kanazawa et al. [174]	Prospective study Japan	PAT	CT	120 no AF 80 PAF 40 PeAF	PAT predictor of AF (OR 1.024; $P < 0.001$) and was independently associated with PeAF (OR = 1.018; $P < 0.018$)
Yorgun et al. [102]	Retrospective study Turkey	EAT Peri-atrial fat	CT	192 no AF 169 PAF 133 PeAF 124 permanent AF	EAT thickness were associated with AF (OR = 1.69; 95% CI, 1.54–2.85; $P = 0.002$) and peri-atrial fat associated with AF (OR 1.76; 95% CI, 1.35–3.22; $P = 0.001$)

AF atrial fibrillation, *CI* confidence interval, *CT* computed tomography, *EAT* epicardial adipose tissue, *LA* left atrial, *OR* odds ratio, *PAF* paroxysmal atrial fibrillation, *PeAF* persistent atrial fibrillation

Another study showed a correlation of pericardial adipose tissue with the severity of AF subtypes. Al Chekakie et al. [80] demonstrated that pericardial fat correlated with paroxysmal (OR = 1.11; 95% CI: 1.01–1.23, $P = 0.04$) and persistent AF (OR = 1.18; 95% CI: 1.05–1.33, $P = 0.004$), independent of traditional AF risk factors including age, hypertension, sex, left atrial (LA) enlargement, valvular heart disease, left ventricular ejection fraction, diabetes mellitus, and BMI. This correlation was further confirmed in a recent meta-analysis that reported that EAT volume is associ-

Table 10.3 Studies showing association between epicardial and pericardial adipose tissue with atrial fibrillation recurrence post-catheter ablation

Study	Study design and location	Fat depot	Imaging	Population	Findings
Wong et al. [65]	Retrospective study Australia	PAT	MRI	20 no AF 38 PAF 34 PeAF 30 permanent AF	PAT predictive long-term AF recurrence post-ablation ($P = 0.035$)
Tsao et al. [85]	Retrospective study Taiwan	EAT	CT	34 no AF 68 AF	EAT multivariate predictor of AF recurrence after ablation ($P = 0.038$)
Murakami et al. [175]	Prospective study Japan	EAT	CT	32 PAF 6 PeAF	EAT a multivariate predictor of AF recurrence post-ablation (HR = 1.36; 95% CI, 1.10–1.66; $P < 0.004$)
Chao et al. [87]	Retrospective study Taiwan	EAT	TTE	227 PAF 56 non-PAF	Independent predictor of AF recurrence Non-PAF HR = 2.361 (95% CI, 1.4–3.98; $P < 0.001$) EAT thickness HR = 2.863 (95% CI, 2.11–3.88; $P < 0.001$)
Kim et al. [83]	Prospective study South Korea	PAT	CT	450 PAF 215 PeAF	PAT a significant predictor for AF recurrence post-ablation in PeAF (HR = 1.1; 95% CI, 1.05–1.16; $P < 0.001$)
Soucek et al. [176]	Prospective USA	EAT	CT	74 PAF 28 PeAF	EAT a predictive of 3 months AF recurrence after PVI (RR 1.01; 95% CI, 1.001–1.018; $P = 0.018$)
Kocyigit et al. [88]	Retrospective study Turkey	Peri-atrial EAT	CT	249 patients with AF	Peri-atrial EAT thickness multivariate predictor of late AF recurrence (HR 1.086; 95% CI, 1.037–1.137; $P = 0.001$)
Masuda et al. [89]	Prospective study Japan	EAT	CT	53 AF	Left atrial EAT multivariate predictor of early AF recurrence (OR 1.02; 95% CI, 1.01–1.03; $P < 0.003$)
Canpolat et al. [177]	Prospective study Turkey	EAT	TTE	190 PAF 44 PeAF	EAT thickness is a multivariate predictor of AF recurrence (HR 1.36; 95% CI, 1.10–1.66, $P < 0.004$)
Ciuffo et al. [178]	Prospective study USA	LA-peri-atrial fat	CT	143 AF	Higher LA-peri-atrial fat attenuation multivariate predictor of AF recurrence (HR 2.65; $P = 0.001$)
Mirolo et al. [179]	Retrospective study France	EAT	Cardiac MRI	231 AF	EAT a multivariate predictor of AF recurrence at 4 months (HR 1.96; 95% CI, 1.20–3.18; $P = 0.007$)

AF atrial fibrillation, *CI* confidence interval, *CT* computed tomography, *EAT* epicardial adipose tissue, *HR* hazard ratio, *LA* left atrial, *MRI* magnetic resonance imaging, *OR* odds ratio, *PAF* paroxysmal atrial fibrillation, *PeAF* persistent atrial fibrillation, *PVI* pulmonary vein isolation, *RR* risk ratio, *TTE* transthoracic echocardiogram

ated with increased risk of AF – one standard deviation was associated with 2.2 higher odds of persistent AF compared to paroxysmal AF (OR = 2.19, 95% CI: 1.66–2.88) [66, 68, 180]. Noteworthy, the strength of associations of AF with EAT was greater than for measures of abdominal or overall adiposity [66]. Increased EAT has also been independently associated with AF after coronary artery bypass grafting [82, 181], electrical cardioversion [182], or ablation [65, 83, 85–89, 176, 177, 183]. Moreover, pericardial fat, when measured by MRI in 130 patients, showed a strong dose-response association with LA volume ($P < 0.001$), AF chronicity ($P < 0.05$), symptom burden ($P < 0.05$), and recurrence of AF after ablation ($P = 0.035$) [65]. However, systemic measures of obesity, including body mass index and body surface area, were not associated with these outcomes. These associations remained valid despite multivariate adjustment and adjustment for body weight.

Recently, Shin et al. also reported that epicardial fat volumes and peri-atrial fat thickness measured by CT scan were significantly associated with the prevalence and persistence of AF [172]. Moreover, a multivariate analysis revealed that only total EAT ($P = 0.004$) and thickness of intraatrial septum ($P = 0.016$) were independently associated with left atrial volume in patients with AF even after adjusting for BMI. These studies have shown that EAT volume may be more predictive of the presence and severity of AF than the conventional measures of obesity.

It is important to note that EAT distribution is often asymmetric and may exert different effects according to its location [184, 185]. As mentioned earlier, it was found that peri-atrial epicardial fat has distinct characteristics and genetic profile compared to peri-ventricular or peri-coronary epicardial fat [90]. Hence, due to its proximity and unique genetic profile, it follows that peri-atrial epicardial fat may be more directly related to the pathogenesis of AF. This was observed in many studies that showed left atrial EAT was significantly increased in patients with AF and may be related to the recurrence of AF after catheter ablation [65, 83, 85–89, 171]. Batal et al. [171] examined 169 patients who underwent CT scans for AF or CAD, measuring EAT thickness. The study found posterior LA fat thickness was a statistically significant predictor of AF burden even after adjusting for age, BMI, or LA area OR = 5.30 (95% CI, 1.39–20.24; $P = 0.015$). On the other hand, what stands true for the left atrial EAT is not necessarily valid for right atrial EAT. Hasebe et al. [186] compared two groups of patients with paroxysmal AF referred for catheter ablation. They reported that EAT volumes around both the RA and LA in the patients whose AF was thought to originate from the RA were significantly smaller than those in the patients whose AF was thought to originate from the LA. Thus, EAT may be more involved in the pathogenesis of AF whose source is the LA. It is important to note that there was no statistical difference in the total volume of EAT surrounding the whole heart between the two groups.

Despite the inability of these studies to demonstrate causation, there is ample evidence of a strong association/correlation between EAT/PAT and AF. This opens the door for questioning about its future clinical implications.

Clinical Implications of EAT in Atrial Fibrillation and Possible Therapeutic Options

EAT as Risk Predictive Biomarker for Atrial Fibrillation

Epicardial adipose tissue is a novel risk prediction marker, and it may have multiple clinical applications in the future. EAT has been linked with various acute coronary syndrome risk prediction scores [187–190]. These include the GRACE (Global Registry of Acute Coronary Events) score, the Syntax score for the severity of coronary lesions, and the TIMI score for the prediction of adverse coronary events. They all have shown positive correlations with increased epicardial fat volume or thickness [187, 189, 191]. Similarly, an increased quantity of adipose tissue surrounding the heart has been shown to predict major adverse cardiac events, including myocardial infarction and death in subjects with acute coronary syndromes, as well as in those with suspected coronary artery disease [192–194]. Like in acute coronary syndromes, multiple studies have established an association between atrial fibrillation and EAT independent of coronary atherosclerosis and classical cardiovascular risk factors [195]. The pericardial adipose tissue was shown to be independently associated with the incidence, severity, recurrence of AF after catheter ablation, and poor ablation outcomes [65, 83].

EAT volume is also associated with stroke and adverse cardiovascular outcomes in AF patients. Akdag et al. [196] calculated the CHA_2DS_2-VASc score and baseline EAT thickness in 96 consecutive patients with AF and 52 age- and sex-matched controls and found that the group with high CHA_2DS_2-VASc score had higher EAT thickness compared to the group with low-intermediate CHA_2DS_2-VASc score;

the CHA_2DS_2-VASc score was positively correlated with EAT. Tsao et al. [197] evaluated whether EAT situated in the vicinity of the LA and the LA appendage (LAA) is correlated with atrial function and the subsequent development of AF-related stroke. They reported that increased accumulation of EAT (OR = 1.12, $P < 0.001$) around the LA was independently associated with stroke in AF patients [197]. Moreover, peri-atrial EAT was negatively correlated with the mechanical function of the LA (LAEF $r = -0.369$, $P < 0.001$). Total EAT was negatively correlated with active EF of the LAA ($r = -0.464$, $P < 0.001$). This contractile dysfunction and the circulatory stasis of the LAA may account for the pathophysiological association of EAT- and AF-related stroke [197]. Similarly, Chu et al. [198] demonstrated that increased EAT thickness per 1 mm is associated with adverse cardiovascular events (cardiovascular mortality, hospitalization for heart failure, myocardial infarction, and stroke) OR = 1.224 (95% CI, 1.096–1.368; $P < 0.001$). Moreover, the addition of EAT thickness to a model containing CHA_2DS_2-VASc score, LA volume index, and left ventricular systolic and diastolic function significantly improved the predictive value for cardiovascular events [198].

Potential Therapeutic Options Targeting EAT

Weight Loss

Weight loss has been recognized to reduce the pericardial fat burden [199]. Weight loss after bariatric surgery in obese subjects has also been associated with a decrease in EAT [200]. A recent meta-analysis showed a significant reduction in EAT with diet and bariatric surgery, but not with exercise [201]. Furthermore, in severe obesity, successful long-term weight reduction was associated with improved left ventricular diastolic function and exercise capacity, while reduction of epicardial fat thickness predicted improved diastolic function [202]. Sustained weight loss, as described in the ARREST-AF study [59] and LEGACY study [60], showed improved arrhythmia free survival and substantial AF burden reduction. Whether a reduction in EAT mediates this effect, at least in part, remains unknown and requires further research.

Medications

Interestingly, statin therapy has been shown to decrease EAT. In hyperlipidemic post-menopausal women, statin therapy caused EAT regression, and intensive therapy was more effective than moderate-intensity therapy [203]. This, however, does not seem linked to low-density lipoprotein lowering and may be secondary to other actions of statins such as their anti-inflammatory effects [203]. A recent meta-analysis reported that perioperative statin therapy in patients with sinus rhythm undergoing cardiac surgery was associated with reduction in the development of postoperative AF, hospital length of stay, and CRP level [204]. This meta-analysis showed that the beneficial effects on AF and CRP were more marked in patients receiving atorvastatin compared to other statins [204]. Another meta-analysis showed that the use of statins is significantly associated with decreased risk of AF in patients with sinus rhythm, but did not examine changes in EAT [205]. Notably, the greatest benefit for statins was seen for postoperative AF prevention, as well as for secondary prevention of the arrhythmia [205]. Whether this effect is partially mediated by a decrease in EAT remains to be seen.

Antidiabetic medications may play a role in targeting EAT, leading to its reduction. In a study performed in type 2 diabetes patients, insulin replacement therapy resulted in a reduction of epicardial fat thickness [206]. EAT was recently collected from 9 patients during cardiac surgery, and it was found that human EAT expresses the GLP-1 receptor (GLP-1R) [207, 208]. Liraglutide is a glucagon-like peptide-1 (GLP-1) receptor agonist; in an interventional case-controlled study, there was a rapid and substantial reduction in EAT thickness when liraglutide was given in addition to metformin vs metformin as monotherapy [209]. In the liraglutide plus metformin group, EAT thickness decreased by 29% and 36% ($P < 0.001$) at 3 and 6 months, respectively, whereas there was no

EAT reduction in the metformin group [209]. Liraglutide is currently being investigated as a potential pharmaceutical therapeutic option as adjunctive therapy to catheter ablation in the Liraglutide Effect in Atrial Fibrillation (LEAF) clinical trial (NCT03856632, https://clinicaltrials.gov/). It is proposed that liraglutide reduces EAT and may thereby stabilize the atrial substrate.

Conclusion

AF is a complex arrhythmia. The initiation and maintenance of AF are dependent on the presence of both trigger and substrate, including electrical and structural atrial remodelling. Obesity has been identified as an important modifiable risk factor for AF, and recent evidence showed that weight loss has a positive impact on AF. Given the growing prevalence of obesity and the expected rise in AF incidence in the future, it is essential to establish a better understanding of the pathogenesis of AF and find alternative therapy that can address the underlying substrate. EAT is also clearly associated with AF. It is reasonable to speculate that the association between obesity and AF may be mediated, at least in part, by EAT. Under pathological condition, EAT could contribute to the pathogenesis of AF via various mechanisms: fatty infiltration, inflammation, oxidative stress, atrial remodelling (electrical and structural), alterations in gene expression, and neuronal mechanisms. EAT could serve as a new risk predictive biomarker of atrial fibrillation and a potential therapeutic target in the future.

References

1. Stewart S, Hart CL, Hole DJ, McMurray JJ. A population-based study of the long-term risks associated with atrial fibrillation: 20-year follow-up of the Renfrew/Paisley study. Am J Med. 2002;113:359–64.
2. Beyerbach DM, Zipes DP. Mortality as an endpoint in atrial fibrillation. Heart Rhythm. 2004;1:8–19.
3. Benjamin EJ, Wolf PA, D'Agostino RB, Silbershatz H, Kannel WB, Levy D. Impact of atrial fibrillation on the risk of death: the Framingham Heart Study. Circulation. 1998;98:946–52.
4. Colilla S, Crow A, Petkun W, Singer DE, Simon T, Liu X. Estimates of current and future incidence and prevalence of atrial fibrillation in the U.S. adult population. Am J Cardiol. 2013;112:1142–7.
5. Kim MH, Johnston SS, Chu B-C, Dalal MR, Schulman KL. Estimation of total incremental health care costs in patients with atrial fibrillation in the United States. Circ Cardiovasc Qual. 2011;4:313–20.
6. Kannel WB, Wolf PA, Benjamin EJ, Levy D. Prevalence, incidence, prognosis, and predisposing conditions for atrial fibrillation: population-based estimates. Am J Cardiol. 1998;82:2n–9n.
7. Feinberg WM, Blackshear JL, Laupacis A, Kronmal R, Hart RG. Prevalence, age distribution, and gender of patients with atrial fibrillation: analysis and implications. Arch Intern Med. 1995;155:469–73.
8. Eldar M, Canetti M, Rotstein Z, Boyko V, Gottlieb S, Kaplinsky E, et al. Significance of paroxysmal atrial fibrillation complicating acute myocardial infarction in the thrombolytic era. Circulation. 1998;97:965–70.
9. Crenshaw BS, Ward SR, Granger CB, Stebbins AL, Topol EJ, Califf RM. Atrial fibrillation in the setting of acute myocardial infarction: the GUSTO-I experience. J Am Coll Cardiol. 1997;30:406–13.
10. Frost L, Hune LJ, Vestergaard P. Overweight and obesity as risk factors for atrial fibrillation or flutter: the Danish Diet, Cancer, and Health Study. Am J Med. 2005;118:489–95.
11. Dublin S, French B, Glazer NL, Wiggins KL, Lumley T, Psaty BM, et al. Risk of new-onset atrial fibrillation in relation to body mass index. Arch Intern Med. 2006;166:2322–8.
12. Kannel WB, Abbott RD, Savage DD, McNamara PM. Epidemiologic features of chronic atrial fibrillation: the Framingham study. N Engl J Med. 1982;306:1018–22.
13. Krahn AD, Manfreda J, Tate RB, Mathewson FA, Cuddy TE. The natural history of atrial fibrillation: incidence, risk factors, and prognosis in the Manitoba Follow-Up Study. Am J Med. 1995;98:476–84.
14. Conen D, Tedrow UB, Koplan BA, Glynn RJ, Buring JE, Albert CM. Influence of systolic and diastolic blood pressure on the risk of incident atrial fibrillation in women. Circulation. 2009;119:2146.
15. Dublin S, Glazer NL, Smith NL, Psaty BM, Lumley T, Wiggins KL, et al. Diabetes mellitus, glycemic control, and risk of atrial fibrillation. J Gen Intern Med. 2010;25:853–8.
16. Benjamin EJ, Levy D, Vaziri SM, D'Agostino RB, Belanger AJ, Wolf PA. Independent risk factors for atrial fibrillation in a population-based cohort. The Framingham Heart Study. JAMA. 1994;271:840–4.
17. Watanabe H, Tanabe N, Watanabe T, Darbar D, Roden DM, Sasaki S, et al. Metabolic syndrome and risk of development of atrial fibrillation: the

Niigata preventive medicine study. Circulation. 2008;117:1255.
18. Maisel WH, Stevenson LW. Atrial fibrillation in heart failure: epidemiology, pathophysiology, and rationale for therapy. Am J Cardiol. 2003;91:2–8.
19. Mehra R, Benjamin EJ, Shahar E, Gottlieb DJ, Nawabit R, Kirchner HL, et al. Association of nocturnal arrhythmias with sleep-disordered breathing: the Sleep Heart Health Study. Am J Respir Crit Care Med. 2006;173:910–6.
20. Mooe T, Gullsby S, Rabben T, Eriksson P. Sleep-disordered breathing: a novel predictor of atrial fibrillation after coronary artery bypass surgery. Coron Arter Dis. 1996;7:475–8.
21. Tanigawa T, Yamagishi K, Sakurai S, Muraki I, Noda H, Shimamoto T, et al. Arterial oxygen desaturation during sleep and atrial fibrillation. Heart. 2006;92:1854–5.
22. Goldberger JJ, Arora R, Green D, Greenland P, Lee DC, Lloyd-Jones DM, et al. Evaluating the atrial myopathy underlying atrial fibrillation: identifying the arrhythmogenic and thrombogenic substrate. Circulation. 2015;132:278–91.
23. Goudis CA, Vasileiadis IE, Liu T. Epicardial adipose tissue and atrial fibrillation: pathophysiological mechanisms, clinical implications, and potential therapies. Curr Med Res Opin. 2018;34:1933–43.
24. Wong CX, Ganesan AN, Selvanayagam JB. Epicardial fat and atrial fibrillation: current evidence, potential mechanisms, clinical implications, and future directions. Eur Heart J. 2017;38:1294–302.
25. Ng Arnold CT, Strudwick M, van der Geest RJ, Ng Austin CC, Gillinder L, Goo Shi Y, et al. Impact of epicardial adipose tissue, left ventricular myocardial fat content, and interstitial fibrosis on myocardial contractile function. Circ Cardiovasc Imaging. 2018;11:e007372.
26. Mazurek T, Zhang L, Zalewski A, Mannion John D, Diehl James T, Arafat H, et al. Human epicardial adipose tissue is a source of inflammatory mediators. Circulation. 2003;108:2460–6.
27. Abed HS, Wittert GA. Obesity and atrial fibrillation. Obes Rev. 2013;14:929–38.
28. Abed HS, Samuel CS, Lau DH, Kelly DJ, Royce SG, Alasady M, et al. Obesity results in progressive atrial structural and electrical remodeling: implications for atrial fibrillation. Heart Rhythm. 2013;10:90–100.
29. Baek YS, Yang PS, Kim TH, Uhm JS, Park J, Pak HN, et al. Associations of abdominal obesity and new-onset atrial fibrillation in the general population. J Am Heart Assoc. 2017;6:e004705.
30. Goudis CA, Korantzopoulos P, Ntalas IV, Kallergis EM, Ketikoglou DG. Obesity and atrial fibrillation: a comprehensive review of the pathophysiological mechanisms and links. J Cardiol. 2015;66:361–9.
31. Wang TJ, Parise H, Levy D, D'Agostino RB Sr, Wolf PA, Vasan RS, et al. Obesity and the risk of new-onset atrial fibrillation. JAMA. 2004;292:2471–7.
32. Gami AS, Hodge DO, Herges RM, Olson EJ, Nykodym J, Kara T, et al. Obstructive sleep apnea, obesity, and the risk of incident atrial fibrillation. J Am Coll Cardiol. 2007;49:565–71.
33. Tedrow UB, Conen D, Ridker PM, Cook NR, Koplan BA, Manson JE, et al. The long- and short-term impact of elevated body mass index on the risk of new atrial fibrillation the WHS (women's health study). J Am Coll Cardiol. 2010;55:2319–27.
34. Knuiman M, Briffa T, Divitini M, Chew D, Eikelboom J, McQuillan B, et al. A cohort study examination of established and emerging risk factors for atrial fibrillation: the Busselton Health Study. Eur J Epidemiol. 2014;29:181–90.
35. Zacharias A, Schwann TA, Riordan CJ, Durham SJ, Shah AS, Habib RH. Obesity and risk of new-onset atrial fibrillation after cardiac surgery. Circulation. 2005;112:3247–55.
36. Wong CX, Sullivan T, Sun MT, Mahajan R, Pathak RK, Middeldorp M, et al. Obesity and the risk of incident, post-operative, and post-ablation atrial fibrillation: a meta-analysis of 626,603 individuals in 51 studies. JACC Clin Electrophysiol. 2015;1:139–52.
37. Lee H, Choi EK, Lee SH, Han KD, Rhee TM, Park CS, et al. Atrial fibrillation risk in metabolically healthy obesity: a nationwide population-based study. Int J Cardiol. 2017;240:221–7.
38. Tsang TS, Barnes ME, Miyasaka Y, Cha SS, Bailey KR, Verzosa GC, et al. Obesity as a risk factor for the progression of paroxysmal to permanent atrial fibrillation: a longitudinal cohort study of 21 years. Eur Heart J. 2008;29:2227–33.
39. Providencia R, Adragao P, de Asmundis C, Chun J, Chierchia G, Defaye P, et al. Impact of body mass index on the outcomes of catheter ablation of atrial fibrillation: a European Observational Multicenter Study. J Am Heart Assoc. 2019;8:e012253.
40. Huxley RR, Lopez FL, Folsom AR, Agarwal SK, Loehr LR, Soliman EZ, et al. Absolute and attributable risks of atrial fibrillation in relation to optimal and borderline risk factors: the Atherosclerosis Risk in Communities (ARIC) study. Circulation. 2011;123:1501–8.
41. Long MJ, Jiang CQ, Lam TH, Xu L, Zhang WS, Lin JM, et al. Atrial fibrillation and obesity among older Chinese: the Guangzhou Biobank Cohort Study. Int J Cardiol. 2011;148:48–52.
42. Karasoy D, Bo Jensen T, Hansen ML, Schmiegelow M, Lamberts M, Gislason GH, et al. Obesity is a risk factor for atrial fibrillation among fertile young women: a nationwide cohort study. Europace. 2013;15:781–6.
43. Berkovitch A, Kivity S, Klempfner R, Segev S, Milwidsky A, Erez A, et al. Body mass index and the risk of new-onset atrial fibrillation in middle-aged adults. Am Heart J. 2016;173:41–8.
44. Foy AJ, Mandrola J, Liu G, Naccarelli GV. Relation of obesity to new-onset atrial fibrillation and atrial flutter in adults. Am J Cardiol. 2018;121:1072–5.

45. Lim YM, Yang PS, Jang E, Yu HT, Kim TH, Uhm JS, et al. Body mass index variability and long-term risk of new-onset atrial fibrillation in the general population: a Korean Nationwide Cohort Study. Mayo Clin Proc. 2019;94:225–35.
46. Sandhu RK, Conen D, Tedrow UB, Fitzgerald KC, Pradhan AD, Ridker PM, et al. Predisposing factors associated with development of persistent compared with paroxysmal atrial fibrillation. J Am Heart Assoc. 2014;3:e000916.
47. Badimon L, Cubedo J. Adipose tissue depots and inflammation: effects on plasticity and resident mesenchymal stem cell function. Cardiovasc Res. 2017;113:1064–73.
48. Guzik TJ, Skiba DS, Touyz RM, Harrison DG. The role of infiltrating immune cells in dysfunctional adipose tissue. Cardiovasc Res. 2017;113:1009–23.
49. Margaritis M, Antonopoulos AS, Digby J, Lee R, Reilly S, Coutinho P, et al. Interactions between vascular wall and perivascular adipose tissue reveal novel roles for adiponectin in the regulation of endothelial nitric oxide synthase function in human vessels. Circulation. 2013;127:2209–21.
50. Antonopoulos AS, Margaritis M, Verheule S, Recalde A, Sanna F, Herdman L, et al. Mutual regulation of epicardial adipose tissue and myocardial redox state by ppar-gamma/adiponectin signalling. Circ Res. 2016;118:842–55.
51. Antonopoulos AS, Margaritis M, Coutinho P, Digby J, Patel R, Psarros C, et al. Reciprocal effects of systemic inflammation and brain natriuretic peptide on adiponectin biosynthesis in adipose tissue of patients with ischemic heart disease. Arterioscler Thromb Vasc Biol. 2014;34:2151–9.
52. Menke A, Muntner P, Wildman RP, Reynolds K, He J. Measures of adiposity and cardiovascular disease risk factors. Obesity. 2007;15:785–95.
53. NCD Risk Factor Collaboration (NCD-RisC). Trends in adult body-mass index in 200 countries from 1975 to 2014: a pooled analysis of 1698 population-based measurement studies with 19.2 million participants. Lancet. 2016;387:1377–96.
54. Hales CM, Carroll MD, Fryar CD, Ogden CL. Prevalence of obesity among adults and youth: United States, 2015–2016. CHS Data Brief. 2017;10(288):1–8.
55. Abed HS, Wittert GA, Leong DP, Shirazi MG, Bahrami B, Middeldorp ME, et al. Effect of weight reduction and cardiometabolic risk factor management on symptom burden and severity in patients with atrial fibrillation: a randomized clinical trial. JAMA. 2013;310:2050–60.
56. Alonso A, Bahnson JL, Gaussoin SA, Bertoni AG, Johnson KC, Lewis CE, et al. Effect of an intensive lifestyle intervention on atrial fibrillation risk in individuals with type 2 diabetes: the Look AHEAD randomized trial. Am Heart J. 2015;170:770–7.e5.
57. Jamaly S, Carlsson L, Peltonen M, Jacobson P, Sjostrom L, Karason K. Bariatric surgery and the risk of new-onset atrial fibrillation in Swedish obese subjects. J Am Coll Cardiol. 2016;68:2497–504.
58. Middeldorp ME, Pathak RK, Meredith M, Mehta AB, Elliott AD, Mahajan R, et al. PREVEntion and regReSsive Effect of weight-loss and risk factor modification on Atrial Fibrillation: the REVERSE-AF study. Europace. 2018;20:1929–35.
59. Pathak RK, Middeldorp ME, Lau DH, Mehta AB, Mahajan R, Twomey D, et al. Aggressive risk factor reduction study for atrial fibrillation and implications for the outcome of ablation: the ARREST-AF cohort study. J Am Coll Cardiol. 2014;64:2222–31.
60. Pathak RK, Middeldorp ME, Meredith M, Mehta AB, Mahajan R, Wong CX, et al. Long-term effect of goal-directed weight management in an atrial fibrillation cohort: a long-term follow-up study (LEGACY). J Am Coll Cardiol. 2015;65:2159–69.
61. January CT, Wann LS, Calkins H, Chen LY, Cigarroa JE, Cleveland JC Jr, et al. 2019 AHA/ACC/HRS focused update of the 2014 AHA/ACC/HRS guideline for the management of patients with atrial fibrillation: a report of the American College of Cardiology/American Heart Association Task Force on Clinical Practice Guidelines and the Heart Rhythm Society. J Am Coll Cardiol. 2019;74:104–32.
62. Hatem SN, Redheuil A, Gandjbakhch E. Cardiac adipose tissue and atrial fibrillation: the perils of adiposity. Cardiovasc Res. 2016;109:502–9.
63. Al-Rawahi M, Proietti R, Thanassoulis G. Pericardial fat and atrial fibrillation: epidemiology, mechanisms and interventions. Int J Cardiol. 2015;195:98–103.
64. Thanassoulis G, Massaro JM, O'Donnell CJ, Hoffmann U, Levy D, Ellinor PT, et al. Pericardial fat is associated with prevalent atrial fibrillation: the Framingham Heart Study. Circ Arrhythm Electrophysiol. 2010;3:345–50.
65. Wong CX, Abed HS, Molaee P, Nelson AJ, Brooks AG, Sharma G, et al. Pericardial fat is associated with atrial fibrillation severity and ablation outcome. J Am Coll Cardiol. 2011;57(17):1745–51.
66. Wong CX, Sun MT, Odutayo A, Emdin CA, Mahajan R, Lau DH, et al. Associations of epicardial, abdominal, and overall adiposity with atrial fibrillation. Circ Arrhythm Electrophysiol. 2016;9(12):e004378.
67. Rabkin SW. The relationship between epicardial fat and indices of obesity and the metabolic syndrome: a systematic review and meta-analysis. Metab Syndr Relat Disord. 2014;12:31–42.
68. Zhu W, Zhang H, Guo L, Hong K. Relationship between epicardial adipose tissue volume and atrial fibrillation: a systematic review and meta-analysis. Herz. 2016;41:421–7.
69. McAninch EA, Fonseca TL, Poggioli R, Panos AL, Salerno TA, Deng Y, et al. Epicardial adipose tissue has a unique transcriptome modified in severe coronary artery disease. Obesity (Silver Spring). 2015;23:1267–78.
70. Iacobellis G. Local and systemic effects of the multifaceted epicardial adipose tissue depot. Nat Rev Endocrinol. 2015;11:363–71.
71. Iacobellis G, Bianco AC. Epicardial adipose tissue: emerging physiological, pathophysiological

and clinical features. Trends Endocrinol Metab. 2011;22:450–7.
72. Iacobellis G, Corradi D, Sharma AM. Epicardial adipose tissue: anatomic, biomolecular and clinical relationships with the heart. Nat Clin Pract Cardiovasc Med. 2005;2:536–43.
73. Iacobellis G, Willens HJ. Echocardiographic epicardial fat: a review of research and clinical applications. J Am Soc Echocardiogr. 2009;22:1311–9; quiz 417–8.
74. Bertaso AG, Bertol D, Duncan BB, Foppa M. Epicardial fat: definition, measurements and systematic review of main outcomes. Arq Bras Cardiol. 2013;101:e18–28.
75. Marchington JM, Mattacks CA, Pond CM. Adipose tissue in the mammalian heart and pericardium: structure, foetal development and biochemical properties. Comp Biochem Physiol B. 1989;94:225–32.
76. Corradi D, Maestri R, Callegari S, Pastori P, Goldoni M, Luong TV, et al. The ventricular epicardial fat is related to the myocardial mass in normal, ischemic and hypertrophic hearts. Cardiovasc Pathol. 2004;13:313–6.
77. Iacobellis G. Epicardial and pericardial fat: close, but very different. Obesity (Silver Spring). 2009;17:625; author reply 6–7.
78. Hatem SN, Sanders P. Epicardial adipose tissue and atrial fibrillation. Cardiovasc Res. 2014;102:205–13.
79. Sacks HS, Fain JN. Human epicardial adipose tissue: a review. Am Heart J. 2007;153:907–17.
80. Al Chekakie MO, Welles CC, Metoyer R, Ibrahim A, Shapira AR, Cytron J, et al. Pericardial fat is independently associated with human atrial fibrillation. J Am Coll Cardiol. 2010;56:784–8.
81. Greif M, von Ziegler F, Wakili R, Tittus J, Becker C, Helbig S, et al. Increased pericardial adipose tissue is correlated with atrial fibrillation and left atrial dilatation. Clin Res Cardiol. 2013;102:555–62.
82. Drossos G, Koutsogiannidis C-P, Ananiadou O, Kapsas G, Ampatzidou F, Madesis A, et al. Pericardial fat is strongly associated with atrial fibrillation after coronary artery bypass graft surgery. Eur J Cardiothorac Surg. 2014;46:1014–20.
83. Kim TH, Park J, Park JK, Uhm JS, Joung B, Lee MH, et al. Pericardial fat volume is associated with clinical recurrence after catheter ablation for persistent atrial fibrillation, but not paroxysmal atrial fibrillation: an analysis of over 600-patients. Int J Cardiol. 2014;176:841–6.
84. Liu J, Taylor HA, Fox CS, Carr JJ, Ding J. Pericardial adipose tissue, atherosclerosis, and cardiovascular disease risk factors: The Jackson Heart Study. Response to Iacobellis and Malavazos. Diabetes Care. 2010;33:e128-e.
85. Tsao HM, Hu WC, Wu MH, Tai CT, Lin YJ, Chang SL, et al. Quantitative analysis of quantity and distribution of epicardial adipose tissue surrounding the left atrium in patients with atrial fibrillation and effect of recurrence after ablation. Am J Cardiol. 2011;107:1498–503.
86. Nagashima K, Okumura Y, Watanabe I, Nakai T, Ohkubo K, Kofune T, et al. Association between epicardial adipose tissue volumes on 3-dimensional reconstructed CT images and recurrence of atrial fibrillation after catheter ablation. Circ J. 2011;75:2559–65.
87. Chao TF, Hung CL, Tsao HM, Lin YJ, Yun CH, Lai YH, et al. Epicardial adipose tissue thickness and ablation outcome of atrial fibrillation. PLoS One. 2013;8:e74926.
88. Kocyigit D, Gurses KM, Yalcin MU, Turk G, Evranos B, Yorgun H, et al. Periatrial epicardial adipose tissue thickness is an independent predictor of atrial fibrillation recurrence after cryoballoon-based pulmonary vein isolation. J Cardiovasc Comput Tomogr. 2015;9:295–302.
89. Masuda M, Mizuno H, Enchi Y, Minamiguchi H, Konishi S, Ohtani T, et al. Abundant epicardial adipose tissue surrounding the left atrium predicts early rather than late recurrence of atrial fibrillation after catheter ablation. J Interv Card Electrophysiol. 2015;44:31–7.
90. Gaborit B, Venteclef N, Ancel P, Pelloux V, Gariboldi V, Leprince P, et al. Human epicardial adipose tissue has a specific transcriptomic signature depending on its anatomical peri-atrial, peri-ventricular, or pericoronary location. Cardiovasc Res. 2015;108:62–73.
91. Prati F, Arbustini E, Labellarte A, Sommariva L, Pawlowski T, Manzoli A, et al. Eccentric atherosclerotic plaques with positive remodelling have a pericardial distribution: a permissive role of epicardial fat? A three-dimensional intravascular ultrasound study of left anterior descending artery lesions. Eur Heart J. 2003;24:329–36.
92. Pezeshkian M, Noori M, Najjarpour-Jabbari H, Abolfathi A, Darabi M, Darabi M, et al. Fatty acid composition of epicardial and subcutaneous human adipose tissue. Metab Syndr Relat Disord. 2009;7:125–31.
93. Iacobellis G, Malavazos AE, Corsi MM. Epicardial fat: from the biomolecular aspects to the clinical practice. Int J Biochem Cell Biol. 2011;43:1651–4.
94. Sacks HS, Fain JN, Holman B, Cheema P, Chary A, Parks F, et al. Uncoupling protein-1 and related messenger ribonucleic acids in human epicardial and other adipose tissues: epicardial fat functioning as brown fat. J Clin Endocrinol Metab. 2009;94:3611–5.
95. Sacks HS, Fain JN. Human epicardial fat: what is new and what is missing? Clin Exp Pharmacol Physiol. 2011;38:879–87.
96. Turer AT, Scherer PE. Adiponectin: mechanistic insights and clinical implications. Diabetologia. 2012;55:2319–26.
97. Fang X, Palanivel R, Cresser J, Schram K, Ganguly R, Thong FS, et al. An APPL1-AMPK signaling axis mediates beneficial metabolic effects of adiponectin in the heart. Am J Physiol Endocrinol Metab. 2010;299:E721–9.

98. Ouchi N, Parker JL, Lugus JJ, Walsh K. Adipokines in inflammation and metabolic disease. Nat Rev Immunol. 2011;11:85–97.
99. Wong HK, Cheung TT, Cheung BM. Adrenomedullin and cardiovascular diseases. JRSM Cardiovasc Dis. 2012;1:1–7.
100. Munger TM, Dong YX, Masaki M, Oh JK, Mankad SV, Borlaug BA, et al. Electrophysiological and hemodynamic characteristics associated with obesity in patients with atrial fibrillation. J Am Coll Cardiol. 2012;60:851–60.
101. Mahajan R, Lau DH, Brooks AG, Shipp NJ, Manavis J, Wood JP, et al. Electrophysiological, electroanatomical, and structural remodeling of the atria as consequences of sustained obesity. J Am Coll Cardiol. 2015;66:1–11.
102. Yorgun H, Canpolat U, Aytemir K, Hazirolan T, Sahiner L, Kaya EB, et al. Association of epicardial and peri-atrial adiposity with the presence and severity of non-valvular atrial fibrillation. Int J Cardiovasc Imaging. 2015;31:649–57.
103. Wong CX, Stiles MK, John B, Brooks AG, Lau DH, Dimitri H, et al. Direction-dependent conduction in lone atrial fibrillation. Heart Rhythm. 2010;7:1192–9.
104. Wong CX, John B, Brooks AG, Chandy ST, Kuklik P, Lau DH, et al. Direction-dependent conduction abnormalities in the chronically stretched atria. Europace. 2012;14:954–61.
105. Eckstein J, Zeemering S, Linz D, Maesen B, Verheule S, van Hunnik A, et al. Transmural conduction is the predominant mechanism of breakthrough during atrial fibrillation: evidence from simultaneous endo-epicardial high-density activation mapping. Circ Arrhythm Electrophysiol. 2013;6:334–41.
106. Haemers P, Hamdi H, Guedj K, Suffee N, Farahmand P, Popovic N, et al. Atrial fibrillation is associated with the fibrotic remodelling of adipose tissue in the subepicardium of human and sheep atria. Eur Heart J. 2017;38:53–61.
107. Guo Y, Lip GY, Apostolakis S. Inflammation in atrial fibrillation. J Am Coll Cardiol. 2012;60:2263–70.
108. Wu N, Xu B, Xiang Y, Wu L, Zhang Y, Ma X, et al. Association of inflammatory factors with occurrence and recurrence of atrial fibrillation: a meta-analysis. Int J Cardiol. 2013;169:62–72.
109. Chung MK, Martin DO, Sprecher D, Wazni O, Kanderian A, Carnes CA, et al. C-reactive protein elevation in patients with atrial arrhythmias: inflammatory mechanisms and persistence of atrial fibrillation. Circulation. 2001;104:2886–91.
110. Malouf JF, Kanagala R, Al Atawi FO, Rosales AG, Davison DE, Murali NS, et al. High sensitivity C-reactive protein: a novel predictor for recurrence of atrial fibrillation after successful cardioversion. J Am Coll Cardiol. 2005;46:1284–7.
111. Aviles RJ, Martin DO, Apperson-Hansen C, Houghtaling PL, Rautaharju P, Kronmal RA, et al. Inflammation as a risk factor for atrial fibrillation. Circulation. 2003;108:3006–10.
112. Rotter M, Jais P, Vergnes MC, Nurden P, Takahashi Y, Sanders P, et al. Decline in C-reactive protein after successful ablation of long-lasting persistent atrial fibrillation. J Am Coll Cardiol. 2006;47:1231–3.
113. Li J, Solus J, Chen Q, Rho YH, Milne G, Stein CM, et al. Role of inflammation and oxidative stress in atrial fibrillation. Heart Rhythm. 2010;7:438–44.
114. Yamashita T, Sekiguchi A, Iwasaki YK, Date T, Sagara K, Tanabe H, et al. Recruitment of immune cells across atrial endocardium in human atrial fibrillation. Circ J. 2010;74:262–70.
115. Acet H, Ertas F, Akil MA, Oylumlu M, Polat N, Yildiz A, et al. New inflammatory predictors for non-valvular atrial fibrillation: echocardiographic epicardial fat thickness and neutrophil to lymphocyte ratio. Int J Cardiovasc Imaging. 2014;30:81–9.
116. Malavazos AE, Ermetici F, Coman C, Corsi MM, Morricone L, Ambrosi B. Influence of epicardial adipose tissue and adipocytokine levels on cardiac abnormalities in visceral obesity. Int J Cardiol. 2007;121:132–4.
117. Chang SL, Tuan TC, Tai CT, Lin YJ, Lo LW, Hu YF, et al. Comparison of outcome in catheter ablation of atrial fibrillation in patients with versus without the metabolic syndrome. Am J Cardiol. 2009;103:67–72.
118. Mazurek T, Kiliszek M, Kobylecka M, Skubisz-Gluchowska J, Kochman J, Filipiak K, et al. Relation of proinflammatory activity of epicardial adipose tissue to the occurrence of atrial fibrillation. Am J Cardiol. 2014;113:1505–8.
119. Kusayama T, Furusho H, Kashiwagi H, Kato T, Murai H, Usui S, et al. Inflammation of left atrial epicardial adipose tissue is associated with paroxysmal atrial fibrillation. J Cardiol. 2016;68:406–11.
120. Sun Y, Xun K, Wang C, Zhao H, Bi H, Chen X, et al. Adiponectin, an unlocking adipocytokine. Cardiovasc Ther. 2009;27:59–75.
121. Kourliouros A, Karastergiou K, Nowell J, Gukop P, Tavakkoli Hosseini M, Valencia O, et al. Protective effect of epicardial adiponectin on atrial fibrillation following cardiac surgery. Eur J Cardiothorac Surg. 2011;39:228–32.
122. Ybarra J, Resmini E, Planas F, Navarro-López F, Webb S, Pou JM, et al. Relationship between adiponectin and left atrium size in uncomplicated obese patients: adiponectin, a link between fat and heart. Obes Surg. 2009;19:1324–32.
123. van Osch D, Dieleman JM, van Dijk D, Jacob KA, Kluin J, Doevendans PA, et al. Dexamethasone for the prevention of postoperative atrial fibrillation. Int J Cardiol. 2015;182:431–7.
124. Liu C, Wang J, Yiu D, Liu K. The efficacy of glucocorticoids for the prevention of atrial fibrillation, or length of intensive care unit or hospital stay after cardiac surgery: a meta-analysis. Cardiovasc Ther. 2014;32:89–96.
125. Lin YK, Chen YC, Chen JH, Chen SA, Chen YJ. Adipocytes modulate the electrophysiology of atrial myocytes: implications in obesity-induced atrial fibrillation. Basic Res Cardiol. 2012;107:293.

126. Friedman DJ, Wang N, Meigs JB, Hoffmann U, Massaro JM, Fox CS, et al. Pericardial fat is associated with atrial conduction: the Framingham Heart Study. J Am Heart Assoc. 2014;3:e000477.
127. Zghaib T, Ipek EG, Zahid S, Balouch MA, Misra S, Ashikaga H, et al. Association of left atrial epicardial adipose tissue with electrogram bipolar voltage and fractionation: electrophysiologic substrates for atrial fibrillation. Heart Rhythm. 2016;13:2333–9.
128. Takahashi Y, Sanders P, Jais P, Hocini M, Dubois R, Rotter M, et al. Organization of frequency spectra of atrial fibrillation: relevance to radiofrequency catheter ablation. J Cardiovasc Electrophysiol. 2006;17:382–8.
129. Atienza F, Calvo D, Almendral J, Zlochiver S, Grzeda KR, Martinez-Alzamora N, et al. Mechanisms of fractionated electrograms formation in the posterior left atrium during paroxysmal atrial fibrillation in humans. J Am Coll Cardiol. 2011;57:1081–92.
130. Li D, Fareh S, Leung TK, Nattel S. Promotion of atrial fibrillation by heart failure in dogs: atrial remodeling of a different sort. Circulation. 1999;100:87–95.
131. Schnabel RB, Larson MG, Yamamoto JF, Kathiresan S, Rong J, Levy D, et al. Relation of multiple inflammatory biomarkers to incident atrial fibrillation. Am J Cardiol. 2009;104:92–6.
132. Kremen J, Dolinkova M, Krajickova J, Blaha J, Anderlova K, Lacinova Z, et al. Increased subcutaneous and epicardial adipose tissue production of proinflammatory cytokines in cardiac surgery patients: possible role in postoperative insulin resistance. J Clin Endocrinol Metab. 2006;91:4620–7.
133. Burstein B, Nattel S. Atrial fibrosis: mechanisms and clinical relevance in atrial fibrillation. J Am Coll Cardiol. 2008;51:802–9.
134. Frustaci A, Chimenti C, Bellocci F, Morgante E, Russo MA, Maseri A. Histological substrate of atrial biopsies in patients with lone atrial fibrillation. Circulation. 1997;96:1180–4.
135. Patella S, Phillips DJ, de Kretser DM, Evans LW, Groome NP, Sievert W. Characterization of serum activin-A and follistatin and their relation to virological and histological determinants in chronic viral hepatitis. J Hepatol. 2001;34:576–83.
136. De Bleser PJ, Niki T, Xu G, Rogiers V, Geerts A. Localization and cellular sources of activins in normal and fibrotic rat liver. Hepatology. 1997;26:905–12.
137. Werner S, Alzheimer C. Roles of activin in tissue repair, fibrosis, and inflammatory disease. Cytokine Growth Factor Rev. 2006;17:157–71.
138. Venteclef N, Guglielmi V, Balse E, Gaborit B, Cotillard A, Atassi F, et al. Human epicardial adipose tissue induces fibrosis of the atrial myocardium through the secretion of adipo-fibrokines. Eur Heart J. 2015;36:795–805a.
139. Greulich S, Maxhera B, Vandenplas G, de Wiza DH, Smiris K, Mueller H, et al. Secretory products from epicardial adipose tissue of patients with type 2 diabetes mellitus induce cardiomyocyte dysfunction. Circulation. 2012;126:2324–34.
140. Oshima Y, Ouchi N, Shimano M, Pimentel David R, Papanicolaou Kyriakos N, Panse Kalyani D, et al. Activin A and follistatin-like 3 determine the susceptibility of heart to ischemic injury. Circulation. 2009;120:1606–15.
141. Greulich S, de Wiza DH, Preilowski S, Ding Z, Mueller H, Langin D, et al. Secretory products of guinea pig epicardial fat induce insulin resistance and impair primary adult rat cardiomyocyte function. J Cell Mol Med. 2011;15:2399–410.
142. Boixel C, Fontaine V, Rucker-Martin C, Milliez P, Louedec L, Michel JB, et al. Fibrosis of the left atria during progression of heart failure is associated with increased matrix metalloproteinases in the rat. J Am Coll Cardiol. 2003;42:336–44.
143. Nagashima K, Okumura Y, Watanabe I, Nakai T, Ohkubo K, Kofune M, et al. Does location of epicardial adipose tissue correspond to endocardial high dominant frequency or complex fractionated atrial electrogram sites during atrial fibrillation? Circ Arrhythm Electrophysiol. 2012;5:676–83.
144. Laxton RC, Hu Y, Duchene J, Zhang F, Zhang Z, Leung KY, et al. A role of matrix metalloproteinase-8 in atherosclerosis. Circ Res. 2009;105:921–9.
145. Xiao Q, Zhang F, Lin L, Fang C, Wen G, Tsai TN, et al. Functional role of matrix metalloproteinase-8 in stem/progenitor cell migration and their recruitment into atherosclerotic lesions. Circ Res. 2013;112:35–47.
146. Felkin LE, Birks EJ, George R, Wong S, Khaghani A, Yacoub MH, et al. A quantitative gene expression profile of matrix metalloproteinases (MMPS) and their inhibitors (TIMPS) in the myocardium of patients with deteriorating heart failure requiring left ventricular assist device support. J Heart Lung Transplant. 2006;25:1413–9.
147. Wang Q, Xi W, Yin L, Wang J, Shen H, Gao Y, et al. Human epicardial adipose tissue cTGF expression is an independent risk factor for atrial fibrillation and highly associated with atrial fibrosis. Sci Rep. 2018;8:3585.
148. Aimé-Sempé C, Folliguet T, Rücker-Martin C, Krajewska M, Krajewski S, Heimburger M, et al. Myocardial cell death in fibrillating and dilated human right atria. J Am Coll Cardiol. 1999;34:1577–86.
149. Ausma J, Wijffels M, Van Eys G, Koide M, Ramaekers F, Allessie M, et al. Dedifferentiation of atrial cardiomyocytes as a result of chronic atrial fibrillation. Am J Pathol. 1997;151:985.
150. Zuk PA, Zhu M, Ashjian P, De Ugarte DA, Huang JI, Mizuno H, et al. Human adipose tissue is a source of multipotent stem cells. Mol Biol Cell. 2002;13:4279–95.
151. Fraser JK, Wulur I, Alfonso Z, Hedrick MH. Fat tissue: an underappreciated source of stem cells for biotechnology. Trends Biotechnol. 2006;24:150–4.

152. Rangappa S, Fen C, Lee EH, Bongso A, Wei ESK. Transformation of adult mesenchymal stem cells isolated from the fatty tissue into cardiomyocytes. Ann Thorac Surg. 2003;75:775–9.
153. Zuk PA, Zhu M, Mizuno H, Huang J, Futrell JW, Katz AJ, et al. Multilineage cells from human adipose tissue: implications for cell-based therapies. Tissue Eng. 2001;7:211–28.
154. Vural M, Talu A, Sahin D, Elalmis OU, Durmaz HA, Uyanik S, et al. Evaluation of the relationship between epicardial fat volume and left ventricular diastolic dysfunction. Jpn J Radiol. 2014;32:331–9.
155. Suffee N, Moore-Morris T, Farahmand P, Rücker-Martin C, Dilanian G, Fradet M, et al. Atrial natriuretic peptide regulates adipose tissue accumulation in adult atria. Proc Natl Acad Sci U S A. 2017;114:E771–E80.
156. Salgado-Somoza A, Teijeira-Fernandez E, Fernandez AL, Gonzalez-Juanatey JR, Eiras S. Proteomic analysis of epicardial and subcutaneous adipose tissue reveals differences in proteins involved in oxidative stress. Am J Physiol Heart Circ Physiol. 2010;299:H202–9.
157. Carnes CA, Chung MK, Nakayama T, Nakayama H, Baliga RS, Piao S, et al. Ascorbate attenuates atrial pacing-induced peroxynitrite formation and electrical remodeling and decreases the incidence of postoperative atrial fibrillation. Circ Res. 2001;89:E32–8.
158. Po SS, Nakagawa H, Jackman WM. Localization of left atrial ganglionated plexi in patients with atrial fibrillation. J Cardiovasc Electrophysiol. 2009;20:1186–9.
159. Coumel P. Paroxysmal atrial fibrillation: a disorder of autonomic tone? Eur Heart J. 1994;15(Suppl A):9–16.
160. Balcioglu AS, Cicek D, Akinci S, Eldem HO, Bal UA, Okyay K, et al. Arrhythmogenic evidence for epicardial adipose tissue: heart rate variability and turbulence are influenced by epicardial fat thickness. Pacing Clin Electrophysiol. 2015;38:99–106.
161. Nakagawa H, Scherlag BJ, Patterson E, Ikeda A, Lockwood D, Jackman WM. Pathophysiologic basis of autonomic ganglionated plexus ablation in patients with atrial fibrillation. Heart Rhythm. 2009;6(12 Suppl):S26–34.
162. Stavrakis S, Nakagawa H, Po SS, Scherlag BJ, Lazzara R, Jackman WM. The role of the autonomic ganglia in atrial fibrillation. JACC Clin Electrophysiol. 2015;1:1–13.
163. Scherlag BJ, Yamanashi W, Patel U, Lazzara R, Jackman WM. Autonomically induced conversion of pulmonary vein focal firing into atrial fibrillation. J Am Coll Cardiol. 2005;45:1878–86.
164. Patterson E, Lazzara R, Szabo B, Liu H, Tang D, Li YH, et al. Sodium-calcium exchange initiated by the Ca2+ transient: an arrhythmia trigger within pulmonary veins. J Am Coll Cardiol. 2006;47:1196–206.
165. Patterson E, Po SS, Scherlag BJ, Lazzara R. Triggered firing in pulmonary veins initiated by in vitro autonomic nerve stimulation. Heart Rhythm. 2005;2:624–31.
166. Chen PS, Chen LS, Fishbein MC, Lin SF, Nattel S. Role of the autonomic nervous system in atrial fibrillation: pathophysiology and therapy. Circ Res. 2014;114:1500–15.
167. Pokushalov E, Kozlov B, Romanov A, Strelnikov A, Bayramova S, Sergeevichev D, et al. Long-term suppression of atrial fibrillation by botulinum toxin injection into epicardial fat pads in patients undergoing cardiac surgery: one-year follow-up of a randomized pilot study. Circ Arrhythm Electrophysiol. 2015;8:1334–41.
168. Chilukoti RK, Giese A, Malenke W, Homuth G, Bukowska A, Goette A, et al. Atrial fibrillation and rapid acute pacing regulate adipocyte/adipositas-related gene expression in the atria. Int J Cardiol. 2015;187:604–13.
169. Chami M, Gozuacik D, Lagorce D, Brini M, Falson P, Peaucellier G, et al. SERCA1 truncated proteins unable to pump calcium reduce the endoplasmic reticulum calcium concentration and induce apoptosis. J Cell Biol. 2001;153:1301–14.
170. Viviano A, Yin X, Zampetaki A, Fava M, Gallagher M, Mayr M, et al. Proteomics of the epicardial fat secretome and its role in post-operative atrial fibrillation. Europace. 2018;20:1201–8.
171. Batal O, Schoenhagen P, Shao M, Ayyad AE, Van Wagoner DR, Halliburton SS, et al. Left atrial epicardial adiposity and atrial fibrillation. Circ Arrhythm Electrophysiol. 2010;3:230–6.
172. Shin SY, Yong HS, Lim HE, Na JO, Choi CU, Choi JI, et al. Total and interatrial epicardial adipose tissues are independently associated with left atrial remodeling in patients with atrial fibrillation. J Cardiovasc Electrophysiol. 2011;22:647–55.
173. Nakanishi K, Fukuda S, Tanaka A, Otsuka K, Sakamoto M, Taguchi H, et al. Peri-atrial epicardial adipose tissue is associated with new-onset nonvalvular atrial fibrillation. Circ J. 2012;76:2748–54.
174. Kanazawa H, Yamabe H, Enomoto K, Koyama J, Morihisa K, Hoshiyama T, et al. Importance of pericardial fat in the formation of complex fractionated atrial electrogram region in atrial fibrillation. Int J Cardiol. 2014;174:557–64.
175. Murakami C, Nagai T, Akira F, Kido T, Nishimura K, Inoue K, et al. Total epicardial fat volume is associated with early recurrence of atrial fibrillation after catheter ablation. J Am Coll Cardiol. 2012;59(13 Suppl):E691.
176. Soucek F, Covassin N, Singh P, Ruzek L, Kara T, Suleiman M, et al. Epicardial adipose tissue volume predicts atrial fibrillation recurrence after pulmonary vein isolation. Eur Heart J. 2014;35:431.
177. Canpolat U, Aytemir K, Yorgun H, Asil S, Dural M, Özer N. The impact of echocardiographic epicardial fat thickness on outcomes of cryoballoon-

based atrial fibrillation ablation. Echocardiography. 2016;33:821–9.
178. Ciuffo L, Nguyen H, Marques MD, Aronis KN, Sivasambu B, et al. Periatrial fat quality predicts atrial fibrillation ablation outcome. Circ Cardiovasc Imaging. 2019;12:e008764.
179. Mirolo A, Viart G, Savouré A, Godin B, Raitière O, Eltchaninoff H, et al. Epicardial fat thickness predicts atrial fibrillation recurrence after a first pulmonary vein isolation procedure using a second-generation cryoballoon. Arch Cardiovasc Dis. 2019;112:314–22.
180. Gaeta M, Bandera F, Tassinari F, Capasso L, Cargnelutti M, Pelissero G, et al. Is epicardial fat depot associated with atrial fibrillation? A systematic review and meta-analysis. Europace. 2017;19:747–52.
181. Opolski MP, Staruch AD, Kusmierczyk M, Witkowski A, Kwiecinska S, Kosek M, et al. Computed tomography angiography for prediction of atrial fibrillation after coronary artery bypass grafting: proof of concept. J Cardiol. 2015;65:285–92.
182. Cho KI, Kim BJ, Cha TJ, Heo JH, Kim HS, Lee JW. Impact of duration and dosage of statin treatment and epicardial fat thickness on the recurrence of atrial fibrillation after electrical cardioversion. Heart Vessel. 2015;30:490–7.
183. Kawakami H, Satomi K, Nakajima I, Miyamoto K, Yamada Y, Okamura H, et al. Total epicardial adipose tissue volume is associated with outcome of pulmonary vein isolation for atrial fibrillation. Europace. 2013;15:ii218.
184. Gorter PM, van Lindert AS, de Vos AM, Meijs MF, van der Graaf Y, Doevendans PA, et al. Quantification of epicardial and peri-coronary fat using cardiac computed tomography; reproducibility and relation with obesity and metabolic syndrome in patients suspected of coronary artery disease. Atherosclerosis. 2008;197:896–903.
185. Abbara S, Desai JC, Cury RC, Butler J, Nieman K, Reddy V. Mapping epicardial fat with multi-detector computed tomography to facilitate percutaneous transepicardial arrhythmia ablation. Eur J Radiol. 2006;57:417–22.
186. Hasebe H, Yoshida K, Iida M, Hatano N, Muramatsu T, Nogami A, et al. Differences in the structural characteristics and distribution of epicardial adipose tissue between left and right atrial fibrillation. Europace. 2017;20:435–42.
187. Altun B, Colkesen Y, Gazi E, Tasolar H, Temiz A, Simsek HY, et al. Could epicardial adipose tissue thickness by echocardiography be correlated with acute coronary syndrome risk scores. Echocardiography. 2013;30:1130–4.
188. Gul I, Zungur M, Aykan AC, Gokdeniz T, Kalaycioğlu E, Turan T, et al. The relationship between GRACE score and epicardial fat thickness in non-STEMI patients. Arq Bras Cardiol. 2016;106:194–200.
189. Özcan F, Turak O, Canpolat U, Kanat S, Kadife İ, Avcı S, et al. Association of epicardial fat thickness with TIMI risk score in NSTEMI/USAP patients. Herz. 2014;39:755–60.
190. Zencirci E, Zencirci AE, Değirmencioğlu A, Karakuş G, Uğurlucan M, Özden K, et al. The relationship between epicardial adipose tissue and ST-segment resolution in patients with acute ST-segment elevation myocardial infarction undergoing primary percutaneous coronary intervention. Heart Vessel. 2015;30:147–53.
191. Wang T, Liu Q, Liu C, Sun L, Li D, Liu A, et al. Correlation of echocardiographic epicardial fat thickness with severity of coronary artery disease in patients with acute myocardial infarction. Echocardiography. 2014;31:1177–81.
192. Tanindi A, Erkan AF, Ekici B. Epicardial adipose tissue thickness can be used to predict major adverse cardiac events. Coron Artery Dis. 2015;26:686–91.
193. Hajsadeghi F, Nabavi V, Bhandari A, Choi A, Vincent H, Flores F, et al. Increased epicardial adipose tissue is associated with coronary artery disease and major adverse cardiovascular events. Atherosclerosis. 2014;237:486–9.
194. Cheng VY, Dey D, Tamarappoo B, Nakazato R, Gransar H, Miranda-Peats R, et al. Pericardial fat burden on ECG-gated noncontrast CT in asymptomatic patients who subsequently experience adverse cardiovascular events. JACC Cardiovasc Imaging. 2010;3:352–60.
195. Bos D, Vernooij MW, Shahzad R, Kavousi M, Hofman A, van Walsum T, et al. Epicardial fat volume and the risk of atrial fibrillation in the general population free of cardiovascular disease. JACC Cardiovasc Imaging. 2017;10:1405–7.
196. Akdag S, Simsek H, Sahin M, Akyol A, Duz R, Babat N. Association of epicardial adipose tissue thickness and inflammation parameters with CHA2DS2-VASc score in patients with nonvalvular atrial fibrillation. Ther Clin Risk Manag. 2015;11:1675.
197. Tsao HM, Hu WC, Tsai PH, Lee CL, Liu FC, Wang HH, et al. The abundance of epicardial adipose tissue surrounding left atrium is associated with the occurrence of stroke in patients with atrial fibrillation. Medicine (Baltimore). 2016;95:e3260.
198. Chu CY, Lee WH, Hsu PC, Lee MK, Lee HH, Chiu CA, et al. Association of increased epicardial adipose tissue thickness with adverse cardiovascular outcomes in patients with atrial fibrillation. Medicine (Baltimore). 2016;95:e2874.
199. Nakazato R, Rajani R, Cheng VY, Shmilovich H, Nakanishi R, Otaki Y, et al. Weight change modulates epicardial fat burden: a 4-year serial study with non-contrast computed tomography. Atherosclerosis. 2012;220:139–44.
200. Gaborit B, Jacquier A, Kober F, Abdesselam I, Cuisset T, Boullu-Ciocca S, et al. Effects of bariatric surgery on cardiac ectopic fat: lesser decrease in epicardial fat compared to visceral fat loss and no

change in myocardial triglyceride content. J Am Coll Cardiol. 2012;60:1381–9.

201. Rabkin S, Campbell H. Comparison of reducing epicardial fat by exercise, diet or bariatric surgery weight loss strategies: a systematic review and meta-analysis. Obes Rev. 2015;16:406–15.
202. Fenk S, Fischer M, Strack C, Schmitz G, Loew T, Lahmann C, et al. Successful weight reduction improves left ventricular diastolic function and physical performance in severe obesity. Int Heart J. 2015;56:196–202.
203. Alexopoulos N, Melek BH, Arepalli CD, Hartlage G-R, Chen Z, Kim S, et al. Effect of intensive versus moderate lipid-lowering therapy on epicardial adipose tissue in hyperlipidemic post-menopausal women: a substudy of the BELLES trial (Beyond Endorsed Lipid Lowering with EBT Scanning). J Am Coll Cardiol. 2013;61:1956–61.
204. Rezaei Y, Gholami-Fesharaki M, Dehghani MR, Arya A, Haghjoo M, Arjmand N. Statin antiarrhythmic effect on atrial fibrillation in statin-naive patients undergoing cardiac surgery: a meta-analysis of randomized controlled trials. J Cardiovasc Pharmacol Ther. 2016;21:167–76.
205. Fauchier L, Clementy N, Babuty D. Statin therapy and atrial fibrillation: systematic review and updated meta-analysis of published randomized controlled trials. Curr Opin Cardiol. 2013;28:7–18.
206. Elisha B, Azar M, Taleb N, Bernard S, Iacobellis G, Rabasa-Lhoret R. Body composition and epicardial fat in type 2 diabetes patients following insulin detemir versus insulin glargine initiation. Horm Metab Res. 2016;48:42–7.
207. Iacobellis G, Camarena V, Sant DW, Wang G. Human epicardial fat expresses glucagon-like peptide 1 and 2 receptors genes. Horm Metab Res. 2017;49:625–30.
208. Iacobellis G. Letter to the Editor: “GLP-1 receptor expression within the human heart”. Endocrinology. 2018;159:1964–5.
209. Iacobellis G, Mohseni M, Bianco SD, Banga PK. Liraglutide causes large and rapid epicardial fat reduction. Obesity. 2017;25:311–6.

Heart Failure and Epicardial Adipose Tissue

11

Gianluca Iacobellis

Key Points
- Epicardial adipose tissue plays a pathogenic role in heart failure. Thermogenic, paracrine, and neural factors seem to be involved.
- Epicardial fat volume is higher in subjects with both systolic and diastolic heart failure.
- Epicardial fat can be reduced in patients with severe heart failure due to fibrotic and apoptotic changes.

Introduction

Heart failure (HF) is a complex clinical syndrome that results from both structural and functional impairment of ventricular pump or filling. The causes leading to HF are multiple, and often co-occurring, such as coronary artery disease (CAD), atrial fibrillation (AF), preexisting cardiomyopathies, myocarditis, metabolic disorders, and acute organ failure. Heart failure can be classified into two types according to the left ventricular ejection fraction (reduced or preserved): systolic heart failure with reduced ejection fraction (HFrEF), and diastolic heart failure with preserved ejection fraction (HFpEF) [1].

Epicardial adipose tissue (EAT) has been investigated in patients with heart failure and suggested to play a pathogenic role. Given its peculiar location and intense metabolic activity, it is plausible to see the role of EAT in the development and progression of EAT. Also, abnormal or excessive EAT has shown to be correlated with both systolic and diastolic functions. Hence, it would be logical to attribute some action of EAT in affecting either the left ventricular pump or the filling phase. However, the results are quite scarce and controversial, also due to the occurrence of other conditions that can affect EAT. Hence, the role of EAT in independently causing or contributing to the development of HF is still uncertain.

Thermogenic Epicardial Fat and Heart Failure

EAT displays genetic and functional features similar to those of the brown fat [2]. Human EAT has the potential to serve as a thermogenic source for the myocardium and therefore protect it against hypothermia. A recent study found that patients with HFrEF expressed significantly lower thermogenic genes in EAT than those

G. Iacobellis (✉)
Division of Endocrinology, Diabetes and Metabolism, Department of Medicine, University of Miami, Miller School of Medicine, Miami, FL, USA
e-mail: giacobellis@med.miami.edu

G. Iacobellis (ed.), *Epicardial Adipose Tissue*, Contemporary Cardiology,
https://doi.org/10.1007/978-3-030-40570-0_11

with HFpEF [3]. In fact, uncoupling protein 1 (UCP1), peroxisome proliferator-activated receptor gamma coactivator 1-alpha (PGC1α), and PR-domain-missing 16 (PRDM16) expression were significantly lower in EAT of patients with HRrEF than those with HFpEF. The correlation of EAT brown fat genes with HF was not independent. In fact, age, male gender, and different cardiovascular diseases were also associated with the levels of thermogenic genes expression. This study suggests that an adequate expression of thermogenic genes could serve a possible protective factor against congestive heart failure. Consequently, a loss of functional EAT brown-like features would contribute to the development of HFrEF. This hypothesis seems to be confirmed by another study in both mice and humans with obesity and heart failure [4]. The authors suggested a role of the epicardial fat heme oxygenase-1 (HO1) PGC-1α in modulating the left ventricle function. HO-1 PGC-1α and PRDM16 were inversely correlated with left ventricular ejection fraction. In summary, these studies suggest a potential protective role of the brown fat features of EAT against systolic heart failure. EAT thermogenic genes could serve as a therapeutic target in patients with HFrEF. Pharmacological manipulation would be certainly challenging as EAT brown fat-like properties tend to significantly decrease with aging [5]. However, these findings should be confirmed in larger and multicenter research trials.

Epicardial Fat Adipokines and Heart Failure

EAT is an active paracrine and endocrine organ. EAT secretome is large and includes both pro- and anti-inflammatory adipokines. Among these, EAT adiponectin has shown to provide potential cardioprotective effects. EAT adiponectin expression is downregulated in patients with coronary artery disease [6]. In a study with patients undergoing cardiac surgery, p53 and adiponectin mRNA expression was measured in frozen fat biopsies or explants culture from both EAT and subcutaneous fat (SAT). p53 expression in adipose tissue is involved in the development of insulin resistance and inflammation [7]. Higher p53 expression was linked to increased production of pro-inflammatory cytokines. p53 mRNA expression levels were higher in EAT of HF patients as compared to SAT. p53 was inversely correlated with adiponectin and regulated by sympathetic activation pathway in patients with HF. A neuromodulatory role of EAT in heart failure will be discussed in details in chap. 12.

Epicardial Fat in Diastolic and Systolic Heart Failure

The relationship between EAT and HF was evaluated by a number of studies, although few of these were focused to specifically address it. In these studies, populations were quite heterogeneous with patients with or without coronary artery disease (CAD) and other confounding factors such as diabetes and hypertension. The role of EAT in the development or progression of HF can be better interpreted if results are adjusted by these factors, and diastolic and systolic functions are factored in the relation. A recent meta-analysis included 26 studies accounting for more than 4000 patients [8]. This analysis was conducted on the basis of diagnosis of left ventricular diastolic and systolic dysfunction and their correlation with EAT. Left ventricular diastolic dysfunction (LVDD) was defined echocardiographically by a ratio of early mitral valve flow velocity (E) to early diastolic lengthening velocity (e'; E/e') during tissue Doppler imaging of ≥10; left ventricular systolic dysfunction (LVSD) was defined with ejection fraction (LVEF) ≤50%. Patients with preserved systolic function (HFpEF) are those with LVDD, whereas those with reduced systolic function (HFrEF) are presenting with LVSD. As previously discussed, EAT can be measured either with standard echocardiography or CT or CMR, as thickness or volume, respectively. The relationship between ultrasound measured EAT thickness and LVDD was reported in eight studies that included 775 cardiac patients with LVDD and 695 controls without LVDD [9–15]. Overall, EAT thickness was significantly higher in patients with LVDD as compared to those without it. The relationship between EAT volume and LVDD was investigated in six studies that included 433 cardiac patients with LVDD and 272 controls without LVDD [16–20]. Overall, EAT volume in cardiac patients with LVDD was increased compared to those without LVDD. One study measured EAT volume with cardiac magnetic resonance in patients with HFpEF defined by an LVEF >40% [21]. EAT volume was significantly higher in HFpEF patients compared to controls (107 mL/m^2 vs. 77 mL/m^2, $P < 0.0001$), despite similar body mass index. HF patients with atrial fibrillation and/or type 2 diabetes mellitus had higher EAT than HF patients without these comorbidities. We can conclude that EAT is higher in patients with LVDD as compared to patients without LVDD, irrespective of whether is measured as volume or thickness. Hence, diastolic heart failure is more commonly associated with increased EAT.

The role of EAT in systolic heart failure (HFrEF) is less consistent, as findings are actually quite conflicting. The association between EAT and LV function was evaluated using either CMR or echocardiography. In some studies, EAT was found higher in subjects with LVSD [22–25]. One study showed that patients with HFrEF had significantly higher indexed EAT volume as measured with cardiac magnetic resonance imaging when compared with patients with HFpEF or the control group [22]. Another study reported an association between EAT and global longitudinal strain, a subclinical measure of myocardial function [23]. An independent correlation between echocardiographic EAT thickness and LVEF was also observed [24]. Epicardial fat thickness is associated with the severity of HF in patients with nonischemic dilated cardiomyopathy [25]. In fact, patients with HF had significantly lower epicardial fat thickness than those in the control group. Some of these results may be confounded by the co-occurrence of diabetes or CAD or obesity. Mechanical restriction from excessive EAT during the diastole may affect the ventricular filling and, consequently, reduce cardiac output in obese subjects [25].

However, some other studies found opposite results. Doesch et al. reported a reduced EAT in patients with congestive, HFrEF [26–28]. When EAT was adjusted by LV end-diastolic mass was significantly reduced in patients with severe HF (EF < 35%) compared to healthy controls (Fig. 11.1). In the analysis performed by Doesch and colleagues, the reduction of EAT was irrespective of the underlying cause of the cardiomyopathy [26]. In fact, there were no differences in EAT between patients with or without CAD. Doesch attributes the reverse correlation between LVEF and indexed EAT to the left ventricular remodeling occurring in heart failure. Lower EAT in patients with poor systolic function was also confirmed in another study [24]. EAT volume, as measured with cardiac magnetic resonance, was also found to be significantly lower in obese patients with HFpEF, and no correlation between EAT and EF was observed [29].

EAT thickness, as measured according to the method first described by Iacobellis et al. [33, 30], was also found to be lower in subjects with HFrEF (EF < 50%) as compared to those without HF, independent of atrial fibrillation and HF [31]. Some mechanisms can be evoked to explain these findings. Epicardial fat reduction in HF subjects may reflect the overall fat mass reduction, commonly observed in these patients. It is also possible to hypothesize that epicardial fat pad may incur in fibrotic changes during chronic cardiac failure [32]. However, the exact interaction of EAT and HF is still unclear. Whether EAT plays a role in the long-term prognosis of HF requires future investigation.

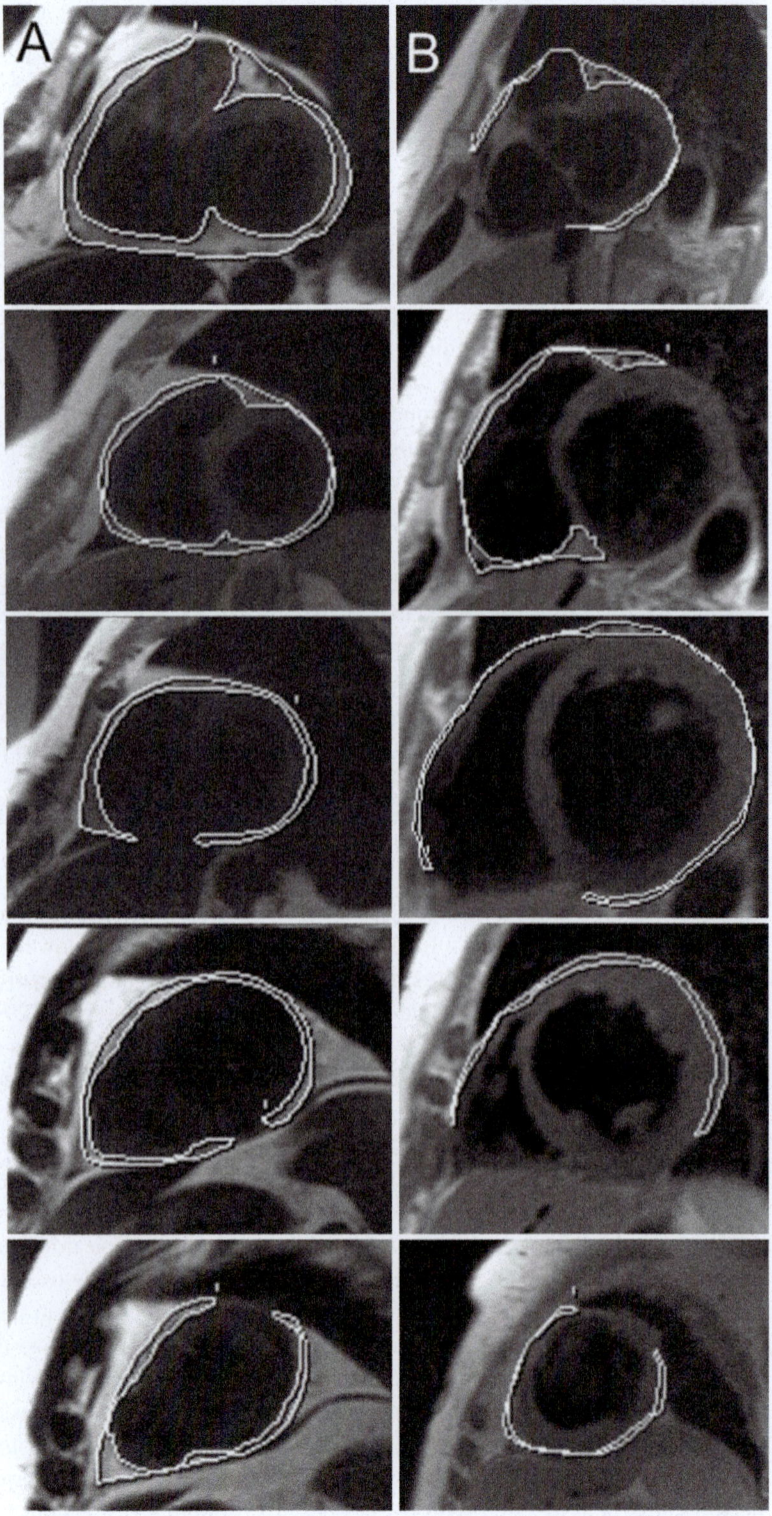

Fig. 11.1 EAT in healthy controls and patients with HFrEF. Volumetric measurement of EAT outlining the contours of EAT in end-diastolic images of short axis covering the left and right ventricles in a healthy control with normal EAT mass (*Panel A*) and in an HFrEF patient with reduced EAT mass (*Panel B*). CHF chronic heart failure, EAT Epicardial adipose tissue, and LV-EDM left ventricular end-diastolic mass. (From Doesch et al. [26], with permission)

References

1. Yancy CW, Jessup M, Bozkurt B, Butler J, Casey DE Jr, Colvin MM, et al. 2017 ACC/AHA/HFSA focused update of the 2013 ACCF/AHA guideline for the management of heart failure: a report of the American College of Cardiology/American Heart Association Task Force on Clinical Practice Guidelines and the Heart Failure Society of America. J Am Coll Cardiol. 2017;70:776–803.
2. Sacks HS, Fain JN, Holman B, Cheema P, Chary A, Parks F. Uncoupling protein-1 and related mRNAs in human epicardial and other adipose tissues: epicardial fat functioning as brown fat. J Clin Endocrinol Metab. 2009;94:3611–5.
3. Pérez-Belmonte LM, Moreno-Santos I, Gómez-Doblas JJ, et al. Expression of epicardial adipose tissue thermogenic genes in patients with reduced and preserved ejection fraction heart failure. Int J Med Sci. 2017;14:891–5.
4. Singh SP, McClung JA, Thompson E, Glick Y, Greenberg M, Acosta-Baez G, et al. Cardioprotective effect of heme oxygenase-1-PGC-1? Signaling in epicardial fat attenuates cardiovascular risk in humans as in obese mice. Obesity. 2019;27:1634–43.
5. Sacks HS, Fain JN. Human epicardial adipose tissue: a review. Am Heart J. 2007;153:907–17.
6. Iacobellis G, Pistilli D, Gucciardo M, Leonetti F, Miraldi F, Brancaccio G, et al. Adiponectin expression in human epicardial adipose tissue in vivo is lower in patients with CAD. Cytokine. 2005;29:251–5.
7. Krstic J, Reinisch I, Schupp M, Schulz TJ, Prokesch A. p53 functions in adipose tissue metabolism and homeostasis. Int J Mol Sci. 2018;19:2622.
8. Nerlekar N, Muthalaly RG, Wong N, Thakur U, Wong DTL, Brown AJ, Marwick TH. Association of volumetric epicardial adipose tissue quantification and cardiac structure and function. J Am Heart Assoc. 2018;7:e009975.
9. Lin HH, Lee JK, Yang CY, Lien YC, Huang JW, Wu CK. Accumulation of epicardial fat rather than visceral fat is an independent risk factor for left ventricular diastolic dysfunction in patients undergoing peritoneal dialysis. Cardiovasc Diabetol. 2013;12:127.
10. Topuz M, Dogan A. The effect of epicardial adipose tissue thickness on left ventricular diastolic functions in patients with normal coronary arteries. Kardiol Pol. 2017;75:196–203.
11. Turak O, Özcan F, Canpolat U, Işleyen A, Cebeci M, Öksüz F, et al. Increased echocardiographic epicardial fat thickness and high-sensitivity CRP level indicate diastolic dysfunction in patients with newly diagnosed essential hypertension. Blood Press Monit. 2013;18:259–64.
12. Lei P, Shi S, Li P, Liu Y, Cheng X, Li Y. Epicardial adipose thickness of hypertension patients correlated with left ventricular diastolic dysfunction (abstract GW25-e4319). J Am Coll Cardiol. 2014;64(16 Suppl C):C172.
13. Kaushik M, Alla VM, Saurav A, Smer A, Madan R, Khan S, et al. Epicardial adipose tissue thickness as assessed by echocardiography & left ventricular diastolic dysfunction (abstract 433). Cardiology. 2013;125(Suppl 2):447.
14. Manka M, Fenk S, Strack C, Kempinger S, Riegger G, Schmitz G, et al. Epicardial fat is related to left ventricular diastolic dysfunction in healthy obese and metabolic syndrome obese (abstract). Circulation. 2014;130:A19045.
15. Jung YH, Yoon SB, Kim WY, Park A. Epicardial fat as a contributing factor to diastolic dysfunction. Korean J Fam Pract. 2016;6:26–31.
16. Fontes-Carvalho R, Fontes-Oliveira M, Sampaio F, Mancio J, Bettencourt N, Teixeira M, et al. Influence of epicardial and visceral fat on left ventricular diastolic and systolic functions in patients after myocardial infarction. Am J Cardiol. 2014;114:1663–9.
17. Konishi M, Sugiyama S, Sugamura K, Nozaki T, Matsubara J, Akiyama E, et al. Accumulation of pericardial fat correlates with left ventricular diastolic dysfunction in patients with normal ejection fraction. J Cardiol. 2012;59:344–51.
18. Vural M, Talu A, Sahin D, Elalmis OU, Durmaz HA, Uyanik S, Dolek BA. Evaluation of the relationship between epicardial fat volume and left ventricular diastolic dysfunction. Jpn J Radiol. 2014;32:331–9.
19. Wu L, Chen W, Chen YJ, Wang KH, Qu KX. Correlation between volume of epicardial adipose tissue measured with MSCT and left ventricular diastolic function in coronary artery disease patients. Chin J Interv Imaging Ther. 2014;11:286–9.
20. Fuzhuang Z, Hong T, Yongmei W, Wenchuan W, Xiuying G, Xianxian Y, et al. Association of epicardial adipose tissue volume with coronary artery atherosclerosis and left ventricular diastolic function. J Cardiovasc Pulmon Dis. 2012;31:58–63.
21. van Woerden G, Gorter TM, Westenbrink BD, Willems TP, van Veldhuisen DJ, Rienstra M. Epicardial fat in heart failure patients with mid-range and preserved ejection fraction. Eur J Heart Fail. 2018;20:1559–66.
22. Wu CK, Tsai HY, Su MM, Wu YF, Hwang JJ, Lin JL, et al. Evolutional change in epicardial fat and its correlation with myocardial diffuse fibrosis in heart failure patients. J Clin Lipidol. 2017;11:1421–31.
23. Ng AC, Goo SY, Roche N, van der Geest RJ, Wang WY. Epicardial adipose tissue volume and left ventricular myocardial function using 3-dimensional speckle tracking echocardiography. Can J Cardiol. 2016;32:1485–92.
24. Khawaja T, Greer C, Chokshi A, Chavarria N, Thadani S, Jones M, et al. Epicardial fat volume in patients with left ventricular systolic dysfunction. Am J Cardiol. 2011;108:397–401.
25. Tabakci MM, Durmuş Hİ, Avci A, Toprak C, Demir S, Arslantaş U, et al. Relation of epicardial fat thickness to the severity of heart failure in patients with non-ischemic dilated cardiomyopathy. Echocardiography. 2015;32:740–8.

26. Doesch C, Haghi D, Fluchter S, Suselbeck T, Schoenberg SO, Michaely H, et al. Epicardial adipose tissue in patients with heart failure. J Cardiovasc Magn Reson. 2010;12:40.
27. Doesch C, Haghi D, Suselbeck T, Schoenberg SO, Borggrefe M, Papavassiliu T. Impact of functional, morphological and clinical parameters on epicardial adipose tissue in patients with coronary artery disease. Circ J. 2012;76:2426–34.
28. Doesch C, Streitner F, Bellm S, Suselbeck T, Haghi D, Heggemann F, et al. Epicardial adipose tissue assessed by cardiac magnetic resonance imaging in patients with heart failure due to dilated cardiomyopathy. Obesity (Silver Spring). 2013;21:E253–61.
29. Haykowsky MJ, Nicklas BJ, Brubaker PH, Hundley WG, Brinkley TE, Upadhya B, et al. Regional adipose distribution and its relationship to exercise intolerance in older obese patients who have heart failure with preserved ejection fraction. JACC Heart Fail. 2018;6:640–9.
30. Iacobellis G, Willens HJ. Echocardiographic epicardial fat: a review of research and clinical applications. J Am Soc Echocardiogr. 2009;22:1311–9.
31. Iacobellis G, Assael F, Ribaudo MC, Zappaterreno A, Alessi G, Di Mario U, et al. Epicardial fat from echocardiography: a new method for visceral adipose tissue prediction. Obes Res. 2003;11:304–10.
32. Iacobellis G, Zaki MC, Garcia D, Willens HJ. Epicardial fat in atrial fibrillation and heart failure. Horm Metab Res. 2014;46:587–90.
33. Ruberg FL, Chen Z, Hua N, Bigornia S, Guo Z, Hallock K, et al. The relationship of ectopic lipid accumulation to cardiac and vascular function in obesity and metabolic syndrome. Obesity (Silver Spring). 2010;18:1116–21.

Autonomic Nervous System Modulation of the Epicardial Adipose Tissue in Heart Failure and Atrial Fibrillation

12

Celina M. Pollard, Jennifer Maning, and Anastasios Lymperopoulos

Key Points

- Epicardial adipose tissue (EAT) receives significant amount of autonomic innervation (both sympathetic and parasympathetic).
- Both autonomic branches modulate EAT transcriptome and secretome, thereby regulating EAT's contribution to cardiac function and dysregulation.
- Targeting of both cholinergic and adrenergic neuronal inputs into EAT can have therapeutic value in heart disease.

Introduction

Epicardial fat is most commonly defined as adipose tissue surrounding the heart, located between the myocardium and the visceral pericardium. Although epicardial fat can be considered as part of total-body visceral adipose tissue, most studies assessing associations of visceral adipose tissue with cardiovascular conditions do not include epicardial (or any intrathoracic) fat with their imaging technique and instead quantify either intra-abdominal fat alone or a combination of intra-abdominal and intrapelvic fat. At the molecular level, fat exists as lipid in the form of triglycerides [1]. While body fat is mostly found in adipose tissue, it also exists within other tissues. EAT, contrary to paracardial fat, separated from the myocardium by the pericardium, has no physical boundaries with the underlying myocardium. Epicardial fat is perfused by the coronary arteries and serves to store energy in the form of lipids for the myocardium, for thermoregulation, to protect autonomic ganglia and neuronal tissue, and regulation of coronary artery vasomotion and luminal size [1]. A range of pathophysiologic mechanisms could contribute to an association between epicardial fat and atrial fibrillation (AF) (Fig. 12.1) [1]. Epicardial fat may lead to AF via structural and electrical remodeling of the atria by both direct (e.g., by the infiltration of adipose tissue leading to altered atrial electrophysiological properties) and indirect mechanisms (e.g., by acting as a source for paracrine modulators of myocardial inflammation and oxidative stress).

Sympathetic Nervous System of the Heart

The sympathetic nervous system (SNS), responsible for orchestrating the body's response to situations of stress or emergency ("fight-or-flight"),

C. M. Pollard · J. Maning · A. Lymperopoulos (✉)
Laboratory for the Study of Neurohormonal Control of the Circulation, Department of Pharmaceutical Sciences, College of Pharmacy, Nova Southeastern University, Fort Lauderdale, FL, USA
e-mail: al806@nova.edu

G. Iacobellis (ed.), *Epicardial Adipose Tissue*, Contemporary Cardiology,
https://doi.org/10.1007/978-3-030-40570-0_12

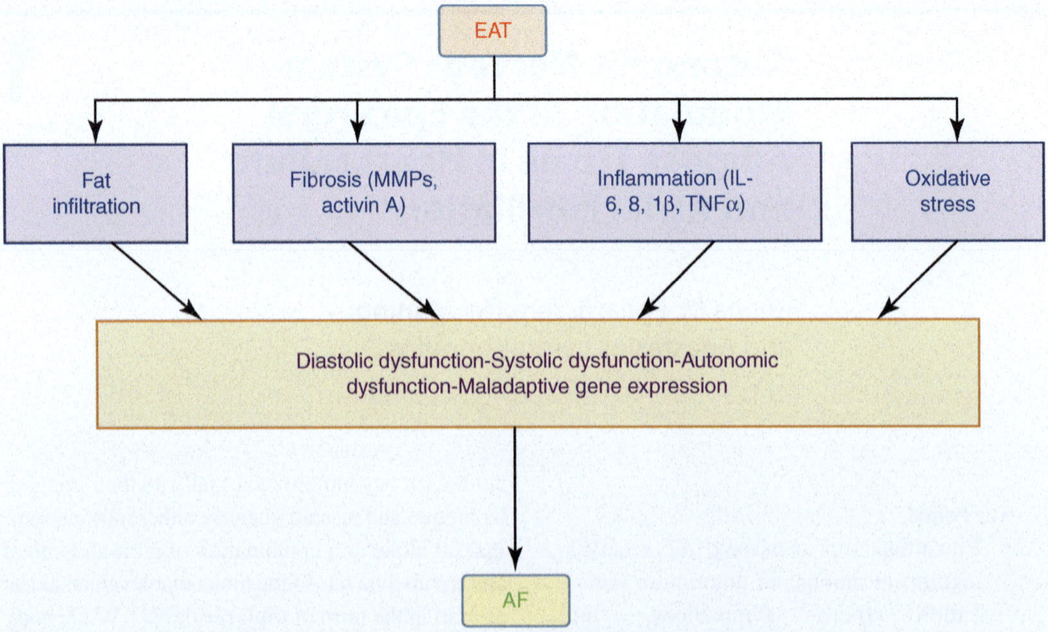

Fig. 12.1 Potential mechanisms underlying EAT involvement in autonomic dysfunction leading to AF pathogenesis. MMP matrix metalloproteinase, IL interleukin, TNF tumor necrosis factor

forms cardiac sympathetic ganglia along the side of the viscera column (paravertebral ganglia) [2]. These ganglia comprise the sympathetic trunks with their connecting fibers. The postganglionic fibers extend to the heart. In general, sympathetic preganglionic neurons are shorter than sympathetic postganglionic neurons [2]. The (postganglionic) sympathetic neurotransmitter is norepinephrine, although the neurotransmitter of the preganglionic neurons of both the sympathetic and parasympathetic systems is acetylcholine (ACh) [2]. Thus, these sympathetic postganglionic fibers are called (nor)adrenergic neurons. Norepinephrine and its close relative epinephrine exert their actions through three α_1, three α_2, and three β adrenergic receptor (AR) subtypes, which are all G protein-coupled receptors (GPCRs) [3–13]. β_1ARs are expressed in the heart (in the sinoatrial and atrioventricular nodes and in atrial and ventricular cardiomyocytes). Their activation increases heart rate (positive chronotropy), contractility (positive inotropy), and atrioventricular node conduction velocity (positive dromotropy) [3–13]. β_1AR is also present in the juxtaglomerular apparatus cells of the kidney where it induces renin release to activate the renin-angiotensin-aldosterone system (RAAS). β_2ARs are mainly expressed in vascular smooth muscle, in skeletal muscle, and in the coronary circulation [5]. Their activation elicits vasodilatation, which, in turn, increases blood perfusion to target organs. These receptors are located in non-sympathetic innervated tissues and thus are primarily stimulated by circulating epinephrine secreted by the adrenal medulla [5]. There are also some low numbers of expression of β_2ARs in cardiomyocytes [14]. α_1ARs are expressed in vascular smooth muscle proximal to sympathetic nerve terminals and they mediate vasoconstriction [15–17]. Cardiac myocytes also express some (minute) levels of α_1ARs [14]. Finally, α_2ARs are expressed in vascular smooth muscle distal from sympathetic nerve terminals, where they also elicit vasoconstriction, but they are also in the central nervous system mediating autoinhibition of sympathetic outflow and in the adrenal medulla mediating autoinhibition of NE and Epi secretion [17–21]. Myocardial contractility represents the ability of the heart to increase force of contraction, determined by the strength of the actomyosin filament interaction, which, in turn, depends on the cytoplasmic Ca^{2+} concentration of the myocyte [22]. Catecholamine binding to the β_1AR is among the most powerful stimuli for elevation of intracellular Ca^{2+} concentration in the cardiomyocyte and, consequently, for contraction of both the atria and ventricles [8, 22]. Of note, the β_3AR subtype mediates atrial contraction but ventricular relaxation, rather than contraction, via nitric oxide generation in the myocardium [23, 24].

Parasympathetic Nervous System of the Heart

The parasympathetic nervous system plays, in most (but not all) cases, an antagonistic, to the sympathetic system, role in regulating heart function [2]. Parasympathetic preganglionic fibers innervate organs of the thorax and upper abdomen as parts of the vagus nerve, which carries ~75% of all parasympathetic nerve fibers passing to the heart and many other visceral organs [2]. The short postganglionic neurons reside essentially inside or very close to the effector organs. Unlike the sympathetic ones, most parasympathetic preganglionic fibers reach the target organs and form the peripheral ganglia in the wall of the organ [2]. The preganglionic fibers synapse within the ganglion, and then short postganglionic fibers leave the ganglia to the target organ. Thus, in the parasympathetic system, preganglionic neurons are generally longer than postganglionic neurons [2]. ACh is the neurotransmitter of both preganglionic and postganglionic parasympathetic neurons (thus, they are called cholinergic neurons). ACh exerts its effects via two types of cholinergic receptors called nicotinic receptors (nAChRs) and muscarinic receptors (mAChRs) [25]. mAChRs are GPCRs located in the membranes of effector cells at the end of postganglionic parasympathetic nerves and at the ends of cholinergic sympathetic fibers. Responses from these receptors are excitatory and relatively slow [2, 9]. The nAChRs are ligand-gated ion channels located at synapses between pre- and postganglionic neurons of the sympathetic and parasympathetic pathways. Exactly because they are ion channels, nAChRs produce rapid, excitatory responses, in contrast to mAChRs [9]. Out of the five different known subtypes of mAChRs, M_2 mAChR is the major cholinergic receptor subtype in the mammalian heart. It is abundantly expressed in the atria and in conductive fibers, such as the sinoatrial and atrioventricular nodes, but, notably, its expression is negligible in the ventricles [26–28]. This means that ACh reduces heart rate via this receptor, shortening both action potential duration and conduction velocity (negative chronotropy and dromotropy) [29–31]. However, given the negligible contribution of the atrial muscle into the overall myocardial contractility, the negative effect of ACh on cardiac inotropy is negligible [2]. M_3 receptors are mainly expressed in vascular endothelium, where they mediate nitric oxide-dependent vasodilatation [2]. In conclusion, the parasympathetic system opposes the effects of the sympathetic nervous system on heart rate and nodal conduction but the effect on myocardial contractility is minimal. Nevertheless, reduced ACh secretion due to decreased neuronal cholinergic activity has been documented to accompany various cardiovascular diseases, such as arrhythmias, hypertension, myocardial infarction, and heart failure [32–40].

Autonomic Dysregulation and EAT: Implications for Human AF and Heart Failure

The autonomic nervous system has ganglions within the heart located in the EAT pads that regulate cardiac autonomic nervous input [41]. Vagal stimulation is modulated through multiple cardiac ganglionic plexi prior to arriving at the sinoatrial (SA) and atrioventricular (AV) nodes [41, 42]. The autonomic dysfunction leading to AF is well documented. The cholinergic system contributes significantly to AF in young, otherwise healthy patients [43]. Significant vagal innervation of the atrial muscle sleeves exists that extends into the pulmonary circulation [44]. As mentioned above (see section "Parasympathetic Nervous System of the Heart"), ACh-activated mAChRs (particularly of the M_2 subtype, which is $G_{i/o}$ protein-coupled) stimulate G protein-gated

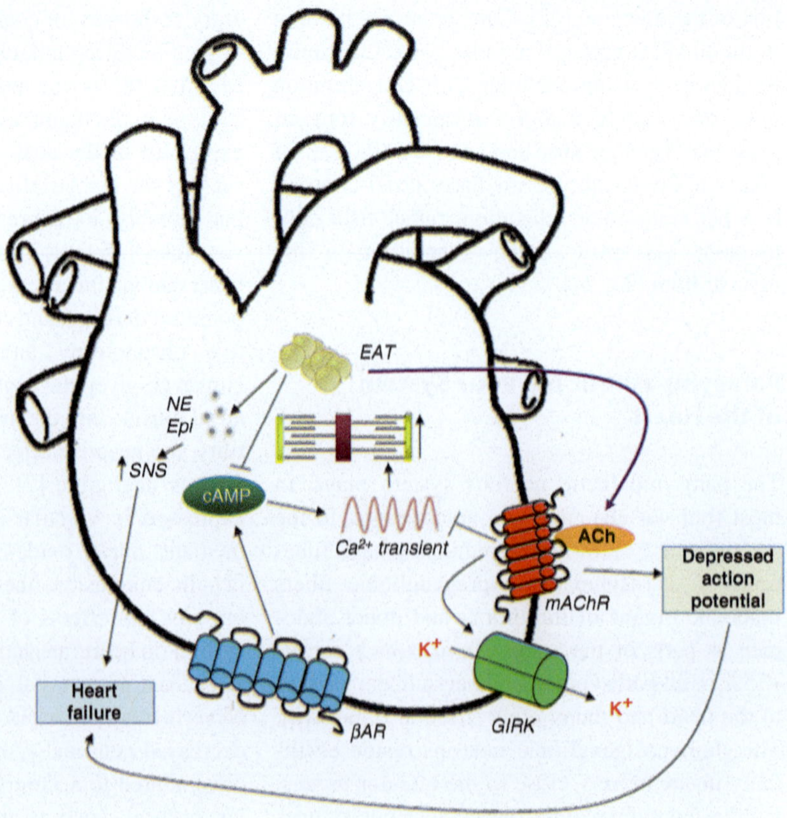

Fig. 12.2 Potential mechanisms underlying EAT involvement in autonomic dysfunction contributing to heart failure pathophysiology. NE norepinephrine, Epi epinephrine, GIRK G protein-gated (coupled) inwardly rectifying K^+ channel, cAMP 3′, 5′-(or cyclic) adenosine monophosphate

atrial K^+ channels (GIRKs) leading to hyperpolarization and indirectly inhibition of cyclic adenosine monophosphate (cAMP), the main second messenger synthesized by the βARs of the cardiac SNS [22, 45, 46]. This results in shortening of the atrial action potential duration with increased spatial heterogeneity [47] allowing for AF occurrence. On the other hand, the SNS can also trigger AF or ventricular arrhythmias by directly eliciting intracellular Ca^{2+} elevations in response to βAR activation [22, 48]. Since autonomic ganglionic plexi are anatomically found within the EAT pads, EAT plays important roles in regulating autonomic nervous system tone. In obese or diabetic individuals, autonomic signals emanating from epicardial fat become dysregulated and cause dysrhythmias. Abnormal increase of pericardial or epicardial fat is associated with abnormal regulation of autonomic nervous system activity, which might lead to increased ventricular arrhythmias and enhanced morbidity and mortality [49].

Since the autonomic nervous system crucially regulates heart rhythm and ganglionated plexi are located in EAT [50, 51], activation of these ganglionated plexi can cause both parasympathetic and sympathetic stimulation, resulting in shortened action potentials and increased calcium transients, respectively (Fig. 12.2) [42]. Thus, several clinical studies have investigated the role that neuromodulation may have in controlling AF, particularly by ablation of ganglionated plexi of the intrinsic cardiac nervous system. It is plausible that EAT influences these encased ganglionated plexi contributing to arrhythmogenesis. Indeed, botulinum toxin injection, which inhibits ACh release from preganglionic nerve terminals, into epicardial fat pads reduces cardiac autonomic nervous activity and AF by potentially suppressing ganglionated plexi [52, 53]. In that particular very recent study, biopsies, explants, or primary cultures were obtained from the EAT of 85 patients that underwent open-heart surgery. M_3 mAChR (a $G_{q/11}$ protein-coupled receptor) was found upregulated after adipogenesis induction and cholinergic fibers in EAT were detected by vesicular ACh transporter levels and acetylcholinesterase activity [54]. ACh treatment modified the secretome of the EAT of these patients, with various EAT-secreted proteins displaying differential levels between patients who developed AF post-surgery compared to those who did not. Thus, cholinergic activity of EAT regulates the interplay among EAT, autonomic nervous system dysfunction, and AF in a clinically meaningful manner [54].

Another interesting recent study examined the relationship between vagal response during cryoballoon catheter ablation for AF and cardiac autonomic nervous system modulation by evaluating EAT locations and heart rate variability analysis [55]. More specifically, the effects of vagal response on the cardiac autonomic nervous system in patients with paroxysmal AF who underwent second-generation cryoballoon ablation were compared between patients receiving vagal stimulation and patients that did not. The vagal response-receiving group exhibited greater EAT volume encasing the left atrium-left superior pulmonary vein junction than the non-vagal stimulated group. Additionally, volume of the EAT occupying this anatomical location correlated well with changes in heart rate variability immediately post-cryoablation. Thus, EAT volume on top of the left atrium-left superior pulmonary vein junction is useful for heart rate variability assessment and autonomic nervous system modulation of the heart [55]. A similar study from a Turkish group demonstrated that patients with higher EAT volume (i.e., thicker EAT) displayed significantly more heart rate variability and turbulence compared to patients with lower volume EAT [56]. The authors concluded that sympathovagal (i.e., autonomic) imbalance is directly related to EAT thickness, and thus, EAT volume and composition may play an important arrhythmogenic role, not necessarily limited to AF. Another piece of evidence supporting this conclusion was provided by a study in Japanese obese subjects, which performed a cross-sectional analysis of their EAT thickness [57]. These authors found that higher EAT thickness correlated with impaired recovery and lower cardiorespiratory fitness compared to subjects with lower EAT thickness. Moreover, higher EAT thickness in men was reported to represent cardiac autonomic dysfunction and poor parasympathetic response to exercise [57, 58].

Of note, an interesting study in dogs reported that a neural pathway from the cervical vagus trunk to the sinoatrial node and left atrium runs through the sinoatrial node-encasing EAT but eventually converges at the atrioventricular node-encasing EAT and suggested that the latter serves as an "integration center" for the former EAT in modulation of sinoatrial node function [59]. In other words, the atrioventricular node-encasing EAT may play a more critical role in the initiation and maintenance of AF. However, a study in patients undergoing coronary artery bypass grafting (CABG) surgery showed that, although maintenance of the EAT pad prevented attenuation of parasympathetic tone after CABG, it did not reduce post-surgery AF or total hospital costs in any appreciable way [60].

As far as EAT involvement in diabetic heart abnormalities is concerned, Burgeiro et al. investigated EAT metabolism in heart failure patients with or without diabetes [61]. They found that the differential between basal and insulin-stimulated glucose uptake was significantly decreased in epicardial vs. control, subcutaneous adipocytes. Moreover, lipolysis stimulated by isoproterenol (a catecholaminergic βAR full agonist) was also decreased in EAT compared to subcutaneous fat, which strongly correlated with lipolysis, lipid storage, and inflammation-related gene expression [61]. Finally, fatty acid composition of both of these fat tissues was significantly altered by diabetes. Thus, significant metabolic differences between EAT and subcutaneous adipose tissue in the presence of diabetic heart failure exist, and EAT metabolism might be a therapeutic target in diabetes-related heart failure [62].

Finally, an Italian study in systolic heart failure patients identified a highly significant correlation between EAT thickness and the extent of cardiac sympathetic denervation [63]. Specifically, EAT thickness was reported to be useful as an independent predictor of SNS dysfunction, since left ventricular mass, EAT thickness, and cardiac sympathetic denervation were found to correlate well with one another in systolic heart failure patients [64]. EAT becomes thicker as cardiac SNS activity decreases and left ventricular mass increases. In addition, this study demonstrated that EAT is a source of catecholamines itself, as both norepinephrine and epinephrine were present in higher concentrations in EAT compared with subcutaneous adipose tissue [64]. In heart failure patients, norepinephrine levels were increased 5.6-fold in EAT compared with subcutaneous adipose tissue and 2-fold compared with plasma. Importantly, these increases were attributed to increased catecholamine biosynthesis within the EAT, since the catecholamine biosynthetic enzymes tyrosine hydroxylase and dopamine beta-hydroxylase were found massively upregulated at both the mRNA and protein levels, compared to the control, subcutaneous adipose tissue of the patients [64]. Although the reported elevations in expression of these enzymes were astonishingly vast (~8-fold for the mRNAs and ~15-fold (!) for the proteins), raising concerns about the accuracy/validity of the assessing techniques employed, this study clearly identified human EAT as a significant source of both norepinephrine and epinephrine, at least in the context of systolic heart failure, and may contribute to the well-documented SNS hyperactivity that accompanies and aggravates human heart failure (see Fig. 12.2). The increased catecholamine biosynthetic activity of EAT in systolic heart failure, which is obviously the result of a thickened EAT (higher volume EAT contains more adipocytes, which express higher levels of biosynthetic enzymes; hence catecholamine synthesis is elevated), adds to the total catecholamine accumulation in the failing heart's EAT. In conclusion, this study provides evidence for EAT thickness being an index of cardiac adrenergic nerve activity and derangement and for use in determining prognosis in systolic heart failure patients. Whether these findings apply also to diastolic heart failure or HFpEF (heart failure with preserved ejection fraction) patients [65–67] remains an open question awaiting an answer in future studies.

Summary

Although our understanding of the relationship between EAT and AF or heart failure has rapidly increased in recent years, this exciting new field of research is still in its infancy. An increasing number of clinical and epidemiological studies demonstrate consistent associations between epicardial fat and AF, but more research is warranted to clarify causation, due to the fact that all these reported associations of epicardial fat with AF (and with heart failure) are confounded by other adipose tissue depots or comorbidities, such as hypertension, diabetes, obesity, metabolic syndrome, and obstructive sleep apnea. Additional evidence from larger, prospective cohort studies is definitely needed, especially for statistically meaningful comparisons of the different visceral adipose tissues and sub-depots of epicardial fat. Both basic science and translational studies will be needed to enhance our understanding of the mechanisms underlying the role of EAT in the autonomic dysfunction that precipitates AF and heart failure. Thanks to its currently rapidly evolving epidemic throughout the Western world, obesity will continue to emerge as a principal risk factor and causative trigger of both AF and heart failure but also of other cardiovascular diseases in the coming years. Thus, investigations into the roles the various human body fat depots, including EAT, play in the pathophysiology of AF and heart failure will continue to be one of the hottest research topics of the biomedical field. The ultimate hope is that they will produce novel weapons to combat heart disease for the cardiologist of the future.

References

1. Wong CX, Ganesan AN, Selvanayagam JB. Epicardial fat and atrial fibrillation: current evidence, potential mechanisms, clinical implications, and future directions. Eur Heart J. 2017;38:1294–302.
2. Lymperopoulos A, Koch WJ. Autonomic pharmacology. In: Waldman SA, Terzic A, editors. Pharmacology

and therapeutics: principles to practice. Philadelphia: Saunders/Elsevier; 2009. p. 115–39.
3. Brodde OE, Michel MC. Adrenergic and muscarinic receptors in the human heart. Pharmacol Rev. 1999;51:651–90.
4. Lymperopoulos A. Introduction/general considerations. In: Lymperopoulos A, editor. The cardiovascular adrenergic system. New York: Springer International Publishing; 2015. p. 3–9.
5. Lymperopoulos A, Rengo G, Koch WJ. Adrenergic nervous system in heart failure: pathophysiology and therapy. Circ Res. 2013;113:739–53.
6. Capote LA, Mendez Perez R, Lymperopoulos A. GPCR signaling and cardiac function. Eur J Pharmacol. 2015;763:143–8.
7. Lymperopoulos A, Garcia D, Walklett K. Pharmacogenetics of cardiac inotropy. Pharmacogenomics. 2014;15:1807–21.
8. Lymperopoulos A, Bathgate A. Pharmacogenomics of the heptahelical receptor regulators G-protein-coupled receptor kinases and arrestins: the known and the unknown. Pharmacogenomics. 2012;13:323–41.
9. Lymperopoulos A, Rengo G, Koch WJ. Adrenal adrenoceptors in heart failure: fine-tuning cardiac stimulation. Trends Mol Med. 2007;13:503–11.
10. Lymperopoulos A. Ischemic emergency? endothelial cells have their own "adrenaline shot" at hand. Hypertension. 2012;60:12–4.
11. Bylund DB, Eikenberg DC, Hieble JP, Langer SZ, Lefkowitz RJ, Minneman KP, et al. International Union of Pharmacology nomenclature of adrenoceptors. Pharmacol Rev. 1994;46(2):121–36.
12. Brodde OE. Beta-adrenoceptors in cardiac disease. Pharmacol Ther. 1993;60:405–30.
13. Yoshikawa T, Port JD, Asano K, Chidiak P, Bouvier M, Dutcher D, et al. Cardiac adrenergic receptor effects of carvedilol. Eur Heart J. 1996;17(Suppl B):8–16.
14. Woodcock EA, Du XJ, Reichelt ME, Graham RM. Cardiac alpha 1-adrenergic drive in pathological remodelling. Cardiovasc Res. 2008;77:452–62.
15. Shannon R, Chaudhry M. Effect of alpha1-adrenergic receptors in cardiac pathophysiology. Am Heart J. 2006;152:842–50.
16. Philipp M, Hein L. Adrenergic receptor knockout mice: distinct functions of 9 receptor subtypes. Pharmacol Ther. 2004;101:65–74.
17. Philipp M, Brede M, Hein L. Physiological significance of alpha(2)-adrenergic receptor subtype diversity: one receptor is not enough. Am J Physiol Regul Integr Comp Physiol. 2002;283:R287–95.
18. Hein L, Altman JD, Kobilka BK. Two functionally distinct alpha2-adrenergic receptors regulate sympathetic neurotransmission. Nature. 1999;402:181–4.
19. Lymperopoulos A, Rengo G, Funakoshi H, Eckhart AD, Koch WJ. Adrenal GRK2 upregulation mediates sympathetic overdrive in heart failure. Nat Med. 2007;13:315–23.
20. Lymperopoulos A, Rengo G, Gao E, Ebert SN, Dorn GW II, Koch WJ. Reduction of sympathetic activity via adrenal-targeted GRK2 gene deletion attenuates heart failure progression and improves cardiac function after myocardial infarction. J Biol Chem. 2010;285:16378–86.
21. Lymperopoulos A, Rengo G, Zincarelli C, Soltys S, Koch WJ. Modulation of adrenal catecholamine secretion by in vivo gene transfer and manipulation of G protein-coupled receptor kinase-2 activity. Mol Ther. 2008;16:302–7.
22. Bers DM. Calcium cycling and signaling in cardiac myocytes. Annu Rev Physiol. 2008;70:23–49.
23. Skeberdis VA, Gendviliene V, Zablockaite D, Treinys R, Macianskiene R, Bogdelis A, et al. Beta3-adrenergic receptor activation increases human atrial tissue contractility and stimulates the L-type Ca^{2+} current. J Clin Invest. 2008;118(9):3219–27.
24. Gauthier C, Leblais V, Kobzik L, Trochu JN, Khandoudi N, Bril A, et al. The negative inotropic effect of beta3-adrenoceptor stimulation is mediated by activation of a nitric oxide synthase pathway in human ventricle. J Clin Invest. 1998;102(7):1377–84.
25. Roy A, Guatimosim S, Prado VF. Cholinergic activity as a new target in diseases of the heart. Mol Med. 2015;20:527–37.
26. Hartzell HC. Regulation of cardiac ion channels by catecholamines, acetylcholine and second messenger systems. Prog Biophys Mol Biol. 1988;52:165–247.
27. Li DL, Liu BH, Sun L, Zhao M, He X, Yu XJ, Zang WJ. Alterations of muscarinic acetylcholine receptors-2, 4 and alpha7-nicotinic acetylcholine receptor expression after ischaemia/reperfusion in the rat isolated heart. Clin Exp Pharmacol Physiol. 2010;37:1114–9.
28. Anderson A, Kulkarni K, Marron Fernandez de Velasco E, Carlblom N, Xia Z, Nakano A, et al. Expression and relevance of the G protein-gated K+ channel in the mouse ventricle. Sci Rep. 2018;8:1192.
29. Giles W, Noble SJ. Changes in membrane currents in bullfrog atrium produced by acetylcholine. J Physiol. 1976;261(1):103–23.
30. Dhein S, van Koppen CJ, Brodde OE. Muscarinic receptors in the mammalian heart. Pharmacol Res. 2001;44:161–82.
31. Caulfield MP. Muscarinic receptors--characterization, coupling and function. Pharmacol Ther. 1993;58:319–79.
32. Agarwal SK, Norby FL, Whitsel EA, Soliman EZ, Chen LY, Loehr LR, et al. Autonomic dysfunction and incidence of atrial fibrillation: results from 20 years follow-up. J Am Coll Cardiol. 2017;69:291–9.
33. Jungen C, Scherschel K, Eickholt C, Kuklik P, Klatt N, Bork N, et al. Disruption of cardiac cholinergic neurons enhances susceptibility to ventricular arrhythmias. Nat Commun. 2017;8:14155.
34. González SA, Forcada P, de Cavanagh EM, Inserra F, Svane JC, Obregón S, et al. Sodium intake is associated with parasympathetic tone and metabolic parameters in mild hypertension. Am J Hypertens. 2012;25:620–4.

35. McAreavey D, Neilson JM, Ewing DJ, Russell DC. Cardiac parasympathetic activity during the early hours of acute myocardial infarction. Br Heart J. 1989;62:165–70.
36. Lombardi F, Sandrone G, Spinnler MT, Torzillo D, Lavezzaro GC, Brusca A, Malliani A. Heart rate variability in the early hours of an acute myocardial infarction. Am J Cardiol. 1996;77:1037–44.
37. Grassi G, Seravalle G, Bertinieri G, Turri C, Stella ML, Scopelliti F, Mancia G. Sympathetic and reflex abnormalities in heart failure secondary to ischaemic or idiopathic dilated cardiomyopathy. Clin Sci (Lond). 2001;101:141–6.
38. Hellermann JP, Jacobsen SJ, Redfield MM, Reeder GS, Weston SA, Roger VL. Heart failure after myocardial infarction: clinical presentation and survival. Eur J Heart Fail. 2005;7:119–25.
39. Lara A, Damasceno DD, Pires R, Gros R, Gomes ER, Gavioli M, et al. Dysautonomia due to reduced cholinergic neurotransmission causes cardiac remodeling and heart failure. Mol Cell Biol. 2010;30:1746–56.
40. Gerber Y, Weston SA, Enriquez-Sarano M, Manemann SM, Chamberlain AM, Jiang R, Roger VL. Atherosclerotic burden and heart failure after myocardial infarction. JAMA Cardiol. 2016;1:156–62.
41. Zhou Q, Zhang L, Wang K, Xu X, Ji M, Zhang F, Wang H, Hou Y. Effect of interconnection between cervical vagus trunk, epicardial fat pad on sinus node function, and atrial fibrillation. Pacing Clin Electrophysiol. 2014;37:356–63.
42. Pabon MA, Manocha K, Cheung JW, Lo JC. Linking arrhythmias and adipocytes: insights, mechanisms, and future directions. Front Physiol. 2018;9:1752.
43. Coumel P. Autonomic influences in atrial tachyarrhythmias. J Cardiovasc Electrophysiol. 1996;7:999–1007.
44. Zipes DP, Knope RF. Electrical properties of the thoracic veins. Am J Cardiol. 1972;29:372–6.
45. Harvey RD, Belevych AE. Muscarinic regulation of cardiac ion channels. Br J Pharmacol. 2003;139:1074–84.
46. Pollard CM, Desimine VL, Wertz SL, Perez A, Parker BM, Maning J, et al. Deletion of osteopontin enhances β_2-adrenergic receptor-dependent anti-fibrotic signaling in cardiomyocytes. Int J Mol Sci. 2019;20:E1396.
47. Rosenshtraukh LV, Zaitsev AV, Fast VG, Pertsov AM, Krinsky VI. Vagally induced block and delayed conduction as a mechanism for circus movement tachycardia in frog atria. Circ Res. 1989;64:213–26.
48. Francis GS. Should asymptomatic ventricular arrhythmias in patients with congestive heart failure be treated with antiarrhythmic drugs? J Am Coll Cardiol. 1988;12:274–83.
49. Wu CK, Tsai HY, Su MY, Wu YF, Hwang JJ, Tseng WY, et al. Pericardial fat is associated with ventricular tachyarrhythmia and mortality in patients with systolic heart failure. Atherosclerosis. 2015;241:607–14.
50. Chen PS, Chen LS, Fishbein MC, Lin SF, Nattel S. Role of the autonomic nervous system in atrial fibrillation: pathophysiology and therapy. Circ Res. 2014;114:1500–15.
51. Oh S, Zhang Y, Bibevski S, Marrouche NF, Natale A, Mazgalev TN. Vagal denervation and atrial fibrillation inducibility: epicardial fat pad ablation does not have long-term effects. Heart Rhythm. 2006;3:701–8.
52. Nakagawa H, Scherlag BJ, Patterson E, Ikeda A, Lockwood D, Jackman WM. Pathophysiologic basis of autonomic ganglionated plexus ablation in patients with atrial fibrillation. Heart Rhythm. 2009;6(12 Suppl):S26–34.
53. Pokushalov E, Kozlov B, Romanov A, Strelnikov A, Bayramova S, Sergeevichev D, et al. Long-term suppression of atrial fibrillation by botulinum toxin injection into epicardial fat pads in patients undergoing cardiac surgery: one year follow up of a randomized pilot study. Circ Arrhythm Electrophysiol. 2015;8:1334–41.
54. Couselo-Seijas M, López-Canoa JN, Agra-Bermejo RM, Díaz-Rodriguez E, Fernandez AL, Martinez-Cereijo JM, et al. Cholinergic activity regulates the secretome of epicardial adipose tissue: association with atrial fibrillation. J Cell Physiol. 2019;234(7):10512–22.
55. Yanagisawa S, Inden Y, Mizutani Y, Fujii A, Kamikubo Y, Kanzaki Y, et al. Vagal response in cryoballoon ablation of atrial fibrillation and autonomic nervous system: Utility of epicardial adipose tissue location. J Arrhythm. 2017;33(4):275–82.
56. Balcioğlu AS, Çiçek D, Akinci S, Eldem HO, Bal UA, Okyay K, Müderrisoğlu H. Arrhythmogenic evidence for epicardial adipose tissue: heart rate variability and turbulence are influenced by epicardial fat thickness. Pacing Clin Electrophysiol. 2015;38:99–106.
57. Kim MK, Tanaka K, Kim MJ, Matsuo T, Tomita T, Ohkubo H, et al. Epicardial fat tissue: relationship with cardiorespiratory fitness in men. Med Sci Sports Exerc. 2010;42:463–9.
58. Quan KJ, Lee JH, Van Hare GF, Biblo LA, Mackall JA, Carlson MD. Identification and characterization of atrioventricular parasympathetic innervation in humans. J Cardiovasc Electrophysiol. 2002;13:735–9.
59. Zhou Q, Zhang L, Wang K, Xu X, Ji M, Zhang F, et al. Effect of interconnection between cervical vagus trunk, epicardial fat pad on sinus node function, and atrial fibrillation. Pacing Clin Electrophysiol. 2014;37:356–63.
60. White CM, Sander S, Coleman CI, Gallagher R, Takata H, Humphrey C, et al. Impact of epicardial anterior fat pad retention on postcardiothoracic surgery atrial fibrillation incidence: the AFIST-III Study. J Am Coll Cardiol. 2007;49:298–303.
61. Burgeiro A, Fuhrmann A, Cherian S, Espinoza D, Jarak I, Carvalho RA, et al. Glucose uptake and lipid metabolism are impaired in epicardial adipose tissue from heart failure patients with or without diabetes. Am J Physiol Endocrinol Metab. 2016;310:E550–64.
62. Katlandur H, Ozbek K, Keser A. Letter to the Editor: the effect of autonomic nervous system on the impairment of glucose uptake and lipid metabolism in epicardial adipose tissue. Am J Physiol Endocrinol Metab. 2016;310:E862.

63. White A. Cardiac sympathetic denervation in the failing heart: a role for epicardial adipose tissue. Circ Res. 2016;118(8):1189–91.
64. Parisi V, Rengo G, Perrone-Filardi P, Pagano G, Femminella GD, Paolillo S, et al. Increased epicardial adipose tissue volume correlates with cardiac sympathetic denervation in patients with heart failure. Circ Res. 2016;118(8):1244–53.
65. Iacobellis G, Leonetti F, Singh N, M Sharma A. Relationship of epicardial adipose tissue with atrial dimensions and diastolic function in morbidly obese subjects. Int J Cardiol. 2007;115:272–3.
66. Iacobellis G, Singh N, Wharton S, Sharma AM. Substantial changes in epicardial fat thickness after weight loss in severely obese subjects. Obesity (Silver Spring). 2008;16:1693–7.
67. Packer M. Leptin-aldosterone-neprilysin axis: identification of its distinctive role in the pathogenesis of the three phenotypes of heart failure in people with obesity. Circulation. 2018;137:1614–31.

Cardiometabolic Risk and Epicardial Adipose Tissue

13

Gianluca Iacobellis
and Alexandra C. Villasante Fricke

Key Points

- Epicardial adipose tissue (EAT) is a quantifiable and modifiable biomarker that can be assessed with standard imaging techniques.
- EAT reflects visceral adiposity and strongly correlates with fatty liver infiltration and insulin resistance. Imaging of EAT can stratify the cardiovascular risk in subjects with type 2 diabetes and pre-diabetes.
- Higher EAT is associated with higher cardiometabolic risk, independently of traditional risk markers. EAT increases the risk of cardiovascular diseases in patients with HIV, psoriasis, and post-menopausal women.

Introduction

Epicardial fat (EAT) is a unique adipose tissue with peculiar anatomical, genetic, and biomolecular features [1–9]. Excessive or abnormal EAT is associated with higher cardiometabolic risk [10, 11]. EAT is a measurable risk factor as it can be detected and assessed with standard imaging techniques [11–13]. Regardless of how it is measured, EAT is a marker of visceral adiposity, rather than overall obesity. EAT correlates with traditional and unconventional risk indicators [10]. Altogether, these features make EAT a novel and appealing risk factor to be used in both clinical and research setting. In this chapter, we review and discuss the role of EAT as biomarker in clinical conditions that increase the cardiometabolic risk.

Metabolic Syndrome

Metabolic syndrome (MetS) is a cluster of metabolic conditions that increase the cardiovascular risk. The first definition was proposed in 1998 by the World Health Organization (WHO) [14], followed by a definition in 2001 by the National Cholesterol Education Program (NCEP) [15]. Other classifications were discussed until the most recent worldwide harmonizing criteria were made in 2009 as a revision to the NCEP criteria

G. Iacobellis (✉)
Division of Endocrinology, Diabetes and Metabolism, Department of Medicine, University of Miami, Miller School of Medicine, Miami, FL, USA
e-mail: giacobellis@med.miami.edu

A. C. Villasante Fricke
Department of Diabetes, Endocrinology, and Metabolism, University of Miami, Miami, FL, USA

G. Iacobellis (ed.), *Epicardial Adipose Tissue*, Contemporary Cardiology,
https://doi.org/10.1007/978-3-030-40570-0_13

[16]. According to the 2009 definition, the five established components of MetS include abdominal obesity defined by ethnicity-specific waist circumference, elevated blood pressure, impaired fasting glucose, increase triglyceride levels, and decreased high-density lipoprotein (HDL) cholesterol levels. However, there is some controversy; for example, the American Diabetes Association and the European Association for the Study of Diabetes stated that the existing criteria for MetS do not actually meet the definition of a syndrome, whereas WHO indicated that the criteria for MetS were an educational concept for a premorbid condition rather than a diagnostic or therapeutic tool [17, 18].

Adipose Tissue Changes in Metabolic Syndrome

The development and progression of the MetS is strongly linked to the adipose tissue inflammation, ectopic lipid infiltration, oxidative stress, and mitochondrial dysfunction, particularly in skeletal muscle and liver [19]. MetS is thought to be a systemic manifestation of adipose tissue disarray [19]. Briefly, adipose tissue secretes many proinflammatory bioactive molecules, such as tumor-necrosis factor-alpha and interleukins. Inflammation leads to changes in VAT including activated lipolysis, release of free fatty acids, hypoxia, oxidative stress, and apoptosis of adipocytes [20]. Specifically, increased secretion of TNF-alpha leads to increased aggregation of activated macrophages from bone marrow and infiltration of macrophages into adipose tissue [21, 22]. Cell oxidative stress within the mitochondria, nucleus, and endoplasmic reticulum due to excess delivery of fuel leads to mitochondrial dysfunction [19, 23, 24].

Epicardial Fat as Marker of Visceral Adiposity

Visceral adipose tissue (VAT) is the adipose tissue that surrounds internal organs, as opposed to subcutaneous adipose tissue that is more superficially located. The separation between these two fat depots is not simply anatomical, but more complex and accounts for genetic and biomolecular differences. Visceral obesity is associated with metabolic disorders including insulin resistance, impaired glucose tolerance, T2DM, and polycystic ovarian syndrome [25]. Increased VAT is known to play a key role in the development of MetS [26–33]. VAT is also associated with cardiovascular disease including hypertension, heart failure, coronary artery disease (CAD), valvular disease, and arrhythmias; pulmonary disease including sleep apnea; brain disease including stroke and dementia; and reduced bone density [25]. Furthermore, VAT is an independent predictor of mortality in males [34].

However, more recently the focus has moved and narrowed to the visceral fat accumulating and infiltrating the internal organs, such as the liver and the heart. There is a growing number of data suggesting that organ-specific fat depots play a direct role in producing organ damages. Because VAT is anatomically and functionally linked to the internal organs, this hypothesis can be likely true. Hence, there is a compelling need of novel markers and not invasive methods for the assessment of local VAT. Anthropomorphic measurements used to estimate VAT are imprecise, with waist circumference being the best anthropomorphic predictor of intra-abdominal fat mass [35, 36]. Given the poor accurateness and sensitivity of the traditional anthropometric markers of body fatness and intra-abdominal fat, such as BMI and waist circumference, there is a great scientific effort in finding reliable and easy markers of the visceral, organ-specific adiposity. Imaging techniques are more precise for measuring VAT, with magnetic resonance imaging (MRI) being the gold standard [37–41]. However, MRI is costly, time intensive, and difficult for patients with claustrophobia to undergo. Computed tomography (CT) imaging is also another method of measuring VAT [42, 43], but it is costly and required exposure to radiation. Abdominal ultrasound has been used to measure abdominal VAT but can be confounded by subcutaneous adipose tissue in obese subjects [44–46]. Iacobellis et al. developed a method of measuring

EAT thickness via transthoracic echocardiographic ultrasound as a proxy for determination of overall VAT [12, 47]. Authors showed that EAT independently and accurately correlates with intra-abdominal VAT as measured by MRI and does so better than waist circumference does [12, 48].

Epicardial Fat and Metabolic Syndrome

VAT is a key component of the MetS. The patients with higher cardiometabolic risk have been historically considered as the one with high intra-abdominal fat. While this is still a correct observation and intra-abdominal fat remains a major predictor of risk and therapeutic target, the interest into less traditional visceral fat depots has grown.

EAT, as marker of VAT, was therefore evaluated in individuals with or without MetS. In healthy subjects without diabetes, hypertension, dyslipidemia, or metabolic disease, those with visceral fat phenotype showed higher EAT thickness than those with predominant peripheral fat distribution [47]. EAT thickness was also higher in subjects with central fat accumulation and at least two clinical and metabolic parameters of MetS than subjects with predominant peripheral fat distribution and no clinical or metabolic alterations [12]. EAT thickness was positively correlated with diastolic blood pressure, fasting insulin, low-density lipoprotein (LDL) cholesterol, glucose, and systolic blood pressure [12]. On the contrary, EAT had a negative linear correlation with plasma adiponectin and HDL cholesterol [12]. Diastolic blood pressure and fasting insulin levels were the variables most strongly correlated with EAT thickness as per multiple regression analysis [12]. No correlation was found with EAT and plasma triglycerides, C-reactive protein, fibrinogen, heart rate, uric acid, or microalbuminuria in this study [12].

In a 2012 meta-analysis of nine studies on echocardiographic EAT thickness in patients with and without MetS pooling 2027 subjects from nine studies, of whom 1030 had MetS, EAT thickness was significantly higher in those with MetS [49]. This meta-analysis found that patients with MetS tended to be older and that MetS was distributed evenly among men and women. It also found that the difference in EAT thickness was more pronounced in non-Hispanic white subjects followed by Hispanic, Turkish, and Asian subjects [49]. In one included study of 246 subjects, 58% of which had MetS, EAT was significantly thicker in both men and women with MetS compared to those without MetS [50].

Some studies sought to propose EAT thickness values to identify high-risk patients. However, there is no consensus yet. The individuals who were enrolled in some of these trials were quite diverse in terms of gender and race. As body fat distribution and visceral adiposity vary by gender and ethnicity, EAT threshold values may be different for ethnic group and not apply well in the general population. Iacobellis et al. provided the reference range and threshold values of high-risk echocardiographic epicardial fat thickness in both white men and women. The reference range was extremely wide with values from 1 mm up to 20 mm indicating a physiological and pathological epicardial fat depot in humans [50].

Higher EAT is likely to be involved in the pathophysiology of the MS, because it produces factors that can influence insulin sensitivity, inflammation, and lipid accumulation. However, a local impact of abnormal and excessive EAT appears more plausible than a systematic effect. EAT thickness is mainly an objective and reproducible indicator of excessive visceral fat accumulation. The measurement of EAT therefore represents an effective approach to identify patients at high risk for MetS and its subsequent consequences.

Epicardial Fat, Diabetes, and Insulin Resistance

Increased VAT, insulin resistance, and chronic inflammation are major factors contributing to the development and progression of type 2 diabetes mellitus (T2DM). Adipose expression of inflammatory markers is directly linked with the development of insulin resistance in obesity and T2DM [51]. EAT is a highly inflammatory and insulin-resistant fat depot. The proinflammatory activity of EAT presents peculiar and unique features in T2DM. Remarkably, recent RNA sequencing analysis showed that diabetic EAT transcriptome is significantly different than not diabetic EAT [52]. Also, when compared to diabetic subcutaneous fat, diabetic EAT is highly enriched with genes involved in inflammation, innate immune response, and endothelium [52]. EAT inflammatory genes expression is upregulated by transcription factors, mainly, primarily activated by the overexpressed advanced glycation end products – receptor advanced glycation end products (AGE-RAGE) signaling [52]. Clinically, EAT is increased in people with T2DM independently of BMI or total body fat [53]. EAT has a greater capacity for uptake and release of free fatty acids compared to other visceral adipose depots, and it also has a lower rate of glucose utilization [1, 17]. Animal studies have shown higher rates of insulin-induced lipogenesis in EAT compared to other visceral adipose depots [1, 17].

In a study of thirty obese subjects without a history of metabolic, cardiovascular, pulmonary, or hepatic disease, EAT thickness was associated with insulin resistance and impaired glucose tolerance [53]. In this study, all subjects underwent transthoracic echocardiography, a euglycemic hyperinsulinemic clamp to estimate insulin sensitivity, and an oral glucose tolerance test to evaluate glucose tolerance [54]. Among these subjects, three were found to have impaired fasting glucose, seven had impaired glucose tolerance, and twenty had no evidence of dysglycemia [54]. In particular, EAT was significantly correlated with waist circumference, fasting insulin, BMI, 120-min insulin, fasting glucose, and area under the curve for insulin even after adjusting for BMI and waist circumference in this study. No correlation was found between EAT thickness and age, area under the curve for glucose, area under the curve for insulin-to-glucose ratio, triglyceride-to-HDL cholesterol ratio, and 120-min glucose levels in this study [55]. Early glucose abnormalities that may precede the development of T2DM have been associated with higher cardiometabolic risk. Excessive VAT can be co-responsible of the higher cardiovascular risk in patients with prediabetes. EAT thickness was therefore measured in patients with impaired fasting (IFG) defined as fasting glucose between 100 and <126 mg/dl and found to be significantly higher in subjects with IFG than in euglycemic subjects [55]. Clinical assessment of EAT thickness or volume can serve as early biomarker of risk in subjects with prediabetes or IFG. Diabetes is often associated with a peculiar and unique cardiomyopathy, although the causes are probably multifactorial. A recent experimental study on rats showed that secretory profile of epicardial fat may contribute to the pathogenesis of diabetes mellitus-related cardiomyopathy [56]. However, larger studies are required to establish an independent correlative or predictive role of epicardial fat in type 2 diabetes. While the link between VAT and T2DM seems to be intuitive and somehow expected, the role of excessive visceral adiposity in subjects with type 1 diabetes has been only recently suggested. Phenotype of type 1 diabetes includes now also patients with central adiposity, as obesity incidence is increasing. Recent evidences pointed out a possible correlation between visceral fat and type 1 diabetes. Few studies showed a relation of EAT with central obesity in type 1 diabetic subjects [57–59]. EAT thickness was higher in type 1 diabetic subjects independently of BMI, HbA1c, and daily insulin requirement [59]. Interestingly, EAT thickness and serum leptin levels are correlated in patients with type 1 diabetes. However, the mechanisms that link EAT to type 1 diabetes remain to be elucidated.

Epicardial Fat and Liver Steatosis

Hepatic steatosis or nonalcoholic fatty liver disease (NAFLD) is the accumulation of adipose tissue in and around the liver. VAT is an independent causative risk factor for liver steatosis, rather than overall obesity [60]. Both liver and visceral fat are independent risk factors for major cardiovascular events. NAFLD is caused by the excessive accumulation of fat in the liver and commonly associated with obesity and MetS. NAFLD can be considered the hepatic expression of the metabolic syndrome. Elevations in alanine aminotransferase [61] and gamma-glutamyltransferase [62] have been found to predict MetS. NAFLD is also known to be associated with increased cardiovascular risk including CAD [63], increased coronary artery calcium score [64], atrial fibrillation [65], and overall cardiovascular risk in diabetics [66, 67].

In 2014, Iacobellis et al. compared 62 obese subjects with ultrasonographic evidence of NAFLD with 62 obese controls and found for the first time that EAT was significantly thicker in subjects with nonalcoholic fatty liver disease [68]. In that study, among waist circumference and BMI, EAT thickness correlated most closely with liver steatosis. At that time, it had been known that EAT was associated with increased alanine transaminase levels [69] and that EAT and hepatic steatosis were correlated with abdominal adiposity and hypertriglyceridemia [70]. Serum transaminases are surrogate markers of fatty liver in subjects with regional fat redistribution and higher visceral fat.

It was also known that patients with fatty liver had abnormal left ventricle energy metabolism [71] and reduced coronary flow reserve [72] and abnormal cardiac geometry [73]. More recently, Turan found that nonalcoholic fatty liver disease fibrosis score is related to EAT thickness and CAD [74]. A recent meta-analysis of thirteen case control studies looking at 2260 subjects found that EAT was significantly increased in subjects with nonalcoholic fatty liver disease compared to controls [75]. The increase in the EAT was associated with the severity of hepatic steatosis, hepatic fibrosis, and cardiovascular disease in patients with nonalcoholic fatty liver disease [75]. Hepatic triglyceride content decreases rapidly during very-low-calorie dietary interventions in morbidly obese subjects who are candidate for bariatric surgery. Interestingly, EAT has shown to quickly and significantly shrink after very-low-calorie diet in morbid obese subjects. The magnitude and responsiveness of both hepatic and cardiac fat to dietary changes highlight the similarities between the two fatty infiltrates.

In fact, the link between EAT and fatty liver can be explained by several mechanisms. Both epicardial and intra-abdominal fat evolve from brown adipose tissue during embryogenesis, suggesting a potential explanation for similar biomolecular properties between the two tissues. Both are organ-specific fat depots and markers of visceral adiposity. EAT and fatty liver share similar biochemical properties with the intra-abdominal visceral fat. EAT is one of the highest sources of free fatty acids and correlates with circulating free fatty acid levels in humans. The increased flux of free fatty acids to the liver impairs hepatic handling of fat inside the hepatocyte. Cardiac and hepatic fat are associated with insulin resistance and lipotoxicity. The accumulation of triglyceride around the myocardium and liver is related to free fatty acids exposure. Although higher EAT free fatty acid breakdown and release unlikely reach the hepatic circulation, all these features underlie the strong clinical correlation between EAT thickness and biomarkers of liver steatosis. An imbalance between cardioprotective and inflammatory cytokines such as adiponectin, transforming growth factors endothelin, and fibroblast growth factors is considered one of the possible mechanisms linking the severity of liver disease and the presence of cardiac alterations [76]. EAT pro-fibrotic and proinflammatory secretome may correlate and possibly contribute, even a systemic effect is likely, to the metabolic components of the hepatic steatosis. EAT sympathetic hyperactivity has been also linked to liver steatosis [77]. While EAT has been correlated with cardiac autonomic function, the evidences that this may interfere and lead to liver damage has not been demonstrated yet.

Epicardial Fat and HIV-Related Cardiovascular Risk

The treatment of HIV-infected patients with HAART has been associated with metabolic dysregulation and changes in body fat deposition. This syndrome, known as HIV/HAART-associated lipodystrophy syndrome, is mainly characterized by increased visceral adiposity, which contributes to an increased cardiovascular risk among these patients. The introduction of highly active antiretroviral therapy (HAART) has significantly improved the clinical outcome of HIV disease with increased survival rates. However, some HAART regimens, especially those including protease inhibitors, have been shown to cause in a high proportion of HIV-infected patients metabolic (dyslipidemia, insulin resistance) and somatic (lipodystrophy/lipoatrophy) changes that are associated with an increased risk of cardiovascular disease (coronary artery disease and stroke). The pathogenesis of HAART-associated metabolic syndrome and of its atherogenic profile is complex, and several factors are involved, including direct effects of HAART on lipid metabolism, endothelial and adipocyte cell function, activation of proinflammatory cytokines, and mitochondrial dysfunction. HAART-associated metabolic syndrome is mainly characterized by increased visceral adiposity, which contributes to an increased cardiovascular risk among these patients.

EAT has been found to be increased in people infected with HIV on highly active antiretroviral therapy [78, 79]. EAT thickness in patients with HIV was correlated with waist circumference, HDL cholesterol level, and plasma triglyceride level [78]. EAT thickness may be related to duration of antiretroviral therapy as well as markers of chronic inflammation [80].

In a 2014 study of 579 HIV-infected and 353 HIV-uninfected men aged 40–70 using CT to measure EAT and coronary artery calcium, HIV-infected men were found to have greater EAT than uninfected men [81]. EAT volume was associated with duration of antiretroviral therapy, specifically azidothymidine. EAT was associated with the presence of coronary artery plaque and noncalcified plaque. In men with positive coronary artery calcium, EAT was associated with the extent of coronary artery calcium [81]. In a 2012 study of 583 HIV-infected men, EAT and VAT but not body mass index were associated with cardiovascular disease [82]. In a cross-sectional study of 876 HIV-infected men and women on antiretroviral therapy, EAT as measured by CT was associated with central fat accumulation, mixed lipodystrophy phenotype, cumulative exposure to antiretroviral therapy, and coronary artery calcium, among other factors [83]. In a study of 78 HIV-infected men and 32 HIV-negative controls, EAT was associated with fasting glucose and plasma insulin levels [84].

The first study looking at EAT in the HIV-infected population was a 2007 study by Iacobellis et al. in which 60 HIV-infected subjects on antiretroviral therapy, MetS, and lipodystrophy were compared with 45 HIV-infected subjects [85]. Their EAT and carotid intima-media thickness were measured by ultrasonography and MRI was used to calculate VAT [85]. EAT by ultrasound was found to correlated with VAT by MRI. Patients with HIV and antiretroviral-associated MetS and lipodystrophy had increased EAT thickness and carotid intima-media thickness as compared with HIV-infected patients without MetS and lipodystrophy [85].

Epicardial Fat and Psoriasis-Related Cardiovascular Risk

Psoriasis is an immune-mediated skin disease associated with increased proinflammatory cytokines and the actions of T-helper-17 and T-helper-1 cells. Patients with psoriasis are at higher risk for cardiovascular diseases. Psoriasis is associated with systemic comorbidities including MetS. There is thought to be a crosstalk between skin inflammation and adipose tissue inflammation [86]. Increased EAT was first described as a marker of cardiovascular disease risk in psoriasis patients in a 2013 cross-sectional and observational study looking at 65 patients with psoriasis and 50 controls [87]. In a 2014 case-control study evaluating patients with psoriasis and 32 control subjects, EAT was found to be significantly higher in patients with psoriasis, and this was independent of preexisting MetS [88]. In a study of 38 patients with psoriasis and 38 controls, EAT as measured by CT was higher in patients with psoriasis and EAT was independently associated with the presence of coronary calcium in all subjects [89]. Another study of 115 adults with psoriasis and 60 matched controls found that EAT as measured by transthoracic echocardiography was higher in the psoriasis group and also found that high-sensitivity CRP was higher in the psoriasis group [90]. A study of 100 patients with severe psoriasis and without ASCVD and 202 controls underwent CT to measure EAT, abdominal VAT, and coronary artery calcification found that psoriasis was associated with subclinical atherosclerosis and with EAT independently of abdominal VAT [91]. A 2016 systematic review and meta-analysis including the five aforementioned trials concluded that psoriasis was associated with increased VAT [92].

Epicardial Fat and Menopause-Related Cardiovascular Risk

It is well established that postmenopausal women have higher risk for developing cardiovascular disease. The role of EAT in increasing the cardiovascular risk in postmenopausal women has been specifically evaluated by few focused studies. The SWAN Cardiovascular Fat Study showed that peri-/postmenopausal women have greater CT measured EAT volumes compared with pre-/early perimenopausal women independent of age and obesity [93]. In menopausal women with endothelial dysfunction, menopausal transition is associated with increased carotid arterial stiffness and ultrasound-measured EAT thickness, independent of age [94]. Vitamin D deficiency is associated with a significant increase in EAT thickness in premenopausal women [95]. Differential EAT pro-inflammatory activity between pre- and postmenopausal women has been also reported. More longitudinal and randomized clinical trials are desirable to evaluate the predictive role of EAT in postmenopausal women.

Racial and Ethnic Differences in Epicardial Fat

The difference in EAT thickness between subjects with and without MetS varies with ethnicity [49, 96, 97]. It is unclear whether this variability depends on racial differences in visceral adipose tissue amount, as reported in some ethnic groups or on differences concerning the extent of visceral fat increase needed to trigger the MetS [96–100]. A 2012 meta-analysis of nine studies on the relationship between EAT and MetS found that the difference in EAT thickness between subjects with or without the MetS was more evident in Caucasian subjects, followed by Hispanic, Turkish, and Asian subjects [49]. In a study of 150 patients admitted to a clinical decision unit in Michigan for chest pain, EAT as measured by echocardiography was significantly greater in non-Hispanic white Caucasians compared with non-Hispanic black African Americans [96]. This was true even when adjusted for age, sex, BMI, and waist circumference [96]. Similar results were found in a study in Miami where EAT was measured by echocardiography [97] and another study in South Carolina where EAT was measured by CT even when adjusted for cardiovascular risk factors [98]. A larger study of 1199 middle-aged men (24.2% white, 7.0% black, 23.6% Japanese Americans, 22.0% Japanese, 23.2% Koreans) found that EAT volumes as measured by CT were highest among Japanese Americans and lowest among blacks [99]. Furthermore, associations of EAT with BMI and VAT differed by racial/ethnic groups. A 2017 Australian study of 150 subjects found that EAT was significantly higher in South Asians and Southeast or East Asians when compared with whites [100]. South Asians were also found to have a higher aggregative plaque volume in the left anterior descending artery compared with whites [100].

Conclusion

EAT is a measurable biomarker and modifiable therapeutic target. Measurement of EAT is an accurate and reproducible method of measuring VAT. Increased EAT is a risk factor for MetS and cardiovascular disease. EAT is associated with T2DM, insulin resistance, and liver steatosis. EAT is elevated in HIV patients on antiretroviral therapy and in psoriasis patients, two groups with increased risk of MetS. Normal EAT varies by race and ethnic group. EAT measurement serves as a powerful potential diagnostic tool in assessing cardiovascular risk. In fact, measurement of VAT via EAT may be a useful diagnostic tool for risk stratification of MetS and its associated conditions including sleep apnea, atrial fibrillation, stroke, dementia, various cancers, and osteoporosis [25]. Furthermore, modification of EAT thickness via weight loss [101] and pharmacologic therapy has therapeutic implications for cardiovascular disease, T2DM, and MetS. It would be useful to measure EAT in patients with high risk of cardiovascular disease and MetS. We also recommend taking into account race and ethnicity when measuring EAT.

References

1. Iacobellis G, Bianco AC. Epicardial adipose tissue: emerging physiological, pathophysiological and clinical features. Trends Endocrinol Metab. 2011;22:450–7.
2. Iacobellis G, Corradi D, Sharma AM. Epicardial adipose tissue: anatomic, biomolecular and clinical relationships with the heart. Nat Clin Pract Cardiovasc Med. 2005;2:536–43.
3. Iacobellis G. Epicardial and pericardial fat: close, but very different. Obesity (Silver Spring). 2009;17:625; author reply: 626–7.
4. Rabkin SW. Epicardial fat: properties, function and relationship to obesity. Obes Rev. 2007;8:253–61.
5. Corradi D, Maestri R, Callegari S, Pastori P, Goldoni M, Luong TV, Bordi C. The ventricular epicardial fat is related to the myocardial mass in normal, ischemic and hypertrophic hearts. Cardiovasc Pathol. 2004;13:313–6.
6. Iacobellis G, Malavazos AE, Corsi MM. Epicardial fat: from the biomolecular aspects to the clinical practice. Int J Biochem Cell Biol. 2011;43:1651–4.
7. Sacks HS, Fain JN, Holman B, Cheema P, Chary A, Parks F, et al. Uncoupling protein-1 and related mRNAs in human epicardial and other adipose tissues: epicardial fat functioning as brown fat. J Clin Endocrinol Metab. 2009;94:3611–5.
8. Mazurek T, Zhang L, Zalewski A, Mannion JD, Diehl JT, Arafat H, et al. Human epicardial adipose tissue is a source of inflammatory mediators. Circulation. 2003;108:2460–6.
9. Iacobellis G, Gao YJ, Sharma AM. Do cardiac and perivascular adipose tissue play a role in atherosclerosis? Curr Diab Rep. 2008;8:20–4.
10. Iacobellis G. Local and systemic effects of the multifaceted epicardial adipose tissue depot. Nat Rev Endocrinol. 2015;11:363–71.
11. Iacobellis G, Ribaudo MC, Assael F, Vecci E, Tiberti C, Zappaterreno A, et al. Echocardiographic epicardial adipose tissue is related to anthropometric and clinical parameters of metabolic syndrome: a new indicator of cardiovascular risk. J Clin Endocrinol Metab. 2003;88:5163–8.
12. Greif M, Becker A, von Ziegler F, Lebherz C, Lehrke M, Broedl UC, et al. Pericardial adipose tissue determined by dual source CT is a risk factor for coronary atherosclerosis. Arterioscler Thromb Vasc Biol. 2009;29:781–6.
13. Gorter PM, van Lindert AS, de Vos AM, Meijs MF, van der Graaf Y, Doevendans PA, et al. Quantification of epicardial and peri-coronary fat using cardiac computed tomography reproducibility and relation with obesity and metabolic syndrome in patients suspected of coronary artery disease. Atherosclerosis. 2008;197:896–903.
14. Alberti KG, Zimmet PZ. Definition, diagnosis and classification of diabetes mellitus and its complications. Part 1: diagnosis and classification of diabetes mellitus provisional report of a WHO consultation. Diabet Med. 1998;15:539–53.
15. Expert Panel on Detection, Evaluation, and Treatment of High Blood Cholesterol in Adults. Executive summary of the third report of the National Cholesterol Education Program (NCEP) expert panel on detection, evaluation, and treatment of high blood cholesterol in adults (Adult Treatment Panel III). JAMA. 2001;285:2486–97.
16. Alberti KG, Eckel RH, Grundy SM, Zimmet PZ, Cleeman JI, Donato KA, et al. Harmonizing the metabolic syndrome: a joint interim statement of the International Diabetes Federation Task Force on Epidemiology and Prevention National Heart, Lung, and Blood Institute American Heart Association World Heart Federation International Atherosclerosis Society and International Association for the Study of Obesity. Circulation. 2009;120:1640–5.
17. Kahn R, Buse J, Ferrannini E, Stern M. American Diabetes Association European Association for the Study of Diabetes. The metabolic syndrome: time for a critical appraisal: joint statement from the American Diabetes Association and the European Association for the Study of Diabetes. Diabetes Care. 2005;28:2289–304.
18. Simmons RK, Alberti KG, Gale EA, Colagiuri S, Tuomilehto J, Qiao Q, et al. The metabolic syndrome: useful concept or clinical tool? Report of a WHO Expert Consultation. Diabetologia. 2010;53:600–5.
19. Oda E. Historical perspectives of the metabolic syndrome. Clin Dermatol. 2018;36:3–8.
20. Berg G, Miksztowicz V, Morales C, Barchuk M. Epicardial adipose tissue in cardiovascular disease. Adv Exp Med Biol. 2019;1127:131–43.
21. Cinti S, Mitchell G, Barbatelli G, Murano I, Ceresi E, Faloia E, et al. Adipocyte death defines macrophage localization and function in adipose tissue of obese mice and humans. J Lipid Res. 2005;46:2347–55.
22. Saberi M, Woods NB, de Luca C, Schenk S, Lu JC, Bandyopadhyay G, et al. Hematopoietic cell-specific deletion of toll-like receptor 4 ameliorates hepatic

and adipose tissue insulin resistance in high-fat-fed mice. Cell Metab. 2009;10:419–29.

23. Anderson EJ, Lustig ME, Boyle KE, Woodlief TL, Kane DA, Lin CT, et al. Mitochondrial H_2O_2 emission and cellular redox state link excess fat intake to insulin resistance in both rodents and humans. J Clin Invest. 2009;119:573–81.
24. Houstis N, Rosen ED, Lander ES. Reactive oxygen species have a causal role in multiple forms of insulin resistance. Nature. 2006;440:944–8.
25. Neeland IJ, Ross R, Després JP, Matsuzawa Y, Yamashita S, Shai I, Seidell J, et al. Visceral and ectopic fat, atherosclerosis, and cardiometabolic disease: a position statement. Lancet Diabetes Endocrinol. 2019;7:715–25.
26. Albu JB, Kovera AJ, Johnson JA. Fat distribution and health in obesity. Ann N Y Acad Sci. 2000;904:491–501.
27. Doll S, Paccaud F, Bovet P, Burnier M, Wietlisbach V. Body mass index, abdominal adiposity and blood pressure: consistency of their association across developing and developed countries. Int J Obes Relat Metab Disord. 2002;26:48–57.
28. Visscher TL, Seidell JC, Molarius A, van der Kuip D, Hofman A, Witteman JC. A comparison of body mass index, waist-hip ratio and waist circumference as predictors of all-cause mortality among the elderly: the Rotterdam study. Int J Obes Relat Metab Disord. 2001;25:1730–5.
29. Rexrode KM, Carey VJ, Hennekens CH, Walters EE, Colditz GA, Stampfer MJ. Abdominal adiposity and coronary heart disease in women. JAMA. 1998;280:1843–8.
30. Rexrode KM, Buring JE, Manson JE. Abdominal and total adiposity and risk of coronary heart disease in men. Int J Obes Relat Metab Disord. 2001;25:1047–56.
31. Folsom AR, Kushi LH, Anderson KE, Mink PJ, Olson JE, Hong CP, et al. Associations of general and abdominal obesity with multiple health outcomes in older women: the Iowa Women's Health Study. Arch Intern Med. 2000;160:2117–28.
32. Peiris AN, Sothmann MS, Hoffmann RG, Hennes MI, Wilson CR, Gustafson AB, Kissebah AH. Adiposity, fat distribution, and cardiovascular risk. Ann Intern Med. 1989;110:867–72.
33. Nakamura T, Tokunaga K, Shimomura I, Nishida M, Yoshida S, Kotani K, et al. Contribution of visceral fat accumulation to the development of coronary artery disease in non-obese men. Atherosclerosis. 1994;107:239–46.
34. Kuk JL, Katzmarzyk PT, Nichaman MZ, Church TS, Blair SN, Ross R. Visceral fat is an independent predictor of all-cause mortality in men. Obesity (Silver Spring). 2006;14:336–41.
35. Wei M, Gaskill SP, Haffner SM, Stern MP. Waist circumference as the best predictor of noninsulin dependent diabetes mellitus (NIDDM) compared to body mass index, waist/hip ratio and other anthropometric measurements in Mexican Americans—a 7-year prospective study. Obes Res. 1997;5:16–23.
36. van der Kooy K, Leenen R, Seidell JC, Deurenberg P, Visser M. Abdominal diameters as indicators of visceral fat: comparison between magnetic resonance imaging and anthropometry. Br J Nutr. 1993;70:47–58.
37. Ross R, Léger L, Morris D, de Guise J, Guardo R. Quantification of adipose tissue by MRI: relationship with anthropometric variables. J Appl Physiol. 1992;72:787–95.
38. Ross R, Shaw KD, Martel Y, de Guise J, Hudson R, Avruch L. Determination of total and regional adipose tissue distribution by magnetic resonance imaging in android women. Basic Life Sci. 1993;60:177–80.
39. Ross R, Shaw KD, Martel Y, de Guise J, Avruch L. Adipose tissue distribution measured by magnetic resonance imaging in obese women. Am J Clin Nutr. 1993;57:470–5.
40. Sharma RC, Kramsch DM, Lee PL, Colletti P, Jiao Q. Quantitation and localization of regional body fat distribution–a comparison between magnetic resonance imaging and somatometry. Obes Res. 1996;4:167–78.
41. Gronemeyer SA, Steen RG, Kauffman WM, Reddick WE, Glass JO. Fast adipose tissue (FAT) assessment by MRI. Magn Reson Imaging. 2000;18:815–8.
42. Armellini F, Zamboni M, Robbi R, Todesco T, Rigo L, Bergamo-Andreis IA, Bosello O. Total and intra-abdominal fat measurements by ultrasound and computerized tomography. Int J Obes Relat Metab Disord. 1993;17:209–14.
43. Koester RS, Hunter GR, Snyder S, Khaled MA, Berland LL. Estimation of computerized tomography derived abdominal fat distribution. Int J Obes Relat Metab Disord. 1992;16:543–54.
44. Ribeiro-Filho FF, Faria AN, Kohlmann O, Ajzen S, Ribeiro AB, Zanella MT, Ferreira SR. Ultrasonography for the evaluation of visceral fat and cardiovascular risk. Hypertension. 2001;38:713–7.
45. Ferrozzi F, Zuccoli G, Tognini G, Castriota-Scanderbeg A, Bacchini E, Bernasconi S, Campani R. An assessment of abdominal fatty tissue distribution in obese children A comparison between echography and computed tomography. Radiol Med. 1999;98:490–4. [Article in Italian].
46. Abe T, Kawakami Y, Sugita M, Yoshikawa K, Fukunaga T. Use of B-mode ultrasound for visceral fat mass evaluation: comparisons with magnetic resonance imaging. Appl Hum Sci. 1995;14:133–9.
47. Iacobellis G, Assael F, Ribaudo MC, Zappaterreno A, Alessi G, Di Mario U, Leonetti F. Epicardial fat from echocardiography: a new method for visceral adipose tissue prediction. Obes Res. 2003;11:304–10.
48. Schejbal V. Epicardial fatty tissue of the right ventricle–morphology, morphometry and functional significance. Pneumologie. 1989;43:490–9. [Article in German].
49. Pierdomenico SD, Pierdomenico AM, Cuccurullo F, Iacobellis G. Meta-analysis of the relation of

echocardiographic epicardial adipose tissue thickness and the metabolic syndrome. Am J Cardiol. 2013;111:73–8.
50. Iacobellis G, Willens HJ, Barbaro G, Sharma AM. Threshold values of high-risk echocardiographic epicardial fat thickness. Obesity (Silver Spring). 2008;16:887–92.
51. Hotamisligil GS, Shargill NS, Spiegelman BM. Adipose expression of tumor necrosis factor-alpha: direct role in obesity-linked insulin resistance. Science. 1993;259:87–91.
52. Camarena V, Sant D, Mohseni M, Salerno T, Zaleski ML, Wang G, Iacobellis G. Novel atherogenic pathways from the differential transcriptome analysis of diabetic epicardial adipose tissue. Nutr Metab Cardiovasc Dis. 2017;27:739–50.
53. Li Y, Liu B, Li Y, Jing X, Deng S, Yan Y, She Q. Epicardial fat tissue in patients with diabetes mellitus: a systematic review and meta-analysis. Cardiovasc Diabetol. 2019;18:3.
54. Iacobellis G, Leonetti F. Epicardial adipose tissue and insulin resistance in obese subjects. J Clin Endocrinol Metab. 2005;90:6300–2.
55. Iacobellis G, Barbaro G, Gerstein HC. Relationship of epicardial fat thickness and fasting glucose. Int J Cardiol. 2008;128:424–6.
56. Greulich S, Maxhera B, Vandenplas G, de Wiza DH, Smiris K, Mueller H, et al. Secretory products from epicardial adipose tissue of patients with type 2 diabetes mellitus induce cardiomyocyte dysfunction. Circulation. 2012;126:2324–34.
57. Yazıcı D, Özben B, Yavuz D, Deyneli O, Aydın H, Tarcin Ö, Akalın S. Epicardial adipose tissue thickness in type 1 diabetic patients. Endocrine. 2011;40:250–5.
58. Momesso DP, Bussade I, Epifanio MA, Schettino CD, Russo LA, Kupfer R. Increased epicardial adipose tissue in type 1 diabetes is associated with central obesity and metabolic syndrome. Diabetes Res Clin Pract. 2011;91:47–53.
59. Iacobellis G, Diaz S, Mendez A, Goldberg R. Increased epicardial fat and plasma leptin in type 1 diabetes independently of obesity. Nutr Metab Cardiovasc Dis. 2014;24:725–9.
60. Kotronen A, Yki-Järvinen H. Fatty liver: a novel component of the metabolic syndrome. Arterioscler Thromb Vasc Biol. 2008;28:27–38.
61. Hanley AJ, Williams K, Festa A, Wagenknecht LE, D'Agostino RB, Haffner SM. Liver markers and development of the metabolic syndrome: the insulin resistance atherosclerosis study. Diabetes. 2005;54:3140–7.
62. Lee DS, Evans JC, Robins SJ, Wilson PW, Albano I, Fox CS, et al. Gamma glutamyl transferase and metabolic syndrome, cardiovascular disease, and mortality risk: the Framingham Heart Study. Arterioscler Thromb Vasc Biol. 2007;27:127–33.
63. Wu S, Wu F, Ding Y, Hou J, Bi J, Zhang Z. Association of non-alcoholic fatty liver disease with major adverse cardiovascular events: a systematic review and meta-analysis. Sci Rep. 2016;6:33386.
64. Jaruvongvanich V, Wirunsawanya K, Sanguankeo A, Upala S. Nonalcoholic fatty liver disease is associated with coronary artery calcification: a systematic review and meta-analysis. Dig Liver Dis. 2016;48:1410–7.
65. Wijarnpreecha K, Boonpheng B, Thongprayoon C, Jaruvongvanich V, Ungprasert P. The association between non-alcoholic fatty liver disease and atrial fibrillation: a meta-analysis. Clin Res Hepatol Gastroenterol. 2017;41:525–32.
66. Zhou YY, Zhou XD, Wu SJ, Hu XQ, Tang B, Poucke S, et al. Synergistic increase in cardiovascular risk in diabetes mellitus with nonalcoholic fatty liver disease: a meta-analysis. Eur J Gastroenterol Hepatol. 2018;30:631–6.
67. Brouha SS, Nguyen P, Bettencourt R, Sirlin CB, Loomba R. Increased severity of liver fat content and liver fibrosis in non-alcoholic fatty liver disease correlate with epicardial fat volume in type 2 diabetes: a prospective study. Eur Radiol. 2018;28:1345–55.
68. Iacobellis G, Barbarini G, Letizia C, Barbaro G. Epicardial fat thickness and nonalcoholic fatty liver disease in obese subjects. Obesity (Silver Spring). 2014;22:332–6.
69. Lai YH, Yun CH, Yang FS, Liu CC, Wu YJ, Kuo JY, et al. Epicardial adipose tissue relating to anthropometrics, metabolic derangements and fatty liver disease independently contributes to serum high-sensitivity C-reactive protein beyond body fat composition: a study validated with computed tomography. J Am Soc Echocardiogr. 2012;25:234–41.
70. Kankaanpää M, Lehto HR, Pärkkä JP, Komu M, Viljanen A, Ferrannini E, et al. Myocardial triglyceride content and epicardial fat mass in human obesity: relationship to left ventricular function and serum free fatty acid levels. J Clin Endocrinol Metab. 2006;91:4689–95.
71. Perseghin G, Lattuada G, De Cobelli F, Esposito A, Belloni E, Ntali G, et al. Increased mediastinal fat and impaired left ventricular energy metabolism in young men with newly found fatty liver. Hepatology. 2008;47:51–8.
72. Yilmaz Y, Kurt R, Gurdal A, Alahdab YO, Yonal O, Senates E, et al. Circulating vaspin levels and epicardial adipose tissue thickness are associated with impaired coronary flow reserve in patients with nonalcoholic fatty liver disease. Atherosclerosis. 2011;217:125–9.
73. Petta S, Argano C, Colomba D, Cammà C, Marco VD, Cabibi D, et al. Epicardial fat, cardiac geometry and cardiac function in patients with nonalcoholic fatty liver disease: association with the severity of liver disease. J Hepatol. 2015;62:928–33.
74. Turan Y. The nonalcoholic fatty liver disease fibrosis score is related to epicardial fat thickness and complexity of coronary artery disease. Angiology. 2020;71(1):77–82.
75. Liu B, Li Y, Li Y, Liu Y, Yan Y, Luo A, et al. Association of epicardial adipose tissue with non-alcoholic fatty liver disease: a meta-analysis. Hepatol Int. 2019;13:757–65.

76. Corrao S, Rinollo C, Scaglione R. Non-alcoholic fatty liver disease: severity of fibrosis and its relationships with clinical and biological variables. J Hepatol. 2015;62:1212–3.
77. Ulucan S, Katlandur H, Kaya Z. Epicardial fat and liver disease; the contribution of cardio autonomic nervous system function. J Hepatol. 2015;62:1214.
78. Devi SB, Chanu KJ, Jeetenkumar T, Lalrinfela H, Lalhmachhuani PC, Das T. Epicardial adipose tissue thickness and its correlation with metabolic risk parameters in people living with HIV: a RIMS Study. Indian J Endocrinol Metab. 2018;22:641–4.
79. Iantorno M, Soleimanifard S, Schär M, Brown TT, Bonanno G, Barditch-Crovo P, et al. Regional coronary endothelial dysfunction is related to the degree of local epicardial fat in people with HIV. Atherosclerosis. 2018;278:7–14.
80. Buggey J, Longenecker CT. Heart fat in HIV: marker or mediator of risk? Curr Opin HIV AIDS. 2017;12:572–8.
81. Brener M, Ketlogetswe K, Budoff M, Jacobson LP, Li X, Rezaeian P, et al. Epicardial fat is associated with duration of antiretroviral therapy and coronary atherosclerosis. AIDS. 2014;28:1635–44.
82. Orlando G, Gabriella O, Guaraldi G, Giovanni G, Zona S, Stefano Z, et al. Ectopic fat is linked to prior cardiovascular events in men with HIV. J Acquir Immune Defic Syndr. 2012;59:494–7.
83. Guaraldi G, Scaglioni R, Zona S, Orlando G, Carli F, Ligabue G, et al. Epicardial adipose tissue is an independent marker of cardiovascular risk in HIV-infected patients. AIDS. 2011;25:1199–205.
84. Lo J, Abbara S, Rocha-Filho JA, Shturman L, Wei J, Grinspoon SK. Increased epicardial adipose tissue volume in HIV-infected men and relationships to body composition and metabolic parameters. AIDS. 2010;24:2127–30.
85. Iacobellis G, Sharma AM, Pellicelli AM, Grisorio B, Barbarini G, Barbaro G. Epicardial adipose tissue is related to carotid intima-media thickness and visceral adiposity in HIV-infected patients with highly active antiretroviral therapy-associated metabolic syndrome. Curr HIV Res. 2007;5:275–9.
86. Chiricozzi A, Raimondo A, Lembo S, Fausti F, Dini V, Costanzo A, et al. Crosstalk between skin inflammation and adipose tissue-derived products: pathogenic evidence linking psoriasis to increased adiposity. Expert Rev Clin Immunol. 2016;12:1299–308.
87. Bulbul Sen B, Atci N, Rifaioglu EN, Ekiz O, Kartal I, Buyukkaya E, et al. Increased epicardial fat tissue is a marker of subclinical atherosclerosis in patients with psoriasis. Br J Dermatol. 2013;169:1081–6.
88. Akyildiz ZI, Seremet S, Emren V, Ozcelik S, Gediz B, Tastan A, Nazlı C. Epicardial fat thickness is independently associated with psoriasis. Dermatology (Basel). 2014;228:55–9.
89. Balci A, Celik M, Balci DD, Karazincir S, Yonden Z, Korkmaz I, et al. Patients with psoriasis have an increased amount of epicardial fat tissue. Clin Exp Dermatol. 2014;39:123–8.
90. Bacaksız A, Tasal A, Sevgili E, Erdoğan E, Onsun N, Sönmez O, et al. Epicardial fat thickness in patients with psoriasis vulgaris. Turk Kardiyol Dern Ars. 2014;42:47–54.
91. Torres T, Bettencourt N, Mendonça D, Vasconcelos C, Gama V, Silva BM, Selores M. Epicardial adipose tissue and coronary artery calcification in psoriasis patients. J Eur Acad Dermatol Venereol. 2015;29:270–7.
92. Wang X, Guo Z, Zhu Z, Bao Y, Yang B. Epicardial fat tissue in patients with psoriasis:a systematic review and meta-analysis. Lipids Health Dis. 2016;15:103.
93. El Khoudary SR, Shields KJ, Janssen I, Hanley C, Budoff MJ, Barinas-Mitchell E, et al. Cardiovascular fat, menopause, and sex hormones in women: the SWAN Cardiovascular Fat Ancillary Study. J Clin Endocrinol Metab. 2015;100:3304–12.
94. Cabrera-Rego JO, Navarro-Despaigne D, Staroushik-Morel L, Díaz-Reyes K, Lima-Martínez MM, Iacobellis G. Association between endothelial dysfunction, epicardial fat and subclinical atherosclerosis during menopause. Clin Investig Arterioscler. 2018;30:21–7.
95. Gurses KM, Tokgozoglu L, Yalcin MU, Kocyigit D, Evranos B, Yorgun H, et al. Epicardial fat thickness is increased in vitamin d deficient premenopausal women and does not decrease after short-term replacement. J Atheroscler Thromb. 2015;22:582–9.
96. Salami SS, Tucciarone M, Bess R, Kolluru A, Szpunar S, Rosman H, Cohen G. Race and epicardial fat: the impact of anthropometric measurements, percent body fat and sex. Ethn Dis. 2013;23:281–5.
97. Willens HJ, Gómez-Marín O, Chirinos JA, Goldberg R, Lowery MH, Iacobelli G. Comparison of epicardial and pericardial fat thickness assessed by echocardiography in African American and non-Hispanic White men: a pilot study. Ethn Dis. 2008;18:311–6.
98. Apfaltrer P, Schindler A, Schoepf UJ, Nance JW, Tricarico F, Ebersberger U, et al. Comparison of epicardial fat volume by computed tomography in black versus white patients with acute chest pain. Am J Cardiol. 2014;113:422–8.
99. El Khoudary SR, Shin C, Masaki K, Miura K, Budoff M, Edmundowicz D, et al. Ectopic cardiovascular fat in middle-aged men: effects of race/ethnicity, overall and central adiposity. The ERA JUMP study. Int J Obes. 2015;39:488–94.
100. Adams DB, Narayan O, Munnur RK, Cameron JD, Wong DT, Talman AH, et al. Ethnic differences in coronary plaque and epicardial fat volume quantified using computed tomography. Int J Cardiovasc Imaging. 2017;33:241–9.
101. Iacobellis G, Singh N, Wharton S, Sharma AM. Substantial changes in epicardial fat thickness after weight loss in severely obese subjects. Obesity (Silver Spring). 2008;16:1693–7.

Adrenal Secretome and Epicardial Adipose Tissue

14

Luigi Petramala, Antonio Concistrè, Gino Iannucci, and Claudio Letizia

Key Points

- Adrenal gland diseases, such as primary aldosteronism and Cushing syndrome, are associated with higher cardiovascular risk.
- Excessive aldosterone can promote the accumulation of epicardial adipose tissue (EAT) and enhance its proinflammatory features.
- EAT thickness is higher in subjects with adrenal incidentaloma as compared to healthy controls.

Introduction

Epicardial adipose tissue (EAT) has specific properties that set it apart from other depots of visceral fat. In healthy people adipocytes in the epicardium have characteristics of brown adipose tissue, inasmuch as it burns fatty acids and nourishes adjacent tissues [1].

During conditions of low oxidative stress, the physiological epicardial adipocytes secrete adiponectin, which protects cardiomyocytes from hypertrophic stimuli and further minimizes inflammation and fibrosis in the heart [2]. On the other hand, in obesity EAT builds up (acting as adipose tissue surrounding visceral organs), modifying its biological features. It takes on many of the characteristics of white adipose tissue, with tendency to lipolysis leading to the release of fatty acids and reactive inflammation [3]. Moreover, in obesity and other metabolic disorders, EAT shifts its profile of adipokine synthesis. The release of adiponectin declines, whereas the fat depot synthesizes a family of proinflammatory adipokines (leptin, interleukin 1-β, tumor necrosis factor-α, resistin, interleukin-6), promoting the infiltration of macrophages, destroying microvascular systems, and activating profibrotic pathways [4, 5].

In addition, the increase in body fat mass corresponds to an increased production of aldosterone, which is synthesized in an excessive way both by the adrenal gland and by adipocytes in obese people [6]. Excess production of aldosterone itself can lead to the accumulation of EAT as well as its shift to a dysfunctional state [7]. Elevated mineralocorticoid signaling is critically involved in the secretion of proinflammatory cytokines by EAT and in the increased traffic of

L. Petramala · A. Concistrè · G. Iannucci
C. Letizia (✉)
Secondary Arterial Hypertension Unit,
Department of Translational and Precision Medicine,
"Sapienza" University of Rome, Rome, Italy
e-mail: claudio.letizia@uniroma1.it

G. Iacobellis (ed.), *Epicardial Adipose Tissue*, Contemporary Cardiology,
https://doi.org/10.1007/978-3-030-40570-0_14

profibrotic mesenchymal stem cells from the epicardium [8]. The activation of these pathways in the contiguous myocardium may explain why heightened levels of aldosterone are strongly associated with cardiac fibrosis in both experimental and clinical models [9]. Enhancement of the actions of aldosterone may explain why obese patients with heart failure are particularly sensitive to mineralocorticoid receptor antagonists [10].

Since aldosterone can promote the accumulation of EAT and enhance its proinflammatory features, mineralocorticoid receptor antagonists may have important benefits in obese people. Eplerenone prevented and reversed obesity-related adipose tissue inflammation [11], and the drug was particularly effective in reducing the risk of cardiovascular death and hospitalization for heart failure in patients with reduced ejection fraction and abdominal obesity [10].

Apart from heart failure model, interaction between EAT and aldosterone is also observed in primary aldosteronism (PA). Moreover, recent studies have highlighted the importance of EAT as a cardiovascular risk marker in adrenal diseases.

Epicardial Adipose Tissue and Primary Aldosteronism

Recent studies show that primary aldosteronism (PA) is one of the most frequent forms of secondary hypertension [12], around 7–10% of hypertensive patients in population-based studies and up to 20% of patients with resistant hypertension attending specialized centers are actually affected by PA [13, 14]. The disease is mainly caused by bilateral adrenal hyperplasia (as idiopathic hyperaldosteronism [IHA]) or aldosterone-producing adenoma (APA), which together account for over 90% of cases. Beyond moderate–severe hypertension and resistant hypertension, PA is associated with increased cardiovascular risk, independent of blood pressure values [15–21]. Early detection and treatment reduces cardiovascular and metabolic comorbidities and mortality of patients affected by PA [15–20]. Recently, it was shown that individuals with PA have greater left ventricular mass (LVM) than patients with essential hypertension and similar blood pressure control [17]. Moreover, several prospective and retrospective observational studies that compared patients with PA and essential hypertension—in order to analyze the association between PA and stroke, coronary artery disease (as co-primary endpoints), atrial fibrillation and heart failure, target organ damage, metabolic syndrome (MS), and diabetes (as secondary endpoints)—showed increased risk of stroke (odds ratio [OR] 2.58), coronary artery disease (OR 1.77), atrial fibrillation (OR 3.52), and heart failure (OR 2.05), as well as increased the risk of diabetes (OR 1.33), MS (1.53), and left ventricular hypertrophy (2.29) [16, 20, 22–34].

Although the causes of these cardiac changes are not clearly understood, an independent effect of aldosterone and locally secreted adipokines has been suggested [17]. In fact, in PA patients it was a significant correlation between aldosterone levels and circulating adipokines levels (increase in leptin and resistin, reduction of adiponectin) was clearly evident, independently of the presence of MS. Given its peculiar biomolecular and anatomic properties EAT, the visceral fat depot of the heart, can cause LV changes and increased LVM, as observed in obese and nonobese population [35–37].

In recent study [7], it was found that ultrasound measured EAT significantly correlates with LVM, plasma aldosterone levels, and plasma renin levels, better than traditional body fat markers such as body mass index (BMI) and waist circumference (WC). This novel finding suggests the emerging concept of an interplay between visceral fat depots and adrenal tumors and hormones [38, 39]. Previous studies suggest an active role of the fat depot surrounding the adrenal gland—paracrine secretion of adipokines [39, 40] from adipose tissue surrounding the adrenal neoplasia being hormonally active.

Echocardiographic EAT is a clear marker of organ-specific visceral fat [37, 41]. In fact, echocardiographic EAT strongly reflects the intra-abdominal visceral fat as measured by magnetic resonance imaging (MRI), better than WC does. Moreover, ultrasound measured EAT is associated with proton magnetic resonance spectroscopy (1H-MRS) intramyocardial lipid content [40, 42]. Myocardial lipid content increases with the degree of adiposity and may contribute to adverse structural and functional cardiac adaptations.

Furthermore, echocardiographic findings were in agreement with autoptic studies. Mechanical and biomolecular mechanisms have been evoked to explain these correlations. Increased EAT, by adding to the mass of the ventricles, may increase the work of pumping. It could be argued that higher LVM could be expected in patients with hypertension, regardless of its cause. Also, EAT has been shown to correlate with blood pressure [38]. However, LV changes in PA may actually be due to an interplay between aldosterone and adipose tissue, independently from the hypertension. For example, it was recently shown that the effect of aldosterone on LV morphology and function could be mediated by elevated circulating levels of resistin [17]. Interestingly, human EAT expresses resistin, and its higher expression was thought to contribute to the postoperative insulin resistance in cardiac surgery patients [43]; additionally, EAT is independently associated with insulin resistance [44]. Hence, the interaction between insulin resistance, aldosterone, and EAT, and their cumulative effect may contribute to cause cardiac and, specifically, LV changes in patients with PA.

Recent studies suggest that activation of the cardiac-specific renin–angiotensin system (RAS) may affect cardiac function and structure, interfering with secretory products from EAT in patients with type 2 diabetes, impairing cardiomyocyte function, through several mechanisms, such as alterations in miRNA expression (i.e., induction of miR-208a), a well-known regulator of energy metabolism [45, 46].

In adult rat, cardiomyocytes generated from EAT biopsies of patients with type 2 diabetes after mechanical stimulus, showed reduced sarcomere shortening and increased miR-208a expression, phenomenon reversed by the angiotensin II receptor type 1 (AGTR1) antagonist losartan. On the other hand, incubation with angiotensin II (Ang II) reduced sarcomere shortening and lowered palmitate-induced mitochondrial respiration and carnitine palmitoyltransferase 1c (CPT1c) expression in cardiomyocytes; locked-nucleic-acid-mediated inhibition of miR208a function reversed the detrimental effects induced by Ang II. It is well known that Ang II levels in EAT-type 2 diabetes were increased by 2.6-fold after culture with cardiomyocytes; these data show that secretory products from EAT-type 2 diabetes impair cardiomyocyte contractile function and mitochondrial β-oxidation via activation of the cardiac-specific RAS system and induction of miR-208a, suggesting that alterations in the secretory profile of EAT may contribute to the development of diabetes-related heart disease [47–49].

Epicardial Adipose Tissue and Adrenal Incidentaloma

Adrenal incidentaloma (AI) is an adrenal mass incidentally detected during a radiologic procedure not directly performed for the evaluation of adrenal disease [50, 51]. AIs are increasingly discovered with the widespread use of thoracic and abdominal imaging. While the majority of AIs are non-functional adenomas, the occurrence of mild Cushing's syndrome has been found in 5–20% of patients [32, 33]. It was recently suggested that patients with AI may have an increased cardiovascular risk [37–40]. Interestingly, abnormal LVM has been described in patients with AI, although the causes of these cardiac changes are not clearly understood [52].

Recent studies have shown that EAT thickness, measured with echocardiography, is higher in subjects with AI when compared to healthy controls [50]; both incidentaloma and mild Cushing's syndrome are associated with increased LVM [51], and EAT thickness correlates with LVM regardless of the hypercortisolism [52].

The clinical significance and management of AIs is the object of recent debate [53, 54]. Interestingly, an higher prevalence of MS and in general a higher cardiovascular risk have been described in patients with AI [55, 56]. Remarkably, early cardiac changes have been reported in subjects with AI, although the mechanisms behind the LV abnormalities remain unknown [56].

It is clear that increased EAT thickness was associated with increased LVM in subjects with a wide range of adiposity [36]. Mechanical and biomolecular mechanisms have been evoked to explain this correlation [38]. Increased EAT by adding to the mass of the ventricles may increase the work of pumping. Based on the previous observations and present findings, it is plausible to affirm that excessive EAT could contribute to cause the early changes in LVM in patients with AIs [41]. These results seem to be consistent with the independent role of visceral adiposity and mostly organ-specific fat depots in causing end-organ damage, as recently suggested [34]. Notably, EAT thickness is stronger than WC and BMI in predicting LVM in our study population [40]. The possibility of the increased visceral fat being evoked to explain the higher prevalence of MS in these individuals is highly suggestive.

Moreover, increased EAT and LVM have been associated with MS and coronary artery disease [34, 40, 57, 58]. Subjects with mild Cushing's syndrome showed higher LVM than those with non-functional adenomas, suggesting that these individuals may be at higher risk. Given that all the study subjects were indeed asymptomatic for cardiovascular disease, the predictive role of EAT thickness in detecting early cardiac changes would be important.

Epicardial Adipose Tissue and Cushing Syndrome

As recently observed in patients with AI and subclinical hypercortisolism [40], EAT measurement may serve as a simple and reliable marker of organ-specific visceral adiposity and cardiac changes in the clinical setting of adrenal disease. In Cushing syndrome important structural and functional modifications of the heart and vessels are present. Detecting the early marker predictors of cardiovascular dysfunction such as EAT and carotid intima-media thickness (cIMT) leads to a better understanding of global risk in patients with Cushing syndrome, also in the first stages of the disease. Moreover, the importance of these markers is easily recognized, the changes before and after treatment of the disease being easy to observe. In fact, in pediatric female patients with Cushing syndrome, there was a significant decrease in EAT after successful surgery, and a strong correlation between EAT and intima media thickness was also found in these patients [59].

Given its objective and readily available measurability, ultrasound measured EAT thickness could be implemented in the routine assessment of patients with endocrine-caused hypertension.

References

1. Fitzgibbons TP, Kogan S, Aouadi M, Hendricks GM, Straubhaar J, Czech MP. Similarity of mouse perivascular and brown adipose tissues and their resistance to diet-induced inflammation. Am J Physiol Heart Circ Physiol. 2011;301:H1425–37.
2. Teijeira-Fernandez E, Eiras S, Salgado Somoza A, Gonzalez-Juanatey JR. Baseline epicardial adipose tissue adiponectin levels predict cardiovascular outcomes: a long-term follow-up study. Cytokine. 2012;60:674–80.
3. van Dam AD, Boon MR, Berbée JFP, Rensen PCN, van Harmelen V. Targeting white, brown and perivascular adipose tissue in atherosclerosis development. Eur J Pharmacol. 2017;816:82–92.
4. Cheng KH, Chu CS, Lee KT, Lin TH, Hsieh CC, Chiu CC, et al. Adipocytokines and proinflammatory mediators from abdominal and epicardial adipose tissue in patients with coronary artery disease. Int J Obes. 2008;32:268–74.
5. Gruzdeva OV, Akbasheva OE, Dyleva YA, Antonova LV, Matveeva VG, Uchasova EG, et al. Adipokine and cytokine profiles of epicardial and subcutaneous adipose tissue in patients with coronary heart disease. Bull Exp Biol Med. 2017;163:608–11.
6. Bentley-Lewis R, Adler GK, Perlstein T, Seely EW, Hopkins PN, Williams GH, Garg R. Body mass index predicts aldosterone production in normotensive adults on a high-salt diet. J Clin Endocrinol Metab. 2007;92:4472–5.
7. Iacobellis G, Petramala L, Marinelli C, Calvieri C, Zinnamosca L, Concistrè A, et al. Epicardial fat

thickness and primary aldosteronism. Horm Metab Res. 2016;48:238–41.
8. Wu C, Zhang H, Zhang J, Xie C, Fan C, Zhang H, et al. Inflammation and fibrosis in perirenal adipose tissue of patients with aldosterone-producing adenoma. Endocrinology. 2018;159:227–37.
9. Essick EE, Sam F. Cardiac hypertrophy and fibrosis in the metabolic syndrome: a role for aldosterone and the mineralocorticoid receptor. Int J Hypertens. 2011;2011:346985.
10. Olivier A, Pitt B, Girerd N, Lamiral Z, Machu JL, McMurray JJ, et al. Effect of eplerenone in patients with heart failure and reduced ejection fraction: potential effect modification by abdominal obesity. Insight from the EMPHASIS-HF trial. Eur J Heart Fail. 2017;19:1186–97.
11. Wada T, Ishikawa A, Watanabe E, Nakamura Y, Aruga Y, Hasegawa H, et al. Eplerenone prevented obesity-induced inflammasome activation and glucose intolerance. J Endocrinol. 2017;235:179–91.
12. Mulatero P, Stowasser M, Loh KC, Fardella CE, Gordon RD, Mosso L, et al. Increased diagnosis of primary aldosteronism, including surgically correctable forms, in centers from five continents. J Clin Endocrinol Metab. 2004;89:1045–50.
13. Rossi GP, Bernini G, Caliumi C, Desideri G, Fabris B, Ferri C, PAPY Study Investigators, et al. A prospective study of the prevalence of primary aldosteronism in 1,125 hypertensive patients. J Am Coll Cardiol. 2006;48:2293–300.
14. Calhoun DA. Hyperaldosteronism as a common cause of resistant hypertension. Annu Rev Med. 2013;64:233–47.
15. Catena C, Colussi G, Nadalini E, Chiuch A, Baroselli S, Lapenna R, Sechi LA. Cardiovascular outcomes in patients with primary aldosteronism after treatment. Arch Intern Med. 2008;168:80–5.
16. Milliez P, Girerd X, Plouin PF, Blacher J, Safar ME, Mourad JJ. Evidence for an increased rate of cardiovascular events in patients with primary aldosteronism. J Am Coll Cardiol. 2005;45:1243–8.
17. Iacobellis G, Petramala L, Cotesta D, Pergolini M, Zinnamosca L, Cianci R, et al. Adipokines and cardiometabolic profile in primary hyperaldosteronism. J Clin Endocrinol Metab. 2010;95:2391–8.
18. Reincke M, Fischer E, Gerum S, Merkle K, Schulz S, Pallauf A, German Conn's Registry-Else Kröner-Fresenius-Hyperaldosteronism Registry, et al. Observational study mortality in treated primary aldosteronism: the German Conn's registry. Hypertension. 2012;60:618–24.
19. Rossi GP, Sacchetto A, Visentin P, Canali C, Graniero GR, Palatini P, Pessina AC. Changes in left ventricular anatomy and function in hypertension and primary aldosteronism. Hypertension. 1996;27:1039–45.
20. Rossi GP, Cesari M, Cuspidi C, Maiolino G, Cicala MV, Bisogni V, et al. Long-term control of arterial hypertension and regression of left ventricular hypertrophy with treatment of primary aldosteronism. Hypertension. 2013;62:62–9.
21. Young M, Fullerton M, Dilley R, Funder J. Mineralocorticoids, hypertension, and cardiac fibrosis. J Clin Invest. 1994;93:2578–83.
22. Savard S, Amar L, Plouin PF, Steichen O. Cardiovascular complications associated with primary aldosteronism: a controlled cross-sectional study. Hypertension. 2013;62:331–6.
23. Mulatero P, Monticone S, Bertello C, Viola A, Tizzani D, Iannaccone A, et al. Long-term cardio- and cerebrovascular events in patients with primary aldosteronism. J Clin Endocrinol Metab. 2013;98:4826–33.
24. Muiesan ML, Rizzoni D, Salvetti M, Porteri E, Monteduro C, Guelfi D, et al. Structural changes in small resistance arteries and left ventricular geometry in patients with primary and secondary hypertension. J Hypertens. 2002;20:1439–44.
25. Reil JC, Hohl M, Selejan S, Lipp P, Drautz F, Kazakow A, et al. Aldosterone promotes atrial fibrillation. Eur Heart J. 2012;33:2098–108.
26. Fischer E, Adolf C, Pallauf A, Then C, Bidlingmaier M, Beuschlein F, et al. Aldosterone excess impairs first phase insulin secretion in primary aldosteronism. J Clin Endocrinol Metab. 2013;98:2513–20.
27. Chen W, Li F, He C, Zhu Y, Tan W. Elevated prevalence of abnormal glucose metabolism in patients with primary aldosteronism: a meta-analysis. Ir J Med Sci. 2014;183:283–91.
28. Matrozova J, Steichen O, Amar L, Zacharieva S, Jeunemaitre X, Plouin PF. Fasting plasma glucose and serum lipids in patients with primary aldosteronism: a controlled cross-sectional study. Hypertension. 2009;53:605–10.
29. Mosso LM, Carvajal CA, Maiz A, Ortiz EH, Castillo CR, Artigas RA, Fardella CE. A possible association between primary aldosteronism and a lower beta-cell function. J Hypertens. 2007;25:2125–30.
30. Goodfriend TL, Egan B, Stepniakowski K, Ball DL. Relationships among plasma aldosterone, high-density lipoprotein cholesterol, and insulin in humans. Hypertension. 1995;25:30–6.
31. Hanslik G, Wallaschofski H, Dietz A, Riester A, Reincke M, Allolio B, Participants of the German Conn's Registry, et al. Increased prevalence of diabetes mellitus and the metabolic syndrome in patients with primary aldosteronism of the German Conn's Registry. Eur J Endocrinol. 2015;173:665–75.
32. Fallo F, Pilon C, Urbanet R. Primary aldosteronism and metabolic syndrome. Horm Metab Res. 2012;44:208–14.
33. Hannemann A, Meisinger C, Bidlingmaier M, Döring A, Thorand B, Heier M, et al. Association of plasma aldosterone with the metabolic syndrome in two German populations. Eur J Endocrinol. 2011;164:751–8.
34. Sowers JR, Whaley-Connell A, Epstein M. Narrative review: the emerging clinical implications of the role of aldosterone in the metabolic syndrome and resistant hypertension. Ann Intern Med. 2009;150:776–83.

35. Iacobellis G, Corradi D, Sharma AM. Epicardial adipose tissue: anatomic, biomolecular and clinical relationships with the heart. Nat Clin Pract Cardiovasc Med. 2005;2:536–43.
36. Iacobellis G, Bianco AC. Epicardial adipose tissue: emerging physiological, pathophysiological and clinical features. Trends Endocrinol Metab. 2011;22:450–7.
37. Iacobellis G, Ribaudo MC, Assael F, Vecci E, Tiberti C, Zappaterreno A, et al. Echocardiographic epicardial adipose tissue is related to anthropometric and clinical parameters of metabolic syndrome: a new indicator of cardiovascular risk. J Clin Endocrinol Metab. 2003;88:5163–8.
38. Letizia C, Petramala L, Di Gioia CR, Chiappetta C, Zinnamosca L, Marinelli C, et al. Leptin and adiponectin mRNA expression from the adipose tissue surrounding the adrenal neoplasia. J Clin Endocrinol Metab. 2015;100:E101–4.
39. Iacobellis G, Petramala L, Barbaro G, Kargi AY, Serra V, Zinnamosca L, et al. Epicardial fat thickness and left ventricular mass in subjects with adrenal incidentaloma. Endocrine. 2013;44:532–6.
40. Iacobellis G, Willens HJ. Echocardiographic epicardial fat: a review of research and clinical applications. J Am Soc Echocardiogr. 2009;22:1311–9.
41. Malavazos AE, Di Leo G, Secchi F, Lupo EN, Dogliotti G, Coman C, et al. Relation of echocardiographic epicardial fat thickness and myocardial fat. Am J Cardiol. 2010;105:1831–5.
42. Kremen J, Dolinkova M, Krajickova J, Blaha J, Anderlova K, Lacinova Z, et al. Increased subcutaneous and epicardial adipose tissue production of proinflammatory cytokines in cardiac surgery patients: possible role in postoperative insulin resistance. J Clin Endocrinol Metab. 2006;91:4620–7.
43. Iacobellis G, Leonetti F. Epicardial adipose tissue and insulin resistance in obese subjects. J Clin Endocrinol Metab. 2005;90:6300–2.
44. Lubrano C, Saponara M, Barbaro G, Specchia P, Addessi E, Costantini D, et al. Relationships between body fat distribution, epicardial fat and obstructive sleep apnea in obese patients with and without metabolic syndrome. PLoS One. 2012;7:e47059.
45. Blumensatt M, Fahlbusch P, Hilgers R, Bekaert M, Herzfeld de Wiza D, Akhyari P, et al. Secretory products from epicardial adipose tissue from patients with type 2 diabetes impair mitochondrial β-oxidation in cardiomyocytes via activation of the cardiac renin-angiotensin system and induction of miR-208a. Basic Res Cardiol. 2017;112:2.
46. Blumensatt M, Greulich S, Herzfeld de Wiza D, Mueller H, Maxhera B, Rabelink MJ, et al. Activin A impairs insulin action in cardiomyocytes via up-regulation of miR-143. Cardiovasc Res. 2013;100:201–10.
47. Bugger H, Abel ED. Molecular mechanisms of diabetic cardiomyopathy. Diabetologia. 2014;57:660–71.
48. Diniz GP, Takano AP, Barreto-Chaves ML. MiRNA-208a and miRNA-208b are triggered in thyroid hormone-induced cardiac hypertrophy - role of type 1 angiotensin II receptor (AT1R) on miRNA-208a/alpha-MHC modulation. Mol Cell Endocrinol. 2013;374:117–24.
49. Goossens GH. The renin-angiotensin system in the pathophysiology of type 2 diabetes. Obes Facts. 2012;5:611–24.
50. Davenport C, Liew A, Doherty B, Win HH, Misran H, Hanna S, et al. The prevalence of adrenal incidentaloma in routine clinical practice. Endocrine. 2011;40:80–3.
51. Mantero F, Terzolo M, Arnaldi G, Osella G, Masini AM, Alì A, et al. A survey on adrenal incidentaloma in Italy. Study Group on Adrenal Tumors of the Italian Society of Endocrinology. J Clin Endocrinol Metab. 2000;85:637–44.
52. Rossi R, Tauchmanova L, Di Luciano A, Martino M, Battista C, Del Viscovo L, et al. Mild Cushing's syndrome in patients with adrenal incidentaloma: clinical and biochemical features. J Clin Endocrinol Metab. 2000;85:1440–8.
53. Terzolo M, Osella G, Alì A, Borretta G, Cesario F, Paccotti P, Angeli A. Mild Cushing's syndrome in adrenal incidentaloma. Clin Endocrinol. 1998;48:89–97.
54. Vassiliadi DA, Tsagarakis S. Subclinical hypercortisolism: debatable or visible on the lightbox? Endocrine. 2012;42:7–8.
55. Giordano R, Guaraldi F, Berardelli R, Karamouzis I, D'Angelo V, Marinazzo E, et al. Glucose metabolism in patients with subclinical Cushing's syndrome. Endocrine. 2012;41:415–23.
56. Ermetici F, Dall'Asta C, Malavazos AE, Morricone L, Dall'Asta C, Corsi MM, Ambrosi B. Echocardiographic alterations in patients with non-functioning adrenal incidentaloma. J Endocrinol Investig. 2008;31:573–7.
57. Nieman LK. Approach to the patient with an adrenal incidentaloma. J Clin Endocrinol Metab. 2010;95:4106–13.
58. Bujawansa S, Bowen-Jones D. Low investigation rate for adrenal incidentalomas. Endocrine. 2011;40:134–6.
59. Bassareo PP, Fanos V, Zaffanello M, Mercuro G. Early markers of cardiovascular dysfunction in young girls affected by Cushing's syndrome before and after successful cure. J Pediatr Endocrinol Metab. 2010;23:627–35.

15 Targeting the Epicardial Adipose Tissue

Gianluca Iacobellis

Key Points

- Epicardial fat can be visualized and measured using standard two-dimensional echocardiography or cardiac computed tomography.
- Given its rapid metabolism, organ fat specificity, and simple objective measurability, epicardial fat can serve as a target for pharmaceutical agents targeting the adipose tissue.
- Newer anti-diabetic drugs, such as glucagon-like peptide-1 receptor (GLP-1R) agonists and sodium-glucose cotransporter 2 inhibitors (SGLT2i), have shown to directly target and decrease excessive epicardial fat. GLP-1R modulation of epicardial fat promotes fatty acids beta-oxidation and white-to-brown adipocyte differentiation, therefore leading to favorable metabolic changes.

G. Iacobellis (✉)
Division of Endocrinology, Diabetes and Metabolism, Department of Medicine, University of Miami, Miller School of Medicine, Miami, FL, USA
e-mail: giacobellis@med.miami.edu

Introduction

Epicardial fat (EAT) can be clinically measured and quantified using standard imaging methodologies [1, 2]. EAT nicely and independently correlates with intra-abdominal visceral fat and intra-organ triglycerides content [3, 4]. However, the quantification of these ectopic fat depots often requires cumbersome and expensive methods. On the contrary, EAT can be easily and not invasively measured with standard echocardiography. More recently, EAT has shown to express the specific receptors of some medications with cardiometabolic effects. All together this makes EAT a measurable risk factor and a modifiable therapeutic target. Given its rapid metabolism, organ fat specificity, and simple objective measurability, EAT can serve as a target for medications commonly used in subjects with diabetes, dyslipidemia, and in general higher cardiovascular risk. The effect on EAT by pharmaceutical drugs or other therapeutic actions directly or indirectly targeting the fat has been evaluated in a good number of studies. The results of these studies are here discussed and summarized in Table 15.1 [5–19].

G. Iacobellis (ed.), *Epicardial Adipose Tissue*, Contemporary Cardiology,
https://doi.org/10.1007/978-3-030-40570-0_15

Table 15.1 Epicardial fat response to pharmaceutical agents

Authors	Drug	Class	EAT change (%)	Weeks
Iacobellis et al. [5]	Liraglutide	GLP-1R agonist	~ −40	24
Morano et al. [6]	Exenatide	GLP-1R agonist	~ −13	18
Lima-Martinez et al. [7]	Sitagliptin	DPP4i	~ −15	24
Sato et al. [8]	Dapagliflozin	SGLT2i	~ −16	24
Yagi et al. [9]	Canagliflozin	SGLT2i	~ −20	24
Fukuda et al. [10]	Ipragliflozin	SGLT2i	~ −13	12
Bouchi et al. [11]	Luseogliflozin	SGLT2i	~ −5	12
Nagai et al. [12]	Pioglitazone	TZD	~ −24	36
Elisha et al. [13]	Detemir	Insulin analogue	~ −20	24
Elisha et al. [13]	Glargine	Insulin analogue	~ −14	24
Park et al. [14]	Atorvastatin	Statin	~ −10	24
Alexopoulos et al. [15]	Atorvastatin	Statin	~ −3	48
Alexopoulos et al. [15]	Pravastatin	Statin	~ −1	48
Raggi et al. [16]	Atorvastatin or pravastatin	Statin	~ −6[a]	48
Park et al. [17]	Simvastatin + ezetimibe	Statin + cholesterol absorption inhibitor	~ −3	24
Ferrante et al. [18]	rGH	Recombinant hormone	~ −29 ~ −40	24 48
Francomano et al. [19]	Testosterone	Replacement hormone		54
Fiore et al. [20]	Sildenafil	PDE5 inhibitor	3	12

EAT epicardial adipose tissue, *GLP1-R* glucagon-like peptide-1 receptor, *DPP4i* dipeptidyl peptidase-4 inhibitor, *SGLT2i* sodium-glucose cotransporter 2 inhibitors, *TZD* thiazolidinedione, and *rGH* recombinant growth hormone

[a]*HUs* Hounsfield units

Weight Loss Interventions Effects on Epicardial Fat

Diet

Earlier and selective visceral fat reduction has been recently thought to be a key factor in the metabolic improvement that follows a weight loss. Diet-induced weight loss may affect visceral fat preferentially, but this effect may be attenuated with greater weight loss. Hence, EAT changes were evaluated after different weight loss interventions. Epicardial fat was also used as a marker of visceral fat changes during not pharmaceutical weight loss procedures. Echocardiographic epicardial fat thickness has been reported to significantly and quickly decrease after a very-low-calorie diet (VLCD) in morbidly obese subjects [20]. The changes in epicardial fat thickness were significantly higher than changes in body mass index and waist circumference after the very-low-calorie diet program. Remarkably, the magnitude of epicardial fat reduction following a low-calorie diet was higher and faster than that of body mass index (BMI) and waist circumference. The changes in epicardial fat thickness were consensually and independently associated with the improvement in cardiac parameters in these subjects. EAT thickness reduction after weight loss intervention was associated with a decrease of plasma inflammatory marker [21]. Another study confirmed the effects of a 16-week VLCD and of subsequent 14 months follow-up on a regular diet on pericardial fat in obese patients with type 2 diabetes [22]. VLCD-induced weight loss in obese diabetic patients is accompanied by a substantial decrease in pericardial fat volume. Interestingly, cardiac fat reduction sustained even after subsequent weight regain.

Bariatric Surgery

Substantial and sustainable weight loss is the primary goal to reduce cardiometabolic risk in obese subjects. Bariatric surgery has proved to be an effective strategy in treating obesity and improving metabolic profile. Nevertheless, whether the proportion changes in overall and visceral adiposity can be different is partially unanswered. Visceral fat reduction is associated with a significant improvement of the cardio-metabolic profile. However, it is unclear how much visceral adipose tissue loss is needed to induce favorable cardiac changes. Bariatric surgery is the most effective treatment for severe and morbid obesity [23–28]. Surgical treatment of obesity generally results in more long-lasting weight loss and a significant reduction of cardiovascular risk than other treatments. In the phase of rapid weight loss after laparoscopic bariatric surgery, a preferential mobilization of visceral abdominal fat, as compared with total and subcutaneous adiposity, was observed [29–32]. However, this preferential visceral fat reduction may occur only in those patients presenting higher levels of visceral fat deposition at baseline. The effects of weight loss on abdominal fat depots induced by nonsurgical and surgical therapies have been reported, although the data and conclusions from these studies are not consistent [29]. Greater reduction in visceral fat than in subcutaneous fat (SAT) 1 year after gastric banding has been reported [29]. Nevertheless, the ratio between visceral and subcutaneous abdominal fat was found constant 6 months following bariatric surgery [29].

The effects of bariatric surgery procedures on EAT have been studied. Undoubtedly, bariatric surgery has shown beneficial effects on cardiac morphology and function. A significant reduction in left ventricular mass indices and improvement in diastolic function have been reported in subjects who undergo bariatric surgery. Bariatric surgery is able to produce a "reverse cardiac remodeling" in morbidly obese subjects [24]. Nevertheless, the mechanisms behind these effects are not completely clear. It is presently unknown whether a decrease of the visceral fat depot of the heart is needed to reverse the cardiac abnormalities observed in morbidly obese subjects. Whether the improvement in cardiac parameters after bariatric surgery is due to a decrease in overall body fat or to an early reduction in the local fat depot of the heart is also unclear.

The evaluation of EAT changes after bariatric surgery-induced weight loss could address these questions. Nevertheless, the results are not univocal. One study showed that epicardial fat decreased significantly after laparoscopic bariatric surgery in 23 severely obese subjects [33]. Epicardial fat thickness decreased from 5.3 ± 2.4 to 4.0 ± 1.6 mm ($p = 0.001$). The change in epicardial fat correlated with initial epicardial fat thickness was measured using echocardiography ($r = 0.71, p < 0.001$) [33].

Although of interest, this study was conducted in a small sample size. In addition, the role of EAT in cardiac reverse remodeling after bariatric surgery was not evaluated.

However, the shrinking effect of bariatric surgery on epicardial fat thickness was confirmed in a larger sample size study. A total of 105 patients (79 women and 26 men) with the mean age of 43.61 ± 12.42 were followed before and after the bariatric surgical procedure [34]. Epicardial fat thickness significantly decreased after sleeve gastrectomy (8.68 ± 1.95 mm vs. 7.41 ± 1.87 mm; $p < 0.001$) concurrently with a reduction of carotid intima-media thickness [34].

Whether EAT reduction is greater or smaller than visceral fat loss after bariatric surgery is an important question that Gaborit et al. sought to address [35]. The relation of post-bariatric surgery EAT and myocardial fat changes was also investigated. Epicardial fat volume, myocardial triglyceride content, cardiac function, and computed tomography visceral abdominal fat measurements at baseline and 6 months after bariatric surgery were calculated [35]. This study found that 6-month bariatric surgery induced a significant decrease in epicardial fat, but no change in myocardial fat. Epicardial fat volume decreased significantly (from 137 ± 37 ml to 98 ± 25 ml, $p < 0.0001$), but in a lower amount than visceral fat diminution (−27 vs. −40%) [35]. Epicardial fat volume variation was not correlated with the percentage of body mass index or visceral fat loss. Epicardial fat volume loss was more prominent in patients with sleep apnea.

Another study found a smaller reduction of EAT compared to other larger fat depots after bariatric surgery [36]. Computed tomography epicardial and paracardial adipose tissue were measured in bariatric surgery and exercise-treated subjects at baseline and 3 months after the intervention. While the authors found that surgery group had a greater loss in abdominal and cardiac visceral adipose tissue as compared to the exercise group, the decrease in EAT was small compared with the other compartments.

The effect of bariatric surgery, mostly Roux-en-Y gastric bypass, or sleeve gastrectomy in shrinking epicardial fat is controversial, with some variability in the percentage of EAT reduction among the studies. Epicardial fat certainly decreases after bariatric surgery, but EAT loss is smaller than larger fat depots. Bariatric surgery causes a large fat mass reduction, whereas EAT seems to be more sensitive to direct intervention. Pharmaceutical intervention directly targeting EAT may be more effective. EAT dysfunction in patients with complicated advanced stage diseases may also explain the smaller response of EAT to bariatric surgery. Hypoxia and fibrosis may affect EAT's capacity to be modulated by large weight loss.

Exercise Effects on Epicardial Fat

The effect of exercise on adipose tissue is complex. Exercise modulates adipokines secretion, improves adipose tissue mitochondrial activity and glucose uptake, and stimulates fat mobilization. These changes can lead to decreases in adipocyte size and lipid content. Exercise also upregulates uncoupling protein 1 (UCP-1) levels and causes a browning or *beiging* change of the white adipose tissue. Overall, fat metabolism and homeostasis improve with physical activity.

The effect of exercise on EAT was investigated, but to date not well established, yet. However, there is a growing evidence that EAT significantly decreases with exercise, although the results are not fully concordant about the extent of this reduction. Nevertheless, the disagreement between recent and previous studies could be attributed to the poor utilization of resistance training and exercise programs meeting weight loss recommendations. It could be also due to the difficulties to quantify and track exercise, or physical activity in general, during a clinical trial.

A recent study showed that both 12-week endurance and resistance training reduced EAT, as measured with cardiac magnetic resonance imaging, in subjects with abdominal obesity [37]. Fifty participants were randomized to a supervised high-intensity interval endurance training (three times a week for 45 min) and resistance training (three times a week for 45 min). Endurance training and resistance training reduced epicardial adipose tissue mass by 32% and 24%, respectively, as compared with the no-exercise controls [37]. Hence, this study on supervised subjects showed a very significant reduction of EAT after exercise. Interestingly, the authors found no significant reduction in pericardial adipose tissue after endurance training. The different effects of exercise further underline the difference between the two fat depots. It may also suggest the idea of customizing the exercise programs based on these functional and anatomical differences. Another study in a smaller population of young obese women found that high-intensity, moderate-volume endurance-resistance training reduced EAT volume [38]. A significant EAT reduction was also reported in patients with major depression and associated metabolic syndrome [39].

How can exercise reduce EAT? Which are the putative mechanisms? A complex study by Company et al. sought to address these questions. The authors evaluated the effects of 16-week aerobic exercise training on the epicardial fat inflammatory transcriptome in peri-coronary epicardial, peri-myocardial epicardial, and visceral and subcutaneous adipose tissues from a castrated male pig model of familial hypercholesterolemia with coronary artery disease (CAD) [40]. The results showed that the inflammatory transcriptome of the myocardial epicardial fat decreased after exercise, whereas peri-coronary epicardial inflammatory gene profile did not change. This suggests that EAT has distinct locations, functions, and heterogeneous response to exercise. Aerobic exercise training reduced a cluster of inflammatory and redox genes in myocardial EAT. Myocardial EAT expression of interleukins (IL1-Ra, IL-6, IL-8), PAI-1, and PGDS and redox genes eNOS and cytochrome c oxidase significantly reduced after exercise in these experimental animals [40]. Notably, aerobic exercise training increased myocardial EAT mass, possibly due to the lack of functional UCP-1 in pigs [40].

The role of interleukin 6 (IL-6) in mediating the effects of exercise on epicardial adipose tissue in humans is under investigation [41].

Hence, the most recent investigations are showing substantial effects of structured and supervised exercise on EAT, much greater than those previously reported [42]. In fact, other studies showed a significant, but modest reduction in EAT thickness (mean change of approximately −0.7 mm) [43, 44]. In one study, patients used a stationary ergometer for 45 min of cycling 3 days/week at a moderate intensity, whereas in another study, patients used a cycling ergometer. Exercise certainly produces EAT changes and significant reduction. The magnitude and the impact of this effect on patient's cardiometabolic profile would require further studies using supervised resistance exercise programs.

Anti-Diabetes Drugs Effects on Epicardial Fat

Glucagon-Like Peptide-1 Receptors Agonists

Glucagon-like peptide-1 receptor (GLP-1R) agonists rapidly emerged as effective anti-diabetic medications with pleiotropic effects. GLP-1R agonists are injectable medications indicated for the treatment of type 2 diabetes mellitus. However, GLP-1R agonists have shown to provide weight loss and cardiovascular protective effects beyond the diabetes control [45–47]. Clinical trials found that overall GLP-1R agonists reduced major adverse cardiovascular events [45–47]. Liraglutide, a daily GLP-1R agonist, improves glycemic control and causes weight loss in type 2 diabetic patients. Liraglutide has shown to reduce the risk of cardiovascular events, as recently reported in the LEADER study [45]. Clinical trials found that weekly GLP-1R agonists, semaglutide, and dulaglutide reduced major adverse cardiovascular events and mortality for all causes by 12% [46, 47]. Weekly GLP-1R agonists are an effective and convenient therapeutic option to improve glycemic control, induce weight loss, and reduce cardiometabolic risk in type 2 diabetics. SUSTAIN 6 trial showed that semaglutide significantly reduced the rate of cardiovascular death, nonfatal myocardial infarction, or nonfatal stroke in patients with type 2 diabetes as compared to those receiving placebo [46].

Whether the GLP-1R agonists could have an effect on EAT has been explored only very recently. Liraglutide effect on epicardial fat was tested in a 24-week interventional case-controlled study in overweight/obese type 2 diabetic subjects on metformin monotherapy [5]. Individuals were randomized in two groups to receive additional liraglutide up to 1.8 mg sc once daily or to remain on metformin up to 1000 mg twice daily. Ultrasound measured EAT thickness decreased from 9.6 ± 2.0 to 6.8 ± 1.5 and 6.2 ± 1.5 mm ($p < 0.001$) after 3 and 6 months, respectively, accounting for a 36% reduction at 24 weeks, whereas there was no significant EAT reduction in the metformin group. Interestingly, EAT decrease was associated with a decrease in indexed left ventricular mass. A milder reduction of EAT thickness was observed after 12 weeks of treatment either with liraglutide or exenatide, a weekly GLP-1R agonist, in a smaller group of patients with type 2 diabetes [6]. There was no significant difference between the two agents.

Another study looked at the effects of exenatide epicardial and other visceral fat depots, such as myocardial, hepatic, and pancreatic adipose pads [48]. Measurements of EAT thickness were performed by magnetic resonance imaging and spectroscopy at baseline and at 26 weeks EAT was reduced by approximately 8.8% after treatment with exenatide. Also, hepatic triglyceride content significantly reduced in patients treated with exenatide.

Whether GLP-1R agonist's effect on EAT is specific or mediated by overall weight loss was the object of very recent investigations. Recent data from the Iacobellis group lab showed that human EAT expresses GLP-1R, supporting a role for a direct effect of GLP-1 agonism on EAT [49]. RNA-sequencing analysis and quantitative real-time RT-PCR were performed to evaluate the presence of GLP-1R in EAT obtained from subjects with CAD and type 2 diabetes mellitus undergoing elective cardiac surgery. The RNA-sequencing analysis showed that EAT expresses GLP-1R genes. Immunofluorescence clearly confirmed the presence of GLP1R protein within EAT whereas the signal was absent in the SAT sample obtained from the same patient [49] (Fig. 15.1).

Given the presence of the GLP-1R within EAT, it is plausible to hypothesize a specific fat-depot effect. However, as GLP-1R agonists induce a substantial body fat loss, the reduction of EAT is likely to be associated with weight loss. However, GLP-1R agonists' effects may be therefore visceral fat-specific and target EAT. The mechanisms behind the fat reduction in response to the GLP-1R activation are unclear. It has been also suggested that GLP-1 promotes EAT preadipocyte differentiation, improves insulin sensitivity, and stimulates EAT thermogenesis and adipocyte browning [50–53]. Central injection of liraglutide, in mice, stimulates brown adipose tissue thermogenesis and adipocyte browning independent of nutrient intake. It has been also suggested that GLP-1 promotes preadipocyte differentiation. The differentiated small adipocytes may have a positive effect on insulin resistance and obesity. Experiments with the 3T3-L1 cell line also showed both lipolytic and lipogenic dose-dependent effects of GLP-1. Iacobellis' group is currently investigating the effects of liraglutide on EAT inflammatory genes in patients with CAD and type 2 diabetes (NCT 03260881). Interestingly, a correlation between epicardial fat GLP-1R and genes encoding for brown fat activity and fatty acid oxidation has been recently

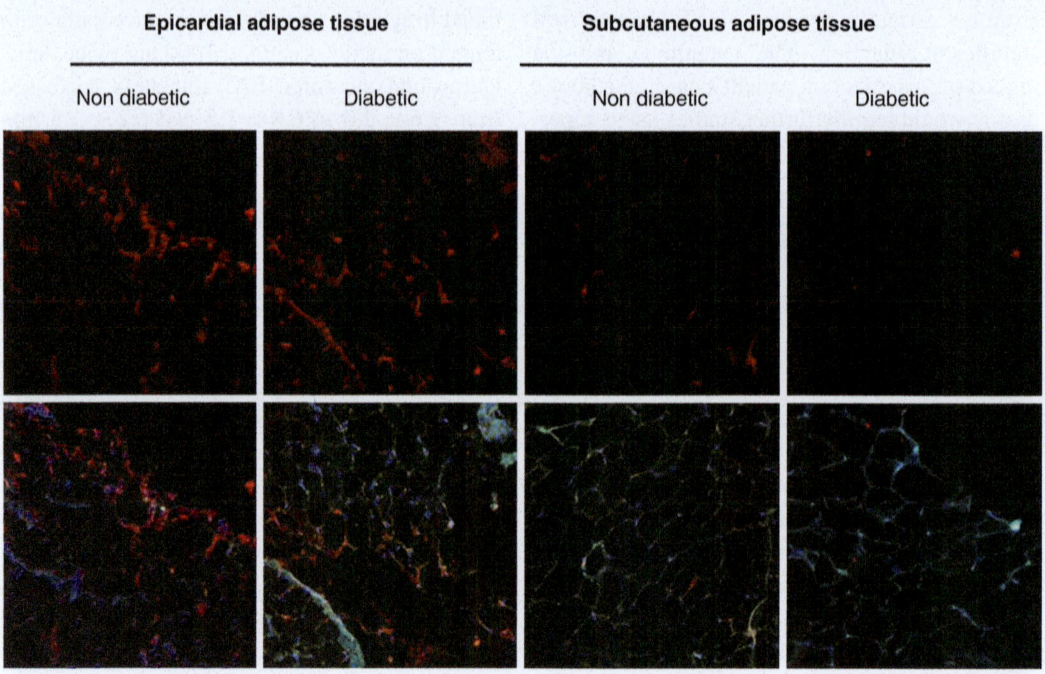

Fig. 15.1 Immunofluorescence signal for glucagon-like peptide-1 receptor (GLP-1R) was present in epicardial adipose tissue (EAT), whereas it was absent in subcutaneous fat (SAT) from the same patient (*top panels*). Interestingly, GLP-1R presence within EAT was irrespective of diabetes. Immunofluorescence analysis performed on EAT and SAT samples from patient who underwent cardiac surgery using Mab3f52 against GLP-1R. GLP1R/488/DAPI control (*lower panels*). (From the lab of Gaofeng Wang, Department of Human Genetics, University of Miami Miller School of Medicine, Miami, FL)

Table 15.2 Positive and negative correlations of glucagon-like peptide-1 receptor (GLP1-R) with genes involved in fatty acid metabolism

Genes positively correlated	Family group	Function	Correlation coefficient, *P*-value
ACAD10	Acyl-CoA dehydrogenases	Promote FA oxidation	0.543, 0.007
ACADL			0.560, 0.006
ACOT6	Acyl-CoA thioesterases	Regulate FA oxidation in mitochondria and peroxisomes	0.861, <0.0001
ACOT 12			0.872, <0.0001
ACSBG2	Acyl-CoA synthetases	Activate long- and medium-chain FA for oxidation	0.915, <0.0001
ACSL6			0.477, 0.021
ACSM3			0.699, 0.0002
ACSM4			0.903, <0.0001
CPT1B	Fatty acid transport	Transport FA into mitochondria for oxidation	0.415, 0.049
FABP1	Fatty acid transport	Facilitate FA transfer across membranes	0.709, 0.0002
FABP2			0.911, <0.0001
FABP6			0.598, 0.003
FABP7			0.918, <0.0001
GK	Triacylglycerol metabolism	Esterification of FA with reduced FA efflux	0.664, 0.0006
GK2			0.930, <0.0001
HMGCS2	Ketogenesis and ketone body metabolism	Synthesis and utilization of lipid-derived energy	0.797, <0.0001
OXCT2			0.694, 0.0002
PRKAA1	Fatty acid biosynthesis regulation	Alpha catalytic subunit of AMPK: switch off ATP-consuming biosynthetic pathways	0.612, 0.0019
PRKAA2			0.799, <0.0001
PRKAG2	Fatty acid biosynthesis regulation	Gamma subunit of AMPK: switch off ATP-consuming biosynthetic pathways	0.430, 0.0403
PRKAG3			0.681, 0.0004
SLC27A1	Fatty acid metabolism	Long-chain FA import into tissue at high levels of beta-oxidation	0.782, <0.0001

Spearman correlation coefficients and corresponding *p*-value are reported. (From Dozio et al. [54], with permission from Elsevier)

reported [54]. EAT GLP-1R was directly correlated with genes promoting beta-oxidation and white-to-brown adipocyte differentiation, and inversely with pro-adipogenic genes (Table 15.2). GLP-1 levels were higher in CAD than controls and in patients with greater EAT thickness. GLP-1 analogs may target EAT GLP-1R and therefore reduce local adipogenesis, improve fat utilization, and induce brown fat differentiation. GLP-1-induced browning effect on EAT is a potential mechanism and certainly warrants further investigations. EAT pathways are then potential targets for intervention strategies, including diet and/or pharmaceuticals designed to promote brown fat function.

Dipeptidyl-4 Inhibitors

GLP-1 is susceptible to cleavage at position 2 (alanine) by the ubiquitous DPP-4, which occurs almost immediately upon the secretion of GLP-1, rendering it a short half-life. DPP-4 inhibitors are a relatively new class of drugs for type 2 diabetes mellitus that exert a hypoglycemic effect by inhibiting the degradation of GLP-1. The add-in therapy with sitagliptin produced a significant and rapid reduction (approximately 15%), of EAT in overweight/obese individuals with type 2 diabetes inadequately controlled on metformin monotherapy [7]. Although it is likely driven by the activation of the GLP-1R, the mechanism behind the effect of sitagliptin on epicardial fat is unknown. A prolonged half-life of GLP-1 mediated by the inhibition of DPP-4 may have an important effect on the EAT reduction shrinkage. Epicardial fat presents a massive macrophages infiltrate; the previously described anti-inflammatory properties of DDP4 inhibition can certainly contribute to modify the fat depot [55, 56]. Interestingly, DDP4 inhibition increased the levels of uncoupling proteins in brown adipose tissue in mice with diet-induced obesity [57].

Sodium-Glucose Cotransporter 2 Inhibitors

Selective sodium-glucose cotransporter 2 inhibitors (SGLT2i) are new oral anti-diabetic agents that reduce hyperglycemia in patients with T2DM by increasing urinary glucose excretion. SGLT2 is responsible for the 80–90% glucose reuptake. Diabetic patients treated with SGLT2i commonly lose weight. Weight loss could result from reduced body fat secondary to caloric loss or from fluid loss secondary to osmotic diuresis or from a combination of both factors. Large clinical trials, the EMPA-REG OUTCOME, CANVAS, and DECLARE-TIMI 58, have recently shown that SGLT2i reduce major adverse cardiovascular events mainly in patients with established atherosclerotic cardiovascular disease [58–60]. SGLT2i reduce the incidence of hospitalization for heart failure and progression of renal disease regardless of existing atherosclerotic cardiovascular disease or a history of heart failure [58]. The effect of SGLT2i on EAT has been investigated only recently.

Dapagliflozin is SGLT2i that improves glucose control and induces weight loss in patients with type 2 diabetes mellitus [61]. Clinical trials showed significant weight loss and visceral fat reduction in type 2 diabetic patients who received additional dapagliflozin [62]. Iacobellis and colleagues are currently leading a randomized clinical trial (NCT 02235298) to evaluate the effects of dapagliflozin on the epicardial fat thickness in patients with type 2 diabetes and obesity.

A recent study showed that 6-month therapy with dapagliflozin caused a significant decrease in the EAT volume and inflammatory markers [8]. To understand the mechanism behind the effects of dapagliflozin on EAT, SGLT2 expression was analyzed by real-time polymerase chain reaction, western blot, and immunohistochemistry from fat samples obtained from patients undergoing cardiac surgery by Díaz-Rodríguez et al. [63]. Fat explants were then treated with dapagliflozin and/or insulin and glucose transporters expression was measured. SGLT2 was expressed in EAT whereas was absent or low in SAT (Fig. 15.2). Of note, the authors found that dapagliflozin increased EAT glucose uptake, reduced the secretion of pro-inflammatory chemokines, improved the differentiation of epicardial adipocytes, and benefited wound healing in endothelial cells [63].

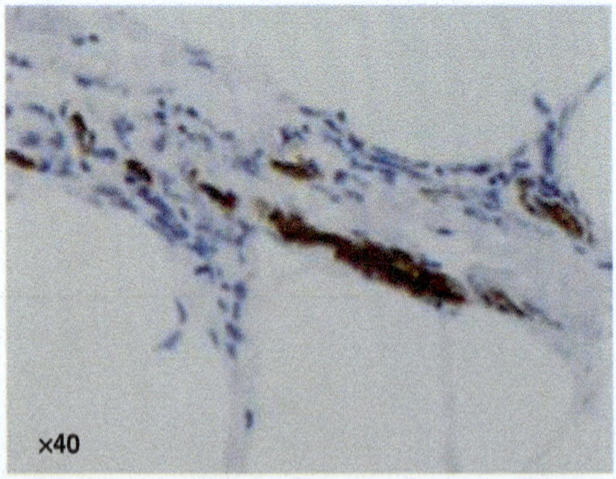

Fig. 15.2 Immunohistochemistry image showing the presence of sodium-glucose transporter 2 (SGLT2) antibody in epicardial adipose tissue (EAT). (From Díaz-Rodríguez et al. [63], with permission from Oxford University Press)

Canagliflozin, another commonly prescribed SGLT2i, decreased EAT thickness after 6 months of treatment in patients with type 2 diabetes [9]. Epicardial fat volume was decreased also in patients treated with two other recently developed SGLT2i agents, ipragliflozin and luseogliflozin [10, 11].

Overall, SGLT2i have shown promising effects on EAT. The exact mechanism is still unknown. Whether this is a direct effect or mediated by the weight loss is unclear. Further studies are warranted to better evaluate the independent effects of SGLT2i on epicardial adipose tissue.

Thiazolidinediones

Thiazolidinediones (TZDs), also known as glitazones, are a group of oral anti-diabetic drugs indicated to treat patients with type 2 diabetes. TZDs are insulin sensitizers that act as agonists of the peroxisome proliferator-activated receptors (PPARs) a group of nuclear receptors. PPARs are the regulator of insulin and glucose levels and lipid profile. TZDs were targeted to the epicardial fat. Treatment with pioglitazone, a commonly used TZD, was associated with a reduction of pro-inflammatory and anti-inflammatory genes in EAT in type 2 diabetic patients with CAD [64].

Interestingly, subjects treated with pioglitazone showed a lower expression of interleukin-1β and other pro-inflammatory genes in epicardial fat. Worthily, PPAR-gamma (PPAR-γ) agonist can induce a rapid browning of the epicardial fat in experimental models. In addition to the beneficial effects on EAT inflammatory transcriptome, pioglitazone has been reported to significantly reduce EAT thickness in type 2 diabetic subjects, with more prominent results in the subjects that had a greater EAT depot at baseline [12]. This finding was not confirmed in a 24-week prospective, double-blind, randomized, controlled study comparing pioglitazone with metformin [65]. In fact, pioglitazone increased pericardial fat volume whereas metformin had no effect on the fat depot. However the effect of piogitazone on the pericardial fat was not associated with changes in left ventricular function. It is should be noted that this study evaluated pericardial rather than epicardial fat.

Rosiglitazone caused a significant upregulation of PPARγ coactivator 1 alpha (PGC1-α), a key precursor of brown fat, in epicardial adipocytes of Zucker rats [66]. Thiazolidinediones may therefore resume or activate the brown fat properties of the epicardial fat, although this hypothetical mechanism would need to be evaluated in humans. Pharmaceutical targeting epicardial fat with TZDs in patients with high cardiovascular risk may result in reducing inflammation and improving metabolic profile through a PPARs stimulation. HIV positive patients who develop metabolic syndrome may particularly benefit from the use of TZDs targeting EAT [67, 68].

Metformin

No randomized controlled trials evaluated the independent effects of metformin on EAT. However, several epicardial fat studies used metformin as a control treatment. None of them found substantial changes in epicardial fat thickness in patients added-on or started on metformin monotherapy. As today, it is reasonable to say that metformin has little or no effects on EAT.

Insulin

Long-acting insulin analogues have shown to provide several and beneficial cardiovascular effects. Insulin detemir was thought to be body weight "neutral" as compared to glargine. A 24-week interventional study was designed to compare the effects of detemir versus glargine on epicardial fat thickness in insulin-naïve inadequately controlled patients with type 2 diabetes [13]. Within the detemir group, epicardial fat thickness change was correlated with truncal fat and total fat mass changes. Detemir resulted in less fat mass gain, a trend for a more pronounced epicardial fat thickness reduction when compared with glargine.

Statins Effects on Epicardial Fat

HMG-CoA reductase pathway inhibitors, commonly known as statins, have pleiotropic effects that go beyond their lipid-lowering effects, including modulation and reduction of adipose tissue inflammation. In light of this effect, statins effects on EAT have been investigated. Epicardial fat thickness reduced more in diabetic subjects treated with atorvastatin than in those who received simvastatin and ezetimibe [14]. EAT decreased by approximately 10% in the atorvastatin group versus 3.1% in the simvastatin/ezetimibe group. Consistently, atorvastatin therapy induced a reduction of computed tomography-measured epicardial fat volume in hyperlipidemic postmenopausal women [15]. At the end of follow-up, epicardial fat regressed more in the atorvastatin than in the pravastatin group (median, −3.38% vs. −0.83%). The effect of atorvastatin on epicardial fat was independent of lipid-lowering or CAD progression. Statins cause inhibition of migration and proliferation of arterial myocytes, inhibition of macrophage growth, inhibition of metalloproteinase secretion, and cell adhesion. EAT overexpresses lipoprotein receptors such as low-density lipoprotein receptor-related protein 1 and very-low-density lipoprotein receptor, recently suggested to play a role in changes of lipid metabolism commonly associated with type 2 diabetes mellitus [69]. More recently, Raggi et al. demonstrated that statins induced a decrease in CT EAT attenuation independent of the low-density lipoprotein cholesterol-lowering effects [16]. One-year treatment with 80 mg of atorvastatin or 40 mg of pravastatin significantly reduced CT EAT density in 420 postmenopausal women [16]. The independent effect of statins on the adipose tissue density suggests a direct modulation of EAT inflammation. Interestingly, pioglitazone, simvastatin, or combination treatment substantially reduced EAT and plasma inflammatory markers in patients with CAD [70] (Fig. 15.3). Pioglitazone alone and simvastatin + pioglitazone treatment were associated with lower CD68+/macrophages, CD45/T-lymphocytes, TNF-α, IL-6, leptin, and resistin in EAT compared to controls. Both pioglitazone and simvastatin modulate and activate the PPARs receptors. Of note, adipocyte development in vivo requires activation of the PPARγ, which is upregulated in human embryonic ventricular epicardial cells [71]. Hence, the PPARs pathway seems to be a likely target of the combined effect on EAT.

Other Drugs Targeting Epicardial Fat

Growth Hormone

Growth hormone deficiency (GHD) syndrome is characterized by an abnormal body fat distribution and increased visceral fat accumulation. Hence, human GH (rhGH) replacement therapy was targeted to EAT, as a marker of visceral fat [72]. Echocardiographic epicardial fat thickness significantly decreased after short-term rhGH replacement therapy, whereas neither waist circumference or body mass index showed significant changes during the replacement treatment [17].

Phosphodiesterase Type 5 Inhibitors

Phosphodiesterase type 5 inhibitors (PDE5i) are used to treat erectile dysfunction, pulmonary hypertension, and benign prostatic hyperplasia. Recent studies suggested an effect of PDE5i on the visceral adipose tissue. Treatment with PDE5i in humans and murine models of diabetes reduces visceral fat by targeting SIRT1 through modulation of miR-22-3p. One study investigated the effects of sildenafil, one of the most common PDE5i, on EAT using microarray-based profiling of pharmacologically modulated microRNA (miRNAs) [19]. Compared with placebo, sildenafil reduced EAT ($P = 0.045$).

Testosterone

Low testosterone levels are associated with an increased amount of visceral fat, particularly in men. Hence, EAT, a marker of visceral adiposity, can well serve as a target for testosterone replacement therapy. One study in patients with Klinefelter syndrome found that epicardial fat thickness was higher in hypogonadal patients than in controls and eugonadal patients [73].

In another observational, parallel-arm, open-label, 54-week study, a severely obese group was allocated either to receive hypocaloric diet plus physical activity or hypocaloric diet plus physical activity plus testosterone injections, followed by 24 weeks of hypocaloric diet plus physical activity alone [18]. At 54 weeks, subjects randomized to hypocaloric diet plus physical activity, and testosterone showed significant improvements in EAT, as well as ejection fraction, diastolic function, carotid intima-media thickness, and endothelial function ($p < 0.01$ vs. controls).

Thyroid

The interaction of thyroid hormones and EAT is still unclear. Small-sized clinical studies reported that EAT thickness was significantly higher either in the hyperthyroid and hypothyroid conditions [74–78]. One study showed an improvement in EAT and overall cardiometabolic profile after levothyroxine replacement therapy. Given the thermogenic function and brown fat-like activity

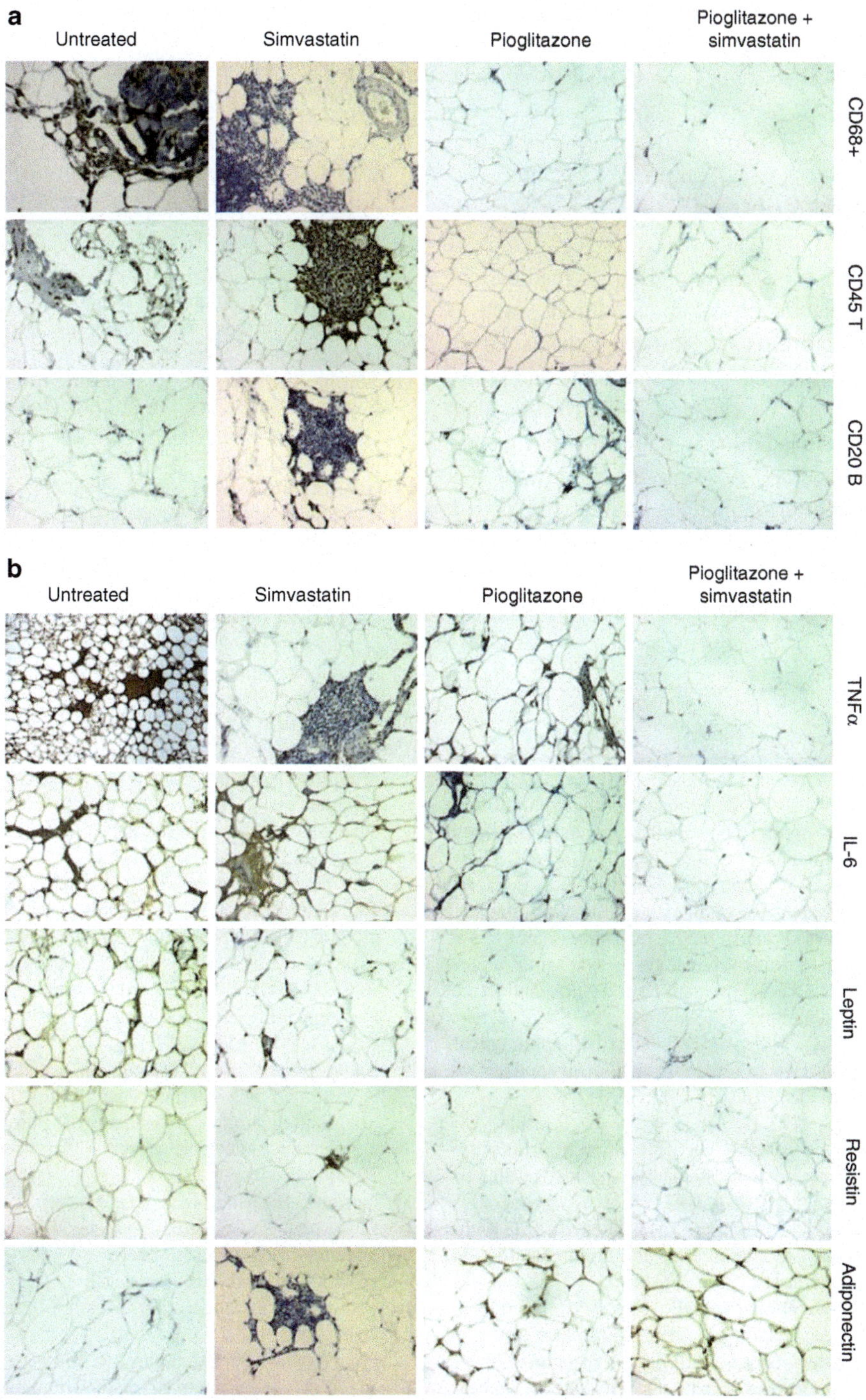

Fig. 15.3 Immunohistochemical staining in the epicardial adipose tissue (EAT) showing the differences between coronary artery disease patients untreated, treated with simvastatin monotherapy, pioglitazone monotherapy, or with the combination of pioglitazone and simvastatin. The combination treatment substantially reduced EAT inflammatory markers and improved anti-inflammatory adipokines. Pioglitazone alone and simvastatin + pioglitazone treatment was associated with a lower mean percentage positive area of CD68+/macrophages, CD45/T-lymphocytes, tumoral necrosis factor-alpha (TNF-α), interleukin 6 (IL-6), leptin and resistin, and higher adiponectin in the EAT samples compared to controls ($p < 0.001$). 200×. (From Grosso et al. [70], with permission)

of EAT, it is possible to hypothesize that the thyroid hormone may modulate this fat depot. However, further studies are needed to evaluate this hypothesis.

TNF Alpha Inhibitors

TNF alpha inhibitors are a group of medications used to treat inflammatory conditions such as rheumatoid arthritis and psoriatic arthritis. Given its highly inflammatory transcriptome and secretome, EAT may be a natural target for this class of drugs. EAT is higher in patients with rheumatoid arthritis [79]. A single study showed that rheumatoid arthritis patients treated with TNF-α inhibitors had significantly lower EAT thickness than those treated with nonbiological Disease-modifying antirheumatic drugs (DMARDs) [80].

References

1. Iacobellis G, Assael F, Ribaudo MC, Zappaterreno A, Alessi G, Di Mario U, Leonetti F. Epicardial fat from echocardiography: a new method for visceral adipose tissue prediction. Obes Res. 2003;11:304–10.
2. Iacobellis G, Ribaudo MC, Assael F, Vecci E, Tiberti C, Zappaterreno A, et al. Echocardiographic epicardial adipose tissue is related to anthropometric and clinical parameters of metabolic syndrome: a new indicator of cardiovascular risk. J Clin Endocrinol Metab. 2003;388:5163–8.
3. Iacobellis G, Willens HJ. Echocardiographic epicardial fat: a review of research and clinical applications. J Am Soc Echocardiogr. 2009;22:1311–9.
4. Malavazos AE, Di Leo G, Secchi F, Lupo EN, Dogliotti G, Coman C, et al. Relation of echocardiographic epicardial fat thickness and myocardial fat. Am J Cardiol. 2010;105:1831–5.
5. Iacobellis G, Mohseni M, Bianco S, Banga PK. Liraglutide causes large and rapid epicardial fat reduction. Obesity. 2017;25:311–6.
6. Morano S, Romagnoli E, Filardi T, Nieddu L, Mandosi E, Fallarino M, et al. Short-term effects of glucagon-like peptide 1 (GLP-1) receptor agonists on fat distribution in patients with type 2 diabetes mellitus: an ultrasonography study. Acta Diabetol. 2015;52:727–32.
7. Lima-Martínez MM, Paoli M, Rodney M, Balladares N, Contreras M, D'Marco L, Iacobellis G. Effect of sitagliptin on epicardial fat thickness in subjects with type 2 diabetes and obesity: a pilot study. Endocrine. 2016;51:448–55.
8. Sato T, Aizawa Y, Yuasa S, Kishi S, Fuse K, Fujita S, Ikeda Y, Kitazawa H, Takahashi M, Sato M, Okabe M. The effect of dapagliflozin treatment on epicardial adipose tissue volume. Cardiovasc Diabetol. 2018;17:6.
9. Yagi S, Hirata Y, Ise T, Kusunose K, Yamada H, Fukuda D, et al. Canagliflozin reduces epicardial fat in patients with type 2 diabetes mellitus. Diabetol Metab Syndr. 2017;9:78.
10. Fukuda T, Bouchi R, Terashima M, Sasahara Y, Asakawa M, Takeuchi T, et al. Ipragliflozin reduces epicardial fat accumulation in non-obese type 2 diabetic patients with visceral obesity: a pilot study. Diabetes Ther. 2017;8:851–61.
11. Bouchi R, Terashima M, Sasahara Y, Asakawa M, Fukuda T, Takeuchi T, et al. Luseogliflozin reduces epicardial fat accumulation in patients with type 2 diabetes: a pilot study. Cardiovasc Diabetol. 2017;16:32.
12. Nagai H, Ito H, Iwakura K. Pioglitazone treatment reduces epicardial fat in patients with type 2 diabetes mellitus and improves left ventricular diastolic function. (Abstract 710). Circulation. 2008;118:S604.
13. Elisha B, Azar M, Taleb N, Bernard S, Iacobellis G, Rabasa-Lhoret R. Body composition and epicardial fat in type 2 diabetes patients following insulin detemir versus insulin glargine initiation. Horm Metab Res. 2016;48:42–7.
14. Park JH, Park YS, Kim YJ, Lee IS, Kim JH, Lee JH, et al. Effects of statins on the epicardial fat thickness in patients with coronary artery stenosis underwent percutaneous coronary intervention: comparison of atorvastatin with simvastatin/ezetimibe. J Cardiovasc Ultrasound. 2010;18:121–6.
15. Alexopoulos N, Melek BH, Arepalli CD, Hartlage GR, Chen Z, Kim S, et al. Effect of intensive versus moderate lipid-lowering therapy on epicardial adipose tissue in hyperlipidemic post-menopausal women: a substudy of the BELLES trial (beyond endorsed lipid lowering with EBT scanning). J Am Coll Cardiol. 2013;61:1956–61.
16. Raggi P, Gadiyaram V, Zhang C, Chen Z, Lopaschuk G, Stillman AE. Statins reduce epicardial adipose tissue attenuation independent of lipid lowering: a potential pleiotropic effect. J Am Heart Assoc. 2019;8:e01310.
17. Ferrante E, Malavazos AE, Giavoli C, Ermetici F, Coman C, Bergamaschi S, et al. Epicardial fat thickness significantly decreases after short-term growth hormone (GH) replacement therapy in adults with GH deficiency. Nutr Metab Cardiovasc Dis. 2013;23:459–65.
18. Francomano D, Bruzziches R, Barbaro G, Lenzi A, Aversa A. Effects of testosterone undecanoate replacement and withdrawal on cardio-metabolic, hormonal and body composition outcomes in severely obese hypogonadal men: a pilot study. J Endocrinol Investig. 2014;37:401–11.
19. Fiore D, Gianfrilli D, Giannetta E, Galea N, Panio G, di Dato C, et al. PDE5 inhibition ameliorates visceral adiposity targeting the miR-22/SIRT1 pathway:

evidence from the CECSID trial. J Clin Endocrinol Metab. 2016;101:1525–34.
20. Iacobellis G, Singh N, Wharton S, Sharma AM. Substantial changes in epicardial fat thickness after weight loss in severely obese subjects. Obesity. 2008;16:1693–7.
21. Fu CP, Sheu WH, Lee IT, Tsai IC, Lee WJ, Liang KW, et al. Effects of weight loss on epicardial adipose tissue thickness and its relationship between serum soluble CD40 ligand levels in obese men. Clin Chim Acta. 2013;421:98–103.
22. Snel M, Jonker JT, Hammer S, Kerpershoek G, Lamb HJ, Meinders AE, et al. Long-term beneficial effect of a 16-week very low calorie diet on pericardial fat in obese type 2 diabetes mellitus patients. Obesity (Silver Spring). 2012;20:1572–6.
23. Dixon JB, Zimmet P, Alberti KG, Rubino F, International Diabetes Federation Taskforce on Epidemiology and Prevention. Bariatric surgery: an IDF statement for obese type 2 diabetes. Diabet Med. 2011;28:628–42.
24. Ashrafian H, le Roux CW, Darzi A, Athanasiou T. Effects of bariatric surgery on cardiovascular function. Circulation. 2008;118:2091–102.
25. De La Cruz-Munoz N, Messiah SE, Lopez-Mitnik G, Arheart KL, Lipshultz SE, Livingstone A. Laparoscopic gastric bypass surgery and adjustable gastric banding significantly decrease the prevalence of type 2 diabetes mellitus and pre-diabetes among morbidly obese multiethnic adults: long-term outcome results. J Am Coll Surg. 2011;212:505–11.
26. De La Cruz-Muñoz N, Lopez-Mitnik G, Arheart KL, Livingstone A, Forno E, Miller TL, et al. Laparoscopic gastric bypass surgery and adjustable gastric banding significantly improves cardiometabolic disease risk among morbidly obese multiethnic adolescents. Circulation. 2010;122(21 Suppl 23):A19842.
27. Pontiroli AE, Pizzocri P, Librenti MC, Vedani P, Marchi M, Cucchi E, et al. Laparoscopic adjustable gastric banding for the treatment of morbid (grade 3) obesity and its metabolic complications: a three-year study. J Clin Endocrinol Metab. 2002;87:3555–61.
28. Chaston TB, Dixon JB. Factors associated with percent change in visceral versus subcutaneous abdominal fat during weight loss: findings from a systematic review. Int J Obes. 2008;32:619–28.
29. Phillips ML, Lewis MC, Chew V, Kow L, Slavotinek JP, Daniels L, et al. The early effects of weight loss surgery on regional adiposity. Obes Surg. 2005;15:1449–55.
30. Weiss R, Appelbaum L, Schweiger C, Matot I, Constantini N, Idan A, et al. Short-term dynamics and metabolic impact of abdominal fat depots after bariatric surgery. Diabetes Care. 2009;32:1910–5.
31. Kim MK, Lee HC, Kwon HS, Baek KH, Kim EK, Lee KW, Song KH. Visceral obesity is a negative predictor of remission of diabetes 1 year after bariatric surgery. Obesity (Silver Spring). 2011;19:1835–9.
32. Heath ML, Kow L, Slavotinek JP, Valentine R, Toouli J, Thompson CH. Abdominal adiposity and liver fat content 3 and 12 months after gastric banding surgery. Metabolism. 2009;58:753–8.
33. Willens HJ, Byers P, Chirinos JA, Labrador E, Hare JM, de Marchena E. Effects of weight loss after bariatric surgery on epicardial fat measured using echocardiography. Am J Cardiol. 2007;99:1242–5.
34. Altin C, Erol V, Aydin E, Yilmaz M, Tekindal MA, Sade LE, et al. Impact of weight loss on epicardial fat and carotid intima media thickness after laparoscopic sleeve gastrectomy: a prospective study. Nutr Metab Cardiovasc Dis. 2018;28:501–9.
35. Gaborit B, Jacquier A, Kober F, Abdesselam I, Cuisset T, Boullu-Ciocca S, et al. Effects of bariatric surgery on cardiac ectopic fat: lesser decrease in epicardial fat compared to visceral fat loss and no change in myocardial triglyceride content. J Am Coll Cardiol. 2012;60:1381–9.
36. Wu FZ, Huang YL, Wu CC, Wang YC, Pan HJ, Huang CK, et al. Differential effects of bariatric surgery versus exercise on excessive visceral fat deposits. Medicine (Baltimore). 2016;95:e2616.
37. Christensen RH, Wedell-Neergaard AS, Lehrskov LL, Legaard GE, Dorph E, Larsen MK, et al. Effect of aerobic and resistance exercise on cardiac adipose tissues: secondary analyses from a randomized clinical trial. JAMA Cardiol. 2019; https://doi.org/10.1001/jamacardio.2019.2074. [Epub ahead of print].
38. Fernandez-del-Valle M, Gonzales JU, Kloiber S, Mitra S, Klingensmith J, Larumbe-Zabala E. Effects of resistance training on MRI-derived epicardial fat volume and arterial stiffness in women with obesity: a randomized pilot study. Eur J Appl Physiol. 2018;118:1231–40.
39. Kahl KG, Kerling A, Tegtbur U, Gützlaff E, Herrmann J, Borchert L, et al. Effects of additional exercise training on epicardial, intra-abdominal and subcutaneous adipose tissue in major depressive disorder: a randomized pilot study. J Affect Disord. 2016;192:91–7.
40. Company JM, Booth FW, Laughlin MH, Arce-Esquivel AA, Sacks HS, Bahouth SW, Fain JN. Epicardial fat gene expression after aerobic exercise training in pigs with coronary atherosclerosis: relationship to visceral and subcutaneous fat. J Appl Physiol. 2010;109:1904–12.
41. Christensen RH, Wedell-Neergaard AS, Lehrskov LL, Legård GE, Dorph EB, Nymand S, et al. The role of exercise combined with tocilizumab in visceral and epicardial adipose tissue and gastric emptying rate in abdominally obese participants: protocol for a randomised controlled trial. Trials. 2018;19:266.
42. Rabkin SW, Campbell H. Comparison of reducing epicardial fat by exercise, diet or bariatric surgery weight loss strategies: a systematic review and meta-analysis. Obes Rev. 2015;16:406–15.
43. Kim MK, Tomita T, Kim MJ, Sasai H, Maeda S, Tanaka K. Aerobic exercise training reduces epicardial fat in obese men. J Appl Physiol. 2009;106:5–11.
44. Wilund KR, Tomayko EJ, Wu PT, Ryong Chung H, Vallurupalli S, Lakshminarayanan B, Fernhall B. Intradialytic exercise training reduces oxidative

stress and epicardial fat: a pilot study. Nephrol Dial Transplant. 2010;25:2695–701.
45. Marso SP, Daniels GH, Brown-Frandsen K, Kristensen P, Mann JF, Nauck MA, LEADER Steering Committee, LEADER Trial Investigators, et al. Liraglutide and cardiovascular outcomes in type 2 diabetes. N Engl J Med. 2016;375:311–22.
46. Marso SP, Bain SC, Consoli A, Eliaschewitz FG, Jódar E, Leiter LA, SUSTAIN-6 Investigators, et al. Semaglutide and cardiovascular outcomes in patients with type 2 diabetes. N Engl J Med. 2016;375:1834–44.
47. Gerstein HC, Colhoun HM, Dagenais GR, Diaz R, Lakshmanan M, Pais P, REWIND Investigators, et al. Dulaglutide and cardiovascular outcomes in type 2 diabetes (REWIND): a double-blind, randomised placebo-controlled trial. Lancet. 2019;394:121–30.
48. Dutour A, Abdesselam I, Ancel P, Kober F, Mrad G, Darmon P, et al. Exenatide decreases liver fat content and epicardial adipose tissue in patients with obesity and type 2 diabetes: a prospective randomized clinical trial using magnetic resonance imaging and spectroscopy. Diabetes Obes Metab. 2016;18:882–91.
49. Iacobellis G, Camarena V, Sant DW, Wang G. Human epicardial fat expresses glucagon-like peptide 1 and 2 receptors genes. Horm Metab Res. 2017;49:625–30.
50. Pyke C, Knudsen LB. The glucagon-like peptide-1 receptor—or not? Endocrinology. 2013;154:4–8.
51. Yang J, Ren J, Song J, Liu F, Wu C, Wang X, et al. Glucagon-like peptide 1 regulates adipogenesis in 3T3-L1 preadipocytes. Int J Mol Med. 2013;31:1429–35.
52. Beiroa D, Imbernon M, Gallego R, Senra A, Herranz D, Villarroya F, et al. GLP-1 agonism stimulates brown adipose tissue thermogenesis and browning through hypothalamic AMPK. Diabetes. 2014;63:3346–58.
53. Vendrell J, El Bekay R, Peral B, García-Fuentes E, Megia A, Macias-Gonzalez M, et al. Study of the potential association of adipose tissue GLP-1 receptor with obesity and insulin resistance. Endocrinology. 2011;152:4072–9.
54. Dozio E, Vianello E, Malavazos AE, Tacchini L, Schmitz G, Iacobellis G, Corsi Romanelli MM. Epicardial adipose tissue GLP-1 receptor is associated with genes involved in fatty acid oxidation and white-to-brown fat differentiation: a target to modulate cardiovascular risk? Int J Cardiol. 2019;292:218–24.
55. Aroor A, McKarns S, Nistala R, DeMarco V, Gardner M, Garcia-Touza M, et al. DPP-4 inhibitors as therapeutic modulators of immune cell function and associated cardiovascular and renal insulin resistance in obesity and diabetes. Cardiorenal Med. 2013;3:48–56.
56. Shah Z, Kampfrath T, Deiuliis JA, Zhong J, Pineda C, Ying Z, et al. Long-term dipeptidyl-peptidase 4 inhibition reduces atherosclerosis and inflammation via effects on monocyte recruitment and chemotaxis. Circulation. 2011;124:2338–49.
57. Shimasaki T, Masaki T, Mitsutomi K, Ueno D, Gotoh K, Chiba S, et al. The dipeptidyl peptidase-4 inhibitor des-fluoro-sitagliptin regulates brown adipose tissue uncoupling protein levels in mice with diet-induced obesity. PLoS One. 2013;8:e63626.
58. Zinman B, Wanner C, Lachin JM, Fitchett D, Bluhmki E, Hantel S, EMPA-REG OUTCOME Investigators, et al. Empagliflozin, cardiovascular outcomes, and mortality in type 2 diabetes. N Engl J Med. 2015;373:2117–28.
59. Mahaffey KW, Neal B, Perkovic V, de Zeeuw D, Fulcher G, Erondu N, CANVAS Program Collaborative Group, et al. Canagliflozin for primary and secondary prevention of cardiovascular events: results from the CANVAS Program (Canagliflozin Cardiovascular Assessment Study). Circulation. 2018;137:323–34.
60. Wiviott SD, Raz I, Bonaca MP, Mosenzon O, Kato ET, Cahn A, DECLARE–TIMI 58 Investigators, et al. Dapagliflozin and cardiovascular outcomes in type 2 diabetes. N Engl J Med. 2019;380:347–57.
61. Guedes EP, Hohl A, de Melo TG, Lauand F. Dapagliflozin: farmacology, efficacy and safety in type 2 diabetes treatment. Diabetol Metab Syndr. 2013;5:25.
62. Bolinder J, Ljunggren Ö, Kullberg J, Johansson L, Wilding J, Langkilde AM, et al. Effects of dapagliflozin on body weight, total fat mass, and regional adipose tissue distribution in patients with type 2 diabetes mellitus with inadequate glycemic control on metformin. J Clin Endocrinol Metab. 2012;97:1020–31.
63. Díaz-Rodríguez E, Agra RM, Fernández ÁL, Adrio B, García-Caballero T, González-Juanatey JR, Eiras S. Effects of dapagliflozin on human epicardial adipose tissue: modulation of insulin resistance, inflammatory chemokine production, and differentiation ability. Cardiovasc Res. 2018;114:336–46.
64. Sacks HS, Fain JN, Cheema P, Bahouth SW, Garrett E, Wolf RY. Inflammatory genes in epicardial fat contiguous with coronary atherosclerosis in the metabolic syndrome and type 2 diabetes: changes associated with pioglitazone. Diabetes Care. 2011;34:730–3.
65. Jonker JT, Lamb HJ, van der Meer RW, Rijzewijk LJ, Menting LJ, Diamant M, et al. Pioglitazone compared with metformin increases pericardial fat volume in patients with type 2 diabetes mellitus. J Clin Endocrinol Metab. 2010;95:456–60.
66. Distel E, Penot G, Cadoudal T, Balguy I, Durant S, Benelli C. Early induction of a brown-like phenotype by rosiglitazone in the epicardial adipose tissue of fatty Zucker rats. Biochimie. 2012;94:1660–7.
67. Iacobellis G, Sharma AM, Pellicelli AM, Grisorio B, Barbarini G, Barbaro G. Epicardial adipose tissue is related to carotid intima-media thickness and visceral adiposity in HIV-infected patients with highly active antiretroviral therapy-associated metabolic syndrome. Curr HIV Res. 2007;5:275–9.
68. Iacobellis G, Pellicelli AM, Sharma AM, Grisorio B, Barbarini G, Barbaro G. Relation of subepicardial

adipose tissue to carotid intima-media thickness in patients with human immunodeficiency virus. Am J Cardiol. 2007;99:1470–2.

69. Nasarre L, Juan-Babot O, Gastelurrutia P, Llucia-Valldeperas A, Badimon L, Bayes-Genis A, Llorente-Cortés V. Low density lipoprotein receptor-related protein 1 is upregulated in epicardial fat from type 2 diabetes mellitus patients and correlates with glucose and triglyceride plasma levels. Acta Diabetol. 2014;51:23–30.
70. Grosso AF, de Oliveira SF, Higuchi Mde L, Favarato D, Dallan LA, da Luz PL. Synergistic anti-inflammatory effect: simvastatin and pioglitazone reduce inflammatory markers of plasma and epicardial adipose tissue of coronary patients with metabolic syndrome. Diabetol Metab Syndr. 2014;6:47.
71. Yamaguchi Y, Cavallero S, Patterson M, Shen H, Xu J, Kumar SR, Sucov HM. Adipogenesis and epicardial adipose tissue: a novel fate of the epicardium induced by mesenchymal transformation and PPARγ activation. Proc Natl Acad Sci U S A. 2015;112:2070–5.
72. Lanes R, Soros A, Flores K, Gunczler P, Carrillo E, Bandel J. Endothelial function, carotid artery intima-media thickness, epicardial adipose tissue, and left ventricular mass and function in growth hormone-deficient adolescents: apparent effects of growth hormone treatment on these parameters. J Clin Endocrinol Metab. 2005;90:3978–82.
73. Granato S, Barbaro G, Di Giorgio MR, Rossi FM, Marzano C, Impronta F, et al. Epicardial fat: the role of testosterone and lipid metabolism in a cohort of patients with Klinefelter syndrome. Metabolism. 2019;95:21–6.
74. Şahin M, Canpolat AG, Çorapçioğlu D, Canpolat U, Emral R, Uysal AR. Association between circulating irisin levels and epicardial fat in patients with treatment-naïve overt hyperthyroidism. Biomarkers. 2018;23:742–7.
75. Altunbaş R, Eren MA, Altıparmak İH, Karaaslan H, Sabuncu T. The relation between epicardial fat tissue thickness and tsh receptor antibody in hyperthyroidism. Exp Clin Endocrinol Diabetes. 2019;127:37–40.
76. Asik M, Sahin S, Ozkul F, Anaforoglu I, Ayhan S, Karagol S, et al. Evaluation of epicardial fat tissue thickness in patients with Hashimoto thyroiditis. Clin Endocrinol. 2013;79:571–6.
77. Kocyigit I, Gungor O, Unal A, Yasan M, Orscelik O, Tunca O, et al. A low serum free triiodothyronine level is associated with epicardial adipose tissue in peritoneal dialysis patients. J Atheroscler Thromb. 2014;21:1066–74.
78. del Busto-Mesa A, Cabrera-Rego JO, Carrero-Fernández L, Hernández-Roca CV, González-Valdés JL, de la Rosa-Pazos JE. Changes in arterial stiffness, carotid intima-media thickness, and epicardial fat after L-thyroxine replacement therapy in hypothyroidism. Endocrinol Nutr. 2015;62:270–6.
79. Fatma E, Bunyamin K, Savas S, Mehmet U, Selma Y, Ismail B, et al. Epicardial fat thickness in patients with rheumatoid arthritis. Afr Health Sci. 2015;15:489–95.
80. Lima-Martínez MM, Campo E, Salazar J, Paoli M, Maldonado I, Acosta C, et al. Epicardial fat thickness as cardiovascular risk factor and therapeutic target in patients with rheumatoid arthritis treated with biological and nonbiological therapies. Arthritis. 2014;2014:782850.

Index

G. Iacobellis (ed.), *Epicardial Adipose Tissue*, Contemporary Cardiology,
https://doi.org/10.1007/978-3-030-40570-0

The manufacturer's authorised representative in the EU is Springer Nature Customer Service Centre GmbH, Europaplatz 3, 69115 Heidelberg, Germany. If you have any concerns regarding our products, please contact ProductSafety@springernature.com

Printed and bound by CPI Group (UK) Ltd, Croydon, CR0 4YY

30/07/2026

02181710-0013